649

Clinical Research Methodology for Complementary Therapies

Edited by George T. Lewith and David Aldridge

Hodder & Stoughton

LONDON SYDNEY AUCKLAND

British Library Cataloguing in Publication Data

Clinical Research Methodology for
Complementary Therapies
  I. Lewith, G. T. II. Aldridge, David
  615.8

  ISBN 0–340–55778–8

First published in Great Britain by
Hodder and Stoughton 1993

Compilation copyright © 1993 George T. Lewith and David Aldridge

Typeset by Wearset, Boldon, Tyne and Wear

Printed in Great Britain for the educational publishing division of Hodder and Stoughton Ltd, Mill Road, Dunton Green, Sevenoaks, Kent by Biddles Ltd, Guildford.

Contents

List of contributors   v

Introduction   vii

Section 1

1   The importance of statistics in research design   3
    Nicola J. Crichton

2   Current issues in the design and interpretation of clinical   21
    trials   *Stuart J. Pocock*

3   Error and bias in single group and controlled data trials   32
    Stuart J. Pocock

4   Every doctor a walking placebo   *George T. Lewith*   38

5   Why measure outcomes?   *Honor M. Anthony and*   46
    Frank M. Parsons

6   Choice of health indicator: the problem of measuring   57
    outcome   *Ann Bowling*

7   The importance of patient selection   *F.A.C. Wiegant,*   77
    C.W. Kramers and R. van Wijk

Section 2

8   Emerging priorities in complementary medical research   93
    David Canter and Lorraine Nanke

9   Some methodological problems in the assessment of   108
    complementary therapy   *Honor M. Anthony*

10 Tactics and practicalities   *Ian James*   122

11 Clinical research: questions to ask and the benefits of   129
    asking them   *Honor M. Anthony*

12 Single case research designs   *David Aldridge*   136

13 The use of health diaries in the field of psychiatric illness in   169
    general practice   *Joanna Murray*

14 The multivariate structure of treatment practices in   189
    complementary medicine   *Lorraine Nanke and David Canter*

15 The use of alternative treatments in the Finnish adult   204
    population   *Tuula Vaskilampi, Pirkko Meriläinen and*
    Sirkka Sinkkonen

16 Medical anthropology as clinical method: the body   230
    paradigm   *Beatrix Pfleiderer*

17 Observational methods: a search for methods in an   241
    ecosystemic paradigm   *David Aldridge*

18 Research strategies in a hospital setting: the development   276
    of appropriate methods   *David Aldridge*

Section 3

19	Acupuncture as a treatment for chronic pain *C.A. Vincent*	289
20	Biofeedback *Sandra Horn*	309
21	Environmental medicine: principles and practice of evaluation *George T. Lewith*	323
22	Research into the homoeopathic treatment of rheumatological disease: why and how? *Peter Fisher*	337
23	Experimentation in hypnosis: towards an adequate methodology *David Kidner*	350
24	The evaluation of herbal medicines: an East Asian perspective *Kiichiro Tsutani*	365
25	Herbal medicines: research strategies *Simon Mills*	394
26	Manipulation and low back pain: an example of principles and practice *T.W. Meade and A.O. Frank*	408

Section 4

27	An introduction to word processing as a research tool *David Aldridge*	425
28	An introduction to electronic data management as a research tool *David Aldridge*	439
29	A guide to preparing a research application *David Aldridge*	459
30	Conclusion: are you ready to begin? *David Aldridge*	473

List of Contributors

George T. Lewith MA, MRCP, MRCGP. Centre for the Study of Complementary Medicine, Southampton.

David Aldridge BEd, BPhil, PhD, PD. Associate Professor, Institute for Music Therapy, Faculty of Medicine, University of Witten Herdecke, Germany.

Honor M. Anthony MB, ChB. Formerly Lecturer, School of Medicine, University of Leeds.

Ann Bowling MSc, PhD. Senior Research Fellow, Departments of Community Medicine and of General Practice and Health Care, St Bartholomews Hospital Medical College, London.

David Canter PhD, FBPsS, FBIM. Director, Health Research Unit, University of Surrey.

Nicola J. Crichton BSc, MSc, PhD. Lecturer in Statistics, Department of Mathematical Statistics and Operational Research, University of Exeter.

Peter Fisher MRCP, FFHom. Consultant Physician, Royal London Homoeopathic Hospital. Honorary Lecturer in Rheumatology and Complementary Medicine, St Bartholomews Hospital Medical College, London.

A. O. Frank FRCP. Consultant Physician in Rheumatology and Rehabilitation, Northwick Park Hospital, Harrow, Middlesex.

Sandra Horn BTech(Hons Physc.), Dip Clin Physc. Lecturer in Health Psychology, University of Southampton.

Ian James MB, PhD, FRCP. Reader in Clinical Pharmacology, Royal Free Hospital, London.

David Kidner BSc, PhD. Lecturer in Clinical Physiology, Fort Lewis College, Durango, Colorado, USA.

C. Willem Kramers MD, PhD. Senior Scientist, Department of Health Sciences and Epidemiology, and participant in the Research Unit for Complementary Medicine, University of Utrecht.

T. W. Meade DM, FRCP. Director, MRC Epidemiology and Medical Care Unit, Wolfson Institute of Preventive Medicine, Medical College of St Bartholomews Hospital, London.

Pirkko Meriläinen Department of Nursing Service, University of Kuopio, Finland.

Simon Y. Mills MA, FNIMH. Co-Director, Centre for Complementary Health Studies, University of Exeter.

Joanna Murray General Practice Research Unit, Institute of Psychiatry, London.

Lorraine Nanke BA, MSc. Research Officer, Health Research Unit, University of Surrey.

Frank M. Parsons BSc, MD, FRCP. Senior Lecturer in Renal Medicine, University of Leeds.

Beatrix Pfleiderer PhD. Professor of Medical Anthropology, University of Hamburg.

Stuart Pocock MSc, PhD. Director, Clinical Trials Research Unit, Royal Free Hospital, London.

Sirkka Sinkkonen Department of Health Administration and Economy, University of Kuopio, Finland.

Kiichiro Tsutani MD, PhD. Associate Professor of Clinical Pharmacology, Division of Information Medicine, Medical Research Institute, Tokyo Medical and Dental University. Former Medical Officer for traditional medicine, WHO Regional Office for the Western Pacific.

Roeland van Wijk PhD. Senior Scientist, Department of Molecular Cell Biology and Coordinator of the Research Unit for Complementary Medicine, University of Utrecht.

Tuula Vaskilampi MA, Lic Sec Sci. Department of Social Policy, University of Jyväskylä, 40100 Jyväskylä, Finland.

Charles A. Vincent PhD. Lecturer in Pyschology Applied to Medicine, Department of Psychology, University College, London.

Fred A.C. Wiegant PhD. Scientist, Department of Molecular Cell Biology, and Research Unit for Complementary Medicine, University of Utrecht.

Introduction

In the early 1980s it became apparent that far more serious thought ought to be given to research within complementary medicine. Until that date there were very few properly trained researchers involved in evaluating techniques such as acupuncture and homoeopathy. The vast bulk of research within these fields was either carried out by complementary therapists with inadequate research training or conventional medical researchers with a limited understanding of the complementary therapy they were investigating.

These major difficulties led to a poor supply of research material, particularly within the field of clinical trials. The research that was published was often methodologically questionable and frequently statistically inept.

The Research Council for Complementary Medicine was formed to rectify this situation and has achieved much over the last five years. At its inception it was designed to fulfil a number of disparate functions. Among these, it aimed to improve the quality and quantity of research within complementary medicine. The constitution of its council and its committees was also designed to bring together conventional medical researchers with an understanding and interest in a variety of different fields within complementary medicine. In order to promulgate the products of its research, and to act as a mouthpiece for the Research Council, it began to publish the journal *Complementary Medical Research.* This journal has formed the basis for many incisive methodological articles and, as a consequence, papers drawn from *Complementary Medical Research* form an important part of our book. We are greatly indebted to the Research Council for Complementary Medicine for both its vision and its journal. Without the enthusiasm, research network and facility for publication provided by the RCCM, this book would not have been possible.

There is little need, we feel, to justify the requirement for research within the complementary therapies. Academics from all over the world have quite rightly demanded support and academic justification for many of the claims made by complementary practitioners. The story of acupuncture perhaps illustrates this most forcefully. During the early 1970s, acupuncture was almost unheard of within the practice of medicine in the United Kingdom and the United States. A strong tradition of Chinese Medicine did exist in France, but even within continental Europe conventional doctors were particularly disdainful of anybody who wasn't practising straightforward conventional medicine. President Nixon's visit to China in 1972, while it raised interest in acupuncture, did nothing to justify or validate its use. Nevertheless, political forces from within the USA began to drive Western physicians to evaluate acupuncture in a more coherent manner.

Along with this political impetus came the need to understand the process of opiate addiction. This again was fired by American money, along with the extent of hard drug addiction experienced by the American forces fighting in South East Asia. Pharmacological and biochemical research revealed that opiate receptors exist within the body and in particular within the nervous system, and soon afterwards natural opiates such as endorphins and encephalins were identified. It soon became clear that the analgesic effect of acupuncture was mediated at least partially through the endorphin and encephalin systems. While the 'gate control theory' had been used previously to justify the analgesic effects of acupuncture, neurological explanations could only partially explain what was happening physiologically. The discovery of a neurohumeral mediator, such as the natural opiates, seemed to fit the bill much more closely. Acupuncture had, at long last, a mechanism that could be understood by conventional pharmacologists. However, this mechanism did not appear to explain the effects of acupuncture in non-painful conditions, such as asthma and irritable bowel; neither did it, in reality, explain the effects of acupuncture in many intractable and chronically painful conditions, which are probably autonomically mediated. The endorphin-acupuncture hypothesis is vital. Despite its inadequacies, it provided the physiological justification which allowed conventional doctors to use acupuncture in the knowledge that at least they understood something about its underlying mechanisms.

A body of clinical research and clinical trial methodology applied to acupuncture soon began to develop. There are now many good clinical papers which justify the use of acupuncture in chronic painful conditions. As a consequence, acupuncture is now widely used as a method of pain relief by conventional physicians throughout the world. The research impetus, both in terms of understanding the basic mechanism and the technique's subsequent clinical evaluation, has resulted in a very substantial change in attitude over the last 15 years. A therapy that was previously derided as no more than a complex placebo effect, or quackery, has become a powerful part of conventional medical practice. This change can be clearly attributed to an increasing academic justification for the use and value of acupuncture.

The situation is not the same, however, with some of the other complementary therapies. Homoeopathy is a good example of this. There is increasing justification within the context of clinical trials for the value of homoeopathy. A number of studies have conclusively demonstrated that pure homoeopathic medicines have a clinical effect far greater than that expected from placebo.[1] Unfortunately, we do not understand the mechanism of homoeopathy. It is apparently still impossible for conventional physicians and pharmacologists to accept that homoeopathic medicines, which must be working through non-pharmacological means, can have a clinical effect, in spite of good clinical trials which demonstrate that these preparations are effective in certain specific conditions. This is a political and conceptual problem which cannot be resolved by research alone, but requires conventional doctors to accept the scientific evidence before them, even though it may at first appear bizarre and in fact contradict many of their inherent assumptions about conventional pharmacology.

In this book, we have tried to lay out the fundamentals required for clinical research. The first section deals largely with statistics and some of the basic concepts involved in research. Its aim is to establish the need for an understanding of conventional clinical trial methodology, and we hope it offers a good initial review of this area, with an appropriate bibliography for those who may wish to follow through specific issues. The second section looks much more specifically at trial methodology, the implication being that the double blind controlled clinical trial is neither necessary nor appropriate in all forms of complementary therapy, and is certainly not the only method for evaluating a coherent therapeutic intervention. In the third section we attempt to tackle certain specific therapeutic methods, offering a review of the major research within these methods, an evaluation of both the positive and negative aspects of the clinical trials already published, and suggestions about the way forward. The final section looks at processing data and applying for research grants. Our aim in this book is to give a complete overview of research within the complementary therapies. Our hope and belief is that this will stimulate better quality research.

Research with complementary medicine is essential if we are to begin to accept a whole variety of safe and effective therapies. The agenda is, however, not only academic but also conceptual and political. The requirement for both clinical and basic research is an important step in helping those practising within the field of complementary medicine to justify the procedures they use, and also to reject those which are ineffective. However, a truly open-minded approach on behalf of conventional and complementary medicine is essential if we are to accept some of the very revolutionary and difficult questions which such research poses.

Reference

[1] Kleijnen, J., Knipschild, P., ter Riet, G. Clinical trials of homoeopathy. *Br Med J* 1991; **303**: 313–23.

Section 1

1 The importance of statistics in research design

Nicola J. Crichton

Summary

This chapter aims to identify the importance of statistical considerations in the planning and design stages of an experimental study. Points are illustrated with examples from published studies on complementary therapies. The need to identify the objective of the study clearly and specifically is stressed, a variety of types of design are discussed and the reasons for careful calculation of sample size are explained.

Introduction

We are confronted by statistics, in the sense of numerical data, every day of our lives. Newspapers may claim that the annual inflation rate is 9%, that there are more deaths on the roads on bank holiday weekends than normal weekends, that 72% of those polled thought that politicians lied. We are expected to assess and understand such material and to make decisions on the basis of this data.

It is important that we all have some understanding of basic statistics in order to avoid being taken in by articles and advertising containing carefully phrased numerical information. Many people are discouraged from the study of statistics by a fear of being overwhelmed by the mathematics. Whilst it is certainly true that many statisticians are also mathematicians, much of statistics can be discussed with minimal use of mathematics, as demonstrated by Huff[1] in his book *How to Lie with Statistics* and in *Statistics, Concepts and Controversies* by Moore.[2]

For researchers in all areas of medicine some knowledge of statistics is essential, firstly so that they can read critically other people's published work and secondly to ensure that their own studies provide convincing evidence. This is especially true for studies of complementary therapies as there may be many sceptics.

There are several stages to any study, as laid out in Figure 1.1. There is a need for statistical input at all stages, not just at the analysis stage. Indeed many serious errors are made at the planning and design stages which introduce biases that cannot be rectified later. For example, one aspect of planning a study is reading up published reports; if published papers are accepted uncritically you might try to verify someone else's spurious result or test a theory with no sound basis. The ethical implications of statistically substandard research are discussed by Altman.[3]

The importance of the design stage cannot be overemphasized and the purpose of this chapter is to discuss some aspects of designing good

PLANNING	**defining the precise purpose of the study**
⇓	
DESIGN	**how to conduct the study**
⇓	
CONDUCT	**doing the experiment**
⇓	
ANALYSIS	**making sense of the data**
⇓	
INTERPRETATION	**drawing conclusions**

Fig. 1.1 The stages of a clinical trial.

studies. The term *design* includes all the structural aspects of the study; notably, definition of study sample, size of the study, method of treatment allocation, type of statistical design and choice of outcome measure. It is not the intention of this chapter to provide detailed guidance about the statistical techniques for analysing studies; however, references are given that may be of help. To assist with understanding and evaluating published work, some notes on commonly used statistical terminology are given in the appendix.

Types of study

Most studies can be classified as either observational studies or experimental studies. In observational studies the researcher simply observes what is happening to a population and has no control over the conditions; epidemiological studies are usually of this type. Such studies may be either cross-sectional, examining disease in a population at one point in time, or longitudinal, studying a fixed group of people over a period of time. In general, observational studies take the form of either surveys or case-control studies. Experimental studies are generally clinical trials, i.e. human, scientific experiments. They are designed to evaluate the effects of various treatments, or preventive measures, and the researcher can specify the conditions under which the study is conducted.

The main characteristic of either type of study is that one uses results based on a limited sample of patients to make inferences or decisions about the population of interest. Supported by a clinical trial using a small number of patients, we make decisions about how to treat the general population of patients who will require treatment in the future. Since future patients are unlikely to be identical in all respects to the patients in our trial, there will be some uncertainty associated with claims we are able to make about the treatment. How confident we can be about claims we make on the basis of our sample depends critically on various features of the study design.

Many of the problems of planning and design biases are common to both observational and experimental studies. In this chapter we will consider designing experimental studies and points will be illustrated with examples from published clinical trials of complementary techniques. For a discussion of design problems in the context of observational studies, see Altman[4] for a brief account or Alderson[5] (particularly Chapters 4, 5 and 6) for a more detailed exposition.

Aim of the study

It is essential that the aims of a study are clearly determined before starting the design. Unless the aims of the study are clearly and precisely stated, it will be difficult to identify suitable patients for the study, devise evaluation scales which will appropriately measure the outcomes of interest, and calculate the necessary sample size for the study. It is not sufficient simply to state that you wish to compare the effectiveness of two treatments; one needs to be more specific about the meaning of 'effectiveness' and about what is to be treated. In general, a study should have only one or possibly two main objectives, which should be clearly and specifically stated.

The aims of the study should be clearly stated when the study is reported. It is surprisingly common to find study reports which fail to state the primary objectives of the research, or which give them in such general terms that one cannot judge whether the design chosen was appropriate or whether the sample size was justified.

The report of Lee et al.[6] is an example of a clearly stated aim; it is posed as two questions, '(1) Does acupuncture decrease the intensity of chronic pain? (2) Does the location of the needle placements alter the result, i.e. are the traditional meridian points crucial, as opposed to non-specific points?'. It is clear from this what treatments are under test, that we need patients with chronic pain and we need to measure pain intensity before and after treatment.

The aim of Reilly et al.[7] is stated as, 'We want to test the assertion that a potency lacking any of the original substance can have other than a placebo action'. The problem with this is that it is not clear what should be measured, the statement is not specific enough. Careful reading of the report suggests that we should append to the aim 'when considering the patient's overall symptoms of hayfever'.

Murphy et al.[8] never state their aim; they simply say that, 'The use of feverfew for migraine prophylaxis was assessed . . .'. Perhaps the best statement of the aim of this work is the title of the paper. However, for this to be a satisfactory statement of aim we really need a more explicit statement of what is meant by prevention, especially as the authors do not seem to mean 'stop completely from happening'.

Patient selection

Who is eligible for inclusion in the study? It is important to ensure that the patients included in the trial are representative of the future class of patients to whom the trial's findings will be applied. We need to give consideration to the source of patient recruitment, the precise definition of the disease state under consideration and any criteria for patient exclusion.

Many trials recruit their patients from hospitals. Generally this provides the advantages of easy monitoring and follow-up, good compliance, and a low drop-out rate. However, it is inappropriate to conduct a study in a hospital population if the treatment is intended for much more general use. For example, a study of depressive illness which recruits hospital inpatients sees a special subset of the population of depressed people, the hospital patients tending to be the more severe cases. Fung *et al.*[9] used children from a special allergy clinic in a study of exercise-induced asthma. This raises doubts about any conclusions concerning the value of their treatment for the wider population of children who suffer from this complaint, but do not attend clinics. Further, the source of patients should be clearly stated in any report to allow readers to judge for themselves the general applicability of the results.

In choosing a source of patients one often has to balance the difficulty of monitoring the progress and compliance of patients in the community against the lack of representativeness of hospitalized patients or special clinic attenders. Reilly *et al.*[7] try to overcome these problems by recruiting some patients from hospital clinics and some from general practices. However, they do not report in the paper the proportion of patients from each source, or whether there were any differences in compliance, drop-out, or response to treatment for the two different sources of patients.

For trials of complementary therapies, it will often be undesirable (or impractical) to use hospital sources; indeed, for many conditions it will be difficult to think of sources of patients. For example, if a study required a large number of women who suffered from premenstrual tension, general practitioners are unlikely to be able to provide lists of such women so the only practical solution might be to advertise for volunteers. In general, this is not a good way to recruit patients simply because volunteers are usually different in important respects from those who do not volunteer. This will raise questions about the generality of the results. Alderson[5] (pp. 196 and 271) gives examples of the problems of using volunteers.

If it is necessary to use volunteers for a study, careful thought should be given to how the volunteers are recruited so as to keep the potential biases to a minimum. Consider, for example, recruitment for a study of a herbal remedy for premenstrual tension. If this is done through advertisement in a health food magazine it is very likely to produce a biased subset of the population of women who suffer premenstrual tension. However, advertisement in a women's magazine with a broader range of readership might be more reasonable. Volunteers from self-help groups are likely to be very compliant and the drop-out rate low, but they are also likely to be an atypical subset of those suffering the disease. Murphy *et al.*[8] used volunteers for their study, but more details of the 'media publicity' and the proportion of volunteers from the self-help group are needed to be able to consider the general applicability of their results.

For many conditions, such as the common cold or premenstrual tension, there is no precise definition of the disease under study; hence it is difficult to determine which patients are eligible. It is an essential part of the trial design to specify what makes a person eligible for the study. For example, Ferley et al.[10] define influenza-like syndrome as 'the association of a rectal temperature equal to or above 38°C, and at least two of the following symptoms: headache, stiffness, lumbar and articular pain, shivers'. Although others may dispute this definition, it is clear to both those running the trial and those reading the report who is eligible and to whom the results apply.

It is often necessary to exclude some patients for practical or clinical reasons. For example, the treatment may be contraindicated because of some other disease the patient suffers or because of potential interaction with other treatments the patient receives. Exclusions should be specified at the design stage so that inappropriate patients are not recruited. Exclusions should also be stated in the report of the study.

Evaluation of patient response

If we are to assess whether the treatment is effective, we will need to decide how we are going to measure the patient's response to treatment. This evaluation needs to be done in an objective, accurate and consistent manner throughout the trial. The precise endpoint of interest depends on the aim of the study. For example, any of the following could be response variables in a trial of a cytotoxic drug: survival time of patient, achievement of tumour response, duration of tumour response, change in performance status of the patient, occurrence of haematological toxicity. Which endpoint is most appropriate depends on the aim of the study. In studies of chronic conditions it must be decided whether to look at short-term or long-term effects of the treatments. In general, it is long-term effects that are of interest to the patients; however, most studies seem to be of short duration!

Whatever response variable and method of measurement is chosen, it will be important to make baseline measurements for each patient before treatment begins, as well as measuring the patient's state after treatment. It will also be necessary to monitor any side effects during the study. Whilst this may be straightforward when the side effects are well known, it can be difficult otherwise and relies heavily on each patient's own assessment of side effects, often prompted by check lists or suggestive questioning.

We need to consider the accuracy of the information collected; ideally it should be precise and reproducible, in the sense that a different person assessing the patient would get the same measurement of treatment effect. This is much easier if we can use objective rather than subjective outcome measures. We can reduce the possibility of errors by training the assessors, by keeping the number of assessors to a minimum, and by taking repeat measurements on each occasion for outcome features such as blood pressure. In studies where the endpoint depends on a subjective measure, such as the patient's assessment of pain, it is certainly preferable to have one assessor dealing with all patients and the assessor should be 'blind'; that is, they should not know which treatment the patient is receiving. Lewith and Machin[11] provide some further discussion on outcome criteria.

Why do we need randomized controlled trials?

The concept of using random allocation when comparing treatments has been considered an important aspect of the design of scientific experiments for many years. The first randomized experiments were in agriculture in which various crops and fertilizers were randomly allocated to plots of land (the experimental units). The purpose of this randomization was twofold: firstly to guard against any use of judgemental or systematic assignment which might lead to one treatment getting experimental units with poorer soil, i.e. to avoid bias; and secondly to provide a basis for standard statistical analyses.

This may be acceptable for agricultural experiments, but the idea that patients should be randomly allocated to one or other form of treatment is not intuitively appealing. So, why should randomization be considered such an important issue in the conduct of clinical trials? This question is discussed in detail by Pocock[12] (Chapter 4) and more briefly by Gore,[13,14] whilst Altman[4] concentrates on the ethical issues associated with randomization.

The main purposes of randomization are to safeguard against selection bias and because the logical foundation of many statistical tests is the premise that each patient could have received any one of the treatments being compared. By selection bias, we mean that consciously or subconsciously the doctor encourages or discourages a patient to take part in the trial because he or she is aware of which treatment the patient will receive. There will be no way of separating the treatment effect and the effect of selection bias, so we must avoid this bias. There is a problem with any method of systematic allocation, such as using date of birth, because by identifying how the system works the doctor will be able to identify which treatment a patient will receive and the study will be liable to selection bias. Thus, only random allocation can protect a study from selection bias.

Studies in which randomization has not been used will fail to provide convincing evidence and often lead to ethical dilemmas. Pocock[15] discusses the problems arising from a non-randomized trial in which pregnant women with a previous neural tube defect birth were given periconceptional multivitamin supplements and were compared to an unsupplemented control group. The trial concluded that there was a significant benefit from using the supplements; however, the control group contained women who elected not to take the supplements. In addition the control group had a much higher proportion of women from high risk areas than did the treated group, thus the comparison may have been severely biased since the treatment and control groups were not initially comparable. There is no way of determining whether the apparent treatment difference is really attributable to bias so there remains uncertainty about the value of the treatment, but there has been considerable opposition on ethical grounds to a proper randomized controlled trial of this treatment. This example is also discussed by Kingman[16] who gives further examples to support the requirement for randomized controlled trials.

When reporting a study you should state whether the trial was randomized and if so, briefly describe the randomization procedure used, so that the reader can properly evaluate the trial. The practical problem of how to conduct randomization is discussed by Gore,[17] including examples of how to use random number tables.

We need to use a control group to provide a comparison of the performance of our new treatment with the current standard treatment. If there is no standard treatment for the condition we are studying then we should use a placebo treatment for the control group. A placebo is an inert substance, and often the primary reason for using a placebo, rather than giving the control group no treatment, is to make patient attitudes to the trial as similar as possible. Altman[4] discusses the use of placebos and points out that comparing a new treatment to a placebo when there is an existing treatment will yield results of no practical importance. One should also question the ethics of treating the control group with a placebo when there is an effective standard treatment. The 'placebo effect' is discussed in detail by Gribbin[18]; this is the psychological effect of 'treating' which we are trying to allow for when we design a trial with a placebo control group. We need to show that the new treatment will cause a larger response than would be expected if it was simply a placebo effect. For some complementary therapies there may be difficulties in devising placebo treatments. This problem is discussed in the case of acupuncture by Lewith.[11,19]

In order to overcome objections to randomization, some studies have used historical controls; that is, they have used patients treated previously as the control group and given all new patients the new treatment. Both Altman[4] and Pocock[12] provide strong arguments against this procedure and point out the potential for both selection bias and experimental bias. Patient selection bias may occur for several reasons; the historical control group is less likely to have clearly defined criteria for patient inclusion since it was not known the patients would be in a trial; the controls were recruited earlier, possibly from a different source; the investigator may be deliberately or subconsciously more restrictive in the choice of patients for the new treatment. Experimental bias may occur because the data recorded for the controls is likely to be inferior and have missing information as it was not known they would be in a trial; also the criteria of response may not be the same for the two groups. The use of historical controls will tend to exaggerate the value of a new treatment.

Nine different trials of complementary therapies are referred to in this chapter[6–10,20–23]; it is encouraging to find that all of these studies were controlled and none used historical controls. Only two of the studies, those of Lee *et al.*[6] and Bullock *et al.*,[20] were not randomized. However, only two of the studies, those of Reilly *et al.*[7] and Lewith *et al.*,[21] give details of the randomization procedure.

Types of design

Throughout this section it will be assumed that we wish to compare two treatments A and B. Most of the designs can be extended to the situation in which more than two treatments are compared. For most of the designs it is theoretically possible for the study to be double blind; that is, both the patient and the practitioner are unaware of which treatment the patient is receiving. This is desirable as it allows assessment of response and side effects to be unbiased. Sometimes it will not be possible for the practitioner to be blind; for example, in a trial of acupuncture the practitioner will know whether they have used correct or incorrect acupuncture points. In such situations it is desirable for the person assessing the patient's response to be different from the person who administered the treatment; the assessor can then be kept blind to the treatment the patient received.

The simplest and most commonly used study design is a **two group comparison** in which patients are randomly allocated, perhaps using random number tables, to one of the treatment groups. One treatment group receives A and the other receives B, and the responses in the two groups are then compared. Six of the nine studies of complementary therapies considered in this chapter use this type of design.[7,10,20,21,22,23]

Sometimes it may be known that a particular variable affects prognosis; for example, the sex of the patient. In such circumstances we would want to make sure that we had proper representation of both sexes in the two treatment groups. To ensure this we might conduct the random allocation into treatment groups for the males separately from the females. This procedure is called *stratification* and was used by Lewith *et al.*[21] As Gore[24] points out, excessive stratification is self-defeating. Suppose for example we have three prognostic factors such as sex, age (in three groups) and duration of illness (in three groups) to take into account. In this case there are $2 \times 3 \times 3 = 18$ subgroups to consider so, unless the study is very large, many of these strata will contain too few patients for meaningful analysis. In such circumstances it may be necessary to consider alternative ways of allowing for prognostic factors. These are discussed by Gore.[24]

If all the patients to be used in the trial are available before the trial starts, then it may be possible to identify for each patient another patient similar in all important prognostic factors; these two patients are called a *matched pair*. For each matched pair we randomly allocate one of the pair to treatment A and the other to treatment B. The reason for doing this is to improve the initial similarity of the two treatment groups. We will need to conduct a matched pair analysis when we analyse the data at the end of the study. Although Jobst *et al.*[23] suggest that they have a matched pairs design, the design section of their paper states that they randomly allocated patients to treatments and after the random allocation they paired similar patients, taking one from each treatment group. Clearly this cannot improve the initial similarity of the two groups. This is an inefficient use of matching since the most appropriate pairing for a particular patient may not be possible because the desired pair may have been allocated to the same treatment group!

For some studies it may be possible to use a simple **within-patient design**. This design, discussed by Gore,[25] is possible if a patient has matched sites; for example, if we are testing eye drops we could use treatment A in one eye and treatment B in the other, selecting at random the eye to be treated with A. The advantage of within-patient designs is that usually far fewer patients are required than for the simple two group design. Fewer patients are needed because the responses by an individual with matched sites are not as variable as the responses compared between individuals. There are unfortunately few occasions when such a design can be used, since even when matched sites exist we will not be able to use a within-patient design if either treatment acts systemically or if there is the possibility of contamination between treatment areas, for example by the patient scratching the site.

Another commonly used approach is the **cross-over design**. In such designs each patient receives both treatments, one after the other, the order in which they receive the treatments being decided randomly. The study of Murphy et al.[8] used a cross-over design; patients received either feverfew or placebo for four months and then received the other treatment for the next four months. Fung et al.[9] measure all patients without any treatment on the first occasion, then use a cross-over design for assessing the effects of sham and real acupuncture. Lee et al.[6] also use a cross-over design for their series I patients, but they have not allocated the patients randomly (or equally) into the two groups.

The advantage of a cross-over trial is that we require fewer patients. Each patient acts as their own control and since within patient variability is much less than between patient variability, we require fewer patients to be able to make reliable assessments of the treatment effect. Again we have a matched pair situation and all analyses should be appropriate to matched data. Such designs are particularly useful when the endpoint is a subjective assessment by the patient, for example pain severity, because the patient can compare their pain experience on the two treatments.

A cross-over design will not be appropriate if a treatment is expected to change the patient's state permanently. Such designs are only possible if we are treating a stable chronic condition, otherwise we will not be applying the two treatments to an equally sick patient. A further problem is the possibility of carry-over effects; that is, the treatment given first continues to have an effect even after it has been stopped. This difficulty could be avoided if it is possible to have a break between the two treatment periods, a so-called 'washout' period. This will not always be practical as it might put the patient at risk to have a period with no treatment. Further problems are the possibility of order effects, that is, systematic changes between the first and subsequent assessments, and period effects, that is, a treatment may be more effective if given in the first period. If there are likely to be any carry-over, order or period effects it would be better to avoid cross-over designs.

It is always a necessary part of the analysis of cross-over designs to check for the presence of carry-over, order and period effects. Two of the three cross-over studies considered in this chapter, those of Lee *et al.*[6] and Fung *et al.*,[9] seem to ignore the possibility that these effects may be present. Murphy *et al.*[8] provide some graphs showing mean values for the treatment groups at four points through the study; these alone are insufficient to rule out the possibility of carry-over, order or period effects. The design and analysis of cross-over studies is reviewed in detail by Hills and Armitage.[26]

Sequential designs are often seen as desirable since they combine the advantage of a randomized study with the attractive feature of taking into account the results so far in determining how long the trial continues. The main advantage over an ordinary two group study is that the required sample size will be smaller if the treatment effect is large, so the bigger the difference between the treatments, the fewer the number of patients who receive the less successful treatment. The major difficulty is that we need the results for each patient to be available quickly, since we will not know whether to recruit more patients until the outcome for the current patient is known. In sequential designs it is difficult to allow for more than one response variable or for more than two treatments and it will be administratively complex if the trial is multicentre. A comprehensive (but mathematical) discussion of sequential designs is provided by Whitehead[27] and a briefer less mathematical account is provided by Gore.[28] Sequential designs are likely to be of limited use for complementary therapies since the treatment results will generally be known too late to limit patient entry; however, if this is not the case a sequential design may provide very efficient use of resources.

Another problem with clinical trials is that of obtaining 'informed consent'. In all the designs so far considered the patient is asked to agree to enter without knowing which of the treatments they will receive; this is often difficult to explain to the patients particularly if they are very sick. Zelen[29] proposed the following design which avoids this problem. He proposed that of the subjects entering a trial, we randomly assign half to group 1 and the rest to group 2. The patients in group 1 all receive the standard treatment, so they are treated as if they were not in a trial apart from the need for standardized assessment and record-keeping. There is no need to obtain special consent or explain about the trial for those in group 1. The patients in group 2 are given a choice; they are offered the new treatment B, which is under investigation, but may have the standard treatment A if they wish. Thus the patient chooses their treatment rather than agreeing to be randomized.

For this so-called 'randomized consent' design to operate successfully it is essential that most of the patients in group 2 accept the new treatment, because in the analysis we will need to compare the whole of group 2 with group 1, the two randomly selected groups. If there are a lot of patients in group 2 rejecting the new treatment, then the group will be 'contaminated' by those undergoing the old treatment and we are unlikely to detect a treatment effect. Such designs cannot be blind since both the patient and practitioner know which treatment is being used. It would be difficult to compare more than two treatments with such a design.

Although 'randomized consent' trials are increasingly used in cancer trials, it is unlikely they will be of widespread use in trials of complementary therapies. It will be difficult to ensure a high take-up for the test treatment, and since many outcome measures are subjective, it is important to try and keep the patient and assessor blind.

Size of the study

Perhaps the question a statistician gets asked most frequently is, 'How large should my study be?'. The approach to answering this question will depend on the complexity of the study design. For the purposes of this discussion we will assume the trial is a simple two group comparison.

The aim of a clinical trial is usually to compare two treatments to determine whether the new treatment is better than the old; where 'better' means there is an improvement in response that is clinically important. Individual patients will vary in their response to the treatments so there is always a possibility that we will draw the wrong conclusion on the basis of our trial because of this variability in response. The more patients we include in the trial the more certain we might expect to be about the existence of any treatment difference. However, our time and resources are limited and we would not wish to deny patients indefinitely a worthwhile treatment. The size of our trial will be decided by balancing statistical and practical considerations.

There are two types of error that we might make. Firstly we could conclude, on the basis of our trial, that the new treatment is significantly better than the old, when in fact there is no difference in response on the two treatments; this is called a type I error. Secondly, we could fail to detect in our trial a clinically important difference, when in fact such a difference exists; this is a type II error. We do not know what the truth is (that is why we need to do a trial), so we need to keep the probability of both types of error as small as possible.

The value we decide is an acceptable probability for the type I error determines the level at which we conduct any significance tests. Commonly this is called α and is often taken as 0.05 and may be written as 5%. In practical terms, α is the probability that we detect a treatment difference, when in fact there is no difference. If we set $\alpha = 0.05$ and our result turns out to be significant, we have a 1 in 20 chance that the result is a false positive. The choice of $\alpha = 0.05$, although used in many published papers, is arbitrary and you should not feel bound to use $\alpha = 0.05$. However, taking α as larger than 0.05 will give too high a chance of a false positive to be widely acceptable, whilst taking α as smaller than 0.05 will increase the sample size required.

In general, people talk about 'power' rather than type II error; power is equal to one minus the type II error probability, so we would like the power to be as close as possible to one. The power is a measure of how likely we are to produce a statistically significant result for a treatment difference of a given magnitude. In practical terms it indicates the ability to detect a true difference of clinical importance. When planning a study it is important that we have a good chance of detecting a clinically significant treatment difference, should it exist. If the power is low, we may well be wasting our time and putting patients at risk for no good reason since, if our study fails to detect a treatment difference, we could not be sure whether that was because there was no treatment difference or because the study was too small to detect the difference.

Precisely how the sample size is determined depends not only on the study design but also on the outcome measure. There are two main types of outcome variable: a continuous measure, in which case we generally wish to compare the mean (average) response for the treatments, or a binary measure (response/no response) in which case we generally compare the proportions responding. In either case we will need to specify the treatment difference we wish to detect. By stating a treatment difference we consider to be of clinical importance, we ensure that 'statistically significant' equates to 'clinically important'.

In order to calculate the sample size for a two group comparison with a continuous outcome variable, you will need to provide the following information: what level of response is expected on the standard treatment, what the variance (measure of variability) of response is on the standard, how large a treatment difference will be considered clinically important, the type I error (α) you find acceptable, and the power to be used. Generally people take α to be equal to 0.05 and the power should be greater than 0.8. Examples of calculating sample sizes for continuous measures are provided by Altman,[30] who also provides a simple nomogram (a graph) to allow calculation of sample size.

To calculate sample size for a two group comparison with a binary response variable, you will need to provide the following information: the proportion expected to respond on the standard treatment, how large a difference in response will be considered clinically important, the type I error and power. This is discussed further by Lewith and Machin[11] who provide tables giving the sample size required for common values of type I error and power. It should be noted that Figure 1 in their paper is not consistent with the values obtained from the tables. The tables are correct; the figure was derived from a less exact approximation.

Before we are able to make sample size calculations we need to decide whether we will be conducting one-sided or two-sided hypothesis tests. A one-sided hypothesis test only allows for the possibility that the new treatment is an improvement on the old treatment. A two-sided hypothesis test allows us to examine whether the new treatment is different from the old (either better or worse). In general I find it difficult to support one-sided tests because if you are confident that the new treatment cannot be worse than the old, thus allowing one-sided tests, is it ethically possible to conduct a trial?

The nomogram given by Altman[30] is for calculating sample sizes assuming two-sided tests. However, the tables given by Lewith and Machin[11] assume a one-sided test; their Table 1a is also approximately appropriate for a two-sided test with $\alpha = 0.1$ and Table 1b is approximately appropriate for a two-sided test with $\alpha = 0.02$. More complete tables for two-sided tests of proportions are given by Fleiss[31] (Table A.3). For those who frequently need to carry out sample size calculations, a computer package called N might be a worthwhile investment.[32]

Perhaps the most common design error is to have too small a sample to get reliable and useful results. Altman[30] points out that power may be calculated retrospectively to see how much chance a completed study had of detecting (as significant) a clinically relevant difference. If the study is reporting a 'negative' finding, retrospective power calculations will indicate whether this is likely to be a true negative result. Even if the finding is positive there is a problem with interpretation because of publication bias.[12] Such bias arises because journals are more likely to publish studies with positive results. Suppose 20 identical low power studies are conducted, all testing with $\alpha = 0.05$ (so a 1 in 20 chance of a false positive); suppose further that 19 of the studies produce negative findings. It is likely that the only study published will be the one with a positive result; indeed, the others might even have been rejected on the grounds of insufficient power. Thus you should always be careful about interpreting the results of studies with low power.

It is necessary to include sufficient information in your study report to allow readers to calculate the power. Of the nine studies reviewed in this chapter, only Reilly *et al.*,[7] Bullock *et al.*[20] and Lewith *et al.*[21] attempt to give the necessary information to calculate the power of their design and hence justify their sample size. Unfortunately Bullock *et al.*[20] fail to state the proportion, p_1 say, that they expect to respond on the control treatment. But, whatever the value of p_1, their calculation that they require 20 patients in each group is wrong. There is no value of p_1 that would provide a sample size as low as 20 per group and be consistent with their other specifications. Bullock *et al.*[20] do, however, try to allow for drop-outs, which they estimate on the basis of a previous study. Unfortunately this seems to have been an underestimate for the control treatment since only one control patient completed the treatment programme.

For studies which fail to justify their sample size we may be able to calculate the power retrospectively, but this will only be possible if the study aim is clear and the outcome variable well defined. We will also need to assume that the response actually measured for the controls is equal to that which the study organizers would have specified, and that the difference observed is equal to that which they would have specified as clinically important. These are perhaps rash assumptions but may provide a reasonable estimate of power since observed treatment differences are rarely as dramatic as those hoped for by the investigators!

For example, Ferley *et al.*[10] had 234 patients receiving placebo and 238 receiving the homoeopathic remedy. The outcome measure was the proportion recovering within 48 hours of treatment; this was 0.10 for the placebo and 0.17 for the active treatment. Taking $\alpha = 0.05$ and assuming two-sided tests, Ferley's study had a power of only 0.55. So a study this size has a probability of only 0.55 of detecting an improvement in treatment effect from 10% response to 17% response, should such a difference exist. This is not a particularly high probability of success; we need to start a study with the assurance of a high probability of detecting clinically important differences.

Jobst et al.[22] had only twelve patients on each treatment; assuming they expected the mean six minute walk distance on placebo to be 240 metres with a standard deviation of 110 metres, the response on active treatment to be 335 metres, and used two-sided tests with $\alpha = 0.05$, then their study had a power of only 0.53. The power for Murphy et al.[8] appears to be almost adequate at about 0.73, assuming that the mean number of migraine sufferers on placebo is 4.7 with a standard deviation of 2.3 and the mean number on feverfew is 3.6. Murphy's study was a cross-over design with 59 people; for the purpose of calculating an approximate power it has been assumed that this is equivalent to a study with 59 people in each group. For the remaining three studies,[6,9,23] either the aim is too vague or the outcome measure unclear or the presented information inadequate for even a retrospective power calculation.

Conclusion

In this chapter, statistical aspects of the planning and design of experimental studies have been discussed. It is imperative that proper consideration be given to the areas identified in this chapter when carrying out studies. Many researchers only seek statistical assistance at the analysis stage, by which time it will be too late to rectify design faults which may render the study useless. Early consultation with a statistician is the best way to prevent catastrophic design errors such as studies that are too small. Researchers should get into the habit of allowing money in their research budget to pay for statistical advice and computer time.

When reading study reports this should be done critically. It is hoped that this chapter provides some guidance about points to watch for in study designs. It is more difficult to criticize statistical results without a reasonable knowledge of statistical techniques, particularly if authors fail to give references for their statistical method. To help understand statistical techniques a good basic textbook written for a medical audience is that by Bland[33] and for more advanced techniques, the book by Armitage and Berry[34] is recommended. Papers by Altman[35,36] and Gore et al.[37] discuss the misuse of statistical methods in medical articles.

In general, it is a good idea to conduct a pilot study before embarking on the real thing. Pilot studies provide an opportunity to find out how easy it is to determine whether a patient is eligible, whether the proposed measure of endpoints is sensible and practical and, in the absence of other data, they can provide estimates of the response values needed for sample size calculations.

It is clear that there have been several serious design flaws in the studies considered in this paper. These studies may not be typical of studies carried out with complementary therapies, but since they are all from major medical journals they are likely to have reached a wide audience. It is probably fair to say that some of these studies are actually no worse than many studies of conventional therapies appearing in major medical journals. Of the studies examined in this paper, the best from a planning and design point of view is the paper by Reilly *et al.*[7]; indeed, their paper would provide a reasonable 'model report'. One of the most important points about their paper is that it provides all the necessary information for the reader to judge for themselves the value of the treatment. Hopefully more studies in the future will be as well reported.

Appendix

Many statistical textbooks will provide further information on the terms listed below. The book by Moore[2] is recommended for clear and predominantly non-mathematical explanations of many of the following terms, whilst the book by Bland[33] provides examples in a more medical context.

Median
Often we wish to summarize the distribution of the values in our sample by one number which is a reasonable representation of the data. The median is the central value of the distribution; half our data values are less than the median and half are more than it. Thus the median is a measure of the central location of the data.[33,2]

Mean
The mean is another single value measure of the location of the data, and tends to be used more often than the median because it has nicer mathematical properties. The mean is affected a lot by extreme data values. Thus if the sample has a small number of cases with values that are very different from the rest of the data, then the median will give a more useful indication of location than the mean.[33,2]

Variance
In addition to knowing the mean, it would also be useful to have some measure of the spread of the distribution. Variance is a measure of spread. The square root of the variance is called the standard deviation (s.d.).[33,2]

Standard error
This is more correctly called the standard error of the mean (s.e.m.), and is a measure of the variability of the mean. That is, if we repeated the experiment with a different sample we will generally get a different value for the sample mean, and the s.e.m. is a measure of this variability. It should be noted that s.e.m. (sometimes denoted by s.e.) is not the same as the standard deviation (s.d.), and s.e.m. for a particular variable will always be smaller than the s.d. Beware of incorrect usage.[33,2]

p value
This is often used in reporting the result of a significance test. It is the

probability of getting a result as extreme, or more extreme, than that observed given the hypothesis under test. If we are conducting significance tests with the type I error set at 0.05, then a result is claimed to be statistically significant if p is less than 0.05. It is more useful to state the actual p value than to simply report $p < 0.05$, since this could result from $p = 0.049$ or from $p = 0.0001$, the second being a much more convincing result.[33,2]

Normal distribution

This probability distribution is also known as the Gaussian distribution and is often regarded as the fundamental probability distribution. The word 'normal' in this context means neither 'ordinary or common' nor 'non-diseased'. Many statistical tests depend on the sample data coming from a Normal distribution, so if we plot a histogram of the values in our sample we hope to see the characteristic symmetrical bell shape of the Normal distribution.[33,2]

t test

Student's t test is a significance test often used to examine hypotheses about the mean, or the difference between two means (perhaps the difference between the mean response on two treatments). The t test is only really appropriate if the data is at least approximately normally distributed. If we are considering the difference between two means and we have paired data (for example from a cross-over trial) then we must use a paired t test.[33,34,36,37]

Chi-squared (χ^2) test

The chi-squared test is often used to test the equality of two proportions, or to test for association between two categorical variables. Often the data used in a chi-squared test will be displayed in the form of a cross-tabulation; if very few cases are expected in a particular cell of such a tabulation, then the validity of the chi-squared test will be in doubt.[33,36,37]

Confidence interval

This is an interval within which we would expect the true population value to lie. For example, if a study reports the 95% confidence interval for the mean to be 7 to 20, then we could be reasonably confident that the true value for the population mean was not zero. A confidence interval is more informative than simply quoting a single value estimate, say the sample mean, because it takes account of variability and the size of the study.[33,2]

References

[1] Huff, D. *How to Lie with Statistics.* Harmondsworth: Penguin, 1973.

[2] Moore, D. S. *Statistics, Concepts and Controversies.* San Francisco: Freeman, 1979.

[3] Altman, D. G. Statistics and ethics in medical research: Misuse of statistics is unethical. *Br Med J* 1980; **281**: 1182–4.

[4] Altman, D. G. Statistics and ethics in medical research: Study design. *Br Med J* 1980; **281**: 1267–9.

5   Alderson, M. *An Introduction to Epidemiology.* 2nd ed. London: Macmillan, 1983.

6   Lee, P. K., Anderson, T. W., Modell, J. H., Saga, S. A. Treatment of chronic pain with acupuncture. *JAMA* 1975; **232**: 1133–75.

7   Reilly, D. T., Taylor, M. A., McSharry, C., Aitchison, T. Is homoeopathy a placebo response? Controlled trial of homoeopathic potency, with pollen in hayfever as model. *Lancet* 1986; **ii**: 881–5.

8   Murphy, J. J., Heptinstall, S., Mitchell, J. R. A. Randomised placebo-controlled trial of feverfew in migraine prevention. *Lancet* 1988; **ii**: 189–92.

9   Fung, K. P., Chow, O. K. W., So, S. Y. Attenuation of exercise-induced asthma by acupuncture. *Lancet* 1986; **ii**: 1419–21.

10 Ferley, J. P., Zmirou, D., D'Adhemar, D., Balducci, F. A controlled evaluation of a homoeopathic preparation in the treatment of influenza-like syndromes. *Br J Clin Pharmacol* 1989; **27**: 329–35.

11 Lewith, G. T., Machin, D. On the evaluation of the clinical effects of acupuncture. *Pain* 1983; **16**: 111–27.

12 Pocock, S. J. *Clinical Trials: A Practical Approach.* Chichester: Wiley, 1983.

13 Gore, S. M. Assessing clinical trials – first steps. *Br Med J* 1981; **282**: 1605–7.

14 Gore, S. M. Assessing clinical trials – why randomise? *Br Med J* 1981; **282**: 1958–60.

15 Pocock, S. J. Current issues in the design and interpretation of clinical trials. *Br Med J* 1985; **290**: 39–42.

16 Kingman, S. Medical research on trial. *New Sci* 1986; **111**: 48–52.

17 Gore, S. M. Assessing clinical trials – simple randomisation. *Br Med J* 1981; **282**: 2036–9.

18 Gribbin, M. Placebos: cheapest medicine in the world. *New Sci* 1981; **89**: 64–5.

19 Lewith, G. T. *Alternative Therapies.* London: Heinemann, 1985.

20 Bullock, M. L., Culliton, P. D., Olander, R. T. Controlled trial of acupuncture for severe recidivist alcoholism. *Lancet* 1989; **i**: 1435–8.

21 Lewith, G. T., Field, J., Machin, D. G. Acupuncture compared with placebo in post-herpetic pain. *Pain* 1983; **17**: 361–8.

22 Jobst, K., Chen, J. H., McPherson, K., Arrowsmith, J., Brown, V., Efthimiou, J., Fletcher, H. J., Maciocia, G., Mole, P., Shifrin, K., Lane, D. J. Controlled trial of acupuncture for dealing with disabling breathlessness. *Lancet* 1986; **ii**: 1416–18.

23 Gaw, A. C., Chang, L. W., Shaw, L. C. Efficacy of acupuncture on osteoarthritic pain. *New Eng J Med* 1975; **293**: 375–8.

24 Gore, S. M. Assessing clinical trials – restricted randomisation. *Br Med J* 1981; **282**: 2114–17.

25 Gore, S. M. Assessing clinical trials – design I. *Br Med J* 1981; **282**: 1780–81.

26 Hills, M., Armitage, P. The two period cross-over clinical trial. *Br J Clin Pharmacol* 1978; **8**: 7–20.

27 Whitehead, J. *The Design and Analysis of Sequential Clinical Trials.* Chichester: Ellis Horwood, 1983.

28 Gore, S. M. Assessing clinical trials – design II. *Br Med J* 1981; **282**: 1861–3.

29 Zelen, M. A new design for randomised clinical trials. *New Eng J Med* 1979; **300**: 1242–5.

30 Altman, D. G. Statistics and ethics in medical research – III How large a sample? *Br Med J* 1980; **281**: 1336–8.

31 Fleiss, J. L. *Statistical Methods for Rates and Proportions.* 2nd ed. New York: Wiley, 1981.

32 Chanter, D. O. Review of N. *App Stat* 1989; **38**: 529–34.

33 Bland, M. *An Introduction to Medical Statistics.* Oxford: OUP, 1987.

34 Armitage, P., Berry, G. *Statistical Methods in Medical Research.* 2nd ed. Oxford: Blackwell, 1987.

35 Altman, D. G. Statistics in medical journals. *Stat Med* 1982; **1**: 59–71.

36 Altman, D. G. Statistics and ethics in medical research – V Analysing data. *Br Med J* 1980; **281**: 1473–5.

37 Gore, S. M., Jones, I. G., Rytter, E. C. Misuse of statistical methods: Critical assessment of articles in BMJ from January to March 1976. *Br Med J* 1977; **1**: 85–7.

2 Current issues in the design and interpretation of clinical trials

Stuart J. Pocock

Summary

Though there have been considerable improvements in the use of statistical methods for clinical trials in recent years, there remain major practical difficulties in the design and interpretation of many trials. This chapter concentrates on problems relating to randomization, the overemphasis on significance testing, and the inadequate size of many trials. Each topic is illustrated by examples from recent trials.

Introduction

This chapter concentrates on three major statistical problems that remain a common cause of difficulty in the design and interpretation of clinical trials.

The first problem is randomization. Many treatments are still being developed without properly randomized controlled trials. Unequal randomization might be used more often in early (phase II) trials for which there exist substantial historical data on the standard treatment. The required degree of stratification in the design of randomized trials is still not clear.

The second topic is an overemphasis on significance testing. Most trial reports in medical journals rely heavily on significance tests and pay inadequate attention to estimating the potential magnitude of treatment differences (for example, confidence limits are under-used). The abundant and selective use of significance tests in clinical trials may greatly increase the risk of false positive claims. Particular problems concern the use of multiple endpoints, interim analyses, and subgroup analyses.

The third problem concerns the size of trials. Many trials remain far too small to provide adequate power to detect relevant treatment differences. When power calculations have been used there is a danger of defining unduly large treatment differences under the alternative hypothesis to achieve the convenient requirement of small sample sizes. Small trials require huge observed differences to be statistically significant, and non-significant small trials are less likely to be published; these two facts lead to major 'publication bias' in reports of clinical trials.

The above problems are practical. Whereas further developments in statistical methods will continue to occur in clinical trials, such theoretical advances may be of secondary importance compared with the need to convey the essentials of good statistical practice to a wider audience. Thus it is important that professional biostatisticians make a greater attempt to communicate effectively with clinicians and other non-statistical collaborators rather than concentrate on mathematically oriented topics of only peripheral relevance to medical and biological research.

The remainder of this chapter includes examples from actual trials in a broader discussion of the three topics.

Randomization

Chaos caused by non-randomized trials

In Britain in the 1980s there was considerable controversy over clinical trials to evaluate periconceptional multivitamin treatment for preventing births of children with neural tube defects to high risk mothers. There were two non-randomized trials in which pregnant women with a previous neural tube defect birth who had had periconceptional multivitamin supplements were compared with an unsupplemented control group.[1,2] The combined results for the two trials were:

	Multivitamin group	Control group	
Total number of births	397	493	$\left.\right\}p < 0.0003$ one-sided test
Number of neural tube defect births	3 (0.8%)	23 (4.7%)	

The authors argued that such a highly significant apparent benefit justified the use of multivitamins for all subsequent such pregnancies, as they considered that bias in the methodology of the trial could not account for the observed treatment difference. In these multicentre trials, however, the control group included some women who had elected not to take supplements and also included more women from high risk areas – for example, Northern Ireland – so that there is ample reason to claim that the treatment comparison may have been severely biased.

The problem is that there is no way of determining whether all or part of the treatment difference is attributable to bias, so that there remains uncertainty whether a subsequent randomized trial is ethically justified. Hence the Medical Research Council Vitamin Study[3] provoked major arguments over whether it was ethically acceptable to randomize some patients to a non-supplemented control group. There was considerable public opposition to this randomized trial. For instance, the *Daily Telegraph* (30 March 1984) carried the headline 'Dummy-pill risk of handicapped babies "immoral"' in an article claiming that the trial was unnecessary. Such views must be regarded with some sympathy: to the layman the results of the earlier trials look impressive. Nevertheless, it is a dangerous precedent to argue that future therapeutic practice should be determined by such inadequate trials.

There is no simple 'right answer' to the question of when a randomized trial is justified in the face of such suggestive (but perhaps grossly exaggerated) prior evidence. The real problem is that non-randomized trials may considerably hinder clarifying therapeutic issues. Undoubtedly the first trial of multivitamins should have been organized properly with a randomized control group. I hope that this unfortunate example will increase awareness of the need to undertake early randomized trials before uncontrolled or poorly controlled data lead to overenthusiastic (and possibly mistaken) support for a new treatment.

Unequal randomization

In many trials of cancer chemotherapy the aim is to assess the value of a new treatment when there is already a standard treatment with substantial experience. The approach is often to conduct an uncontrolled (phase II) trial of the new agent and then to consider a randomized (phase III) trial later. Nevertheless, this may pose problems: uncontrolled trials may produce wildly overoptimistic results and hence decisions on which drugs to put in phase III trials are based on inadequate data.

A useful compromise is to undertake a randomized controlled phase II trial in which most patients (say, two-thirds) are assigned to the new treatment. Compared with the conventional randomized trial, such an unbalanced design permits greater experience of the new treatment, an important consideration in the early stage of testing drugs. At the same time the element of randomization helps to ensure that patient selection, ancillary care, and evaluation of response conform to accepted standards.

Some recent experience of this approach has been in the design of trials for advanced breast cancer. One commonly accepted combination treatment is VAC (vincristine, adriamycin, and cyclophosphamide), and apparently investigators are encouraged to undertake trials of new single agents or combinations that also randomize one-third of patients to VAC. Randomization ratios of $3:2$ or $2:1$ preserve adequate power if comparative analyses are to be undertaken. For instance, if a trial adopts a $2:1$ rather than $1:1$ randomization ratio (while preserving the same total number of patients) then type II errors of 0.05 and 0.5 would be increased to 0.075 and 0.55 respectively.[4] Nevertheless, in such randomized phase II trials the observed response and toxicity rates with the new treatment are of interest in their own right.

A further issue is that response data for the randomized control group might potentially be supplemented by response data from a larger body of historical controls. Given the potential bias in historical controls, caution is needed before undertaking any formal analysis pooling the two sets of control data. If the historical controls were collected in a similar fashion, however – that is, from a previous randomized trial with the same eligibility and response criteria – then some formal combining of control data may be worth considering. In these circumstances it is still appropriate to give greater weight to the randomized controls.

Stratified randomization

Despite the considerable developments in the past decade in statistical methods for stratified randomization,[4,5] there has also been controversy over whether stratification is necessary. The diversity of approaches has been illustrated in an international survey of randomization in major cancer trial centres.[6] For example, ten centres had a current trial in primary breast cancer; two of these trials had no stratification factors (except for institution), whereas one trial had five stratification factors, with a total of $2 \times 2 \times 2 \times 2 \times 3 = 48$ strata. The most common decision was to have two stratification factors, each at two levels.

All of these centres were experienced at coordinating multicentre trials, so that the different approaches were due to conscious decisions rather than to oversight. Should it be argued that the two trials without stratification were inferior? Probably not: as trials in breast cancer require a substantial number of patients, the risk of serious imbalance between randomized groups with respect to prognostic factors is negligible. On the other hand, close prognostic comparability of randomized groups achievable by extensive stratification enhances the acceptability of simple unstratified analyses. To achieve such closely matched groups, however, may require so-called minimization procedures. These are straightforward conceptually (they aim at minimizing some overall measure of the treatment difference in prognostic factor distributions when registering patients but they increase the administrative burden).

It may be sensible to avoid stratifying if there is uncertainty over the relevance or reliability of prognostic factors or if the trial has a simple organization that might not cope well with complex randomization. Nevertheless, for trials with a sophisticated and experienced organization that have well defined prognostic factors the slight gains in statistical efficiency and the appeal of closely matching groups make it sensible to use stratified randomization. The newer, more complex methods based on a minimization approach may enable effective balancing for more prognostic factors than would the conventional random permuted blocks within strata.

To take an overall view of the statistical design of clinical trials, it appears that stratification is a minor issue, particularly in large trials. For most trials it may be more directly profitable to use some form of stratified analysis – that is, adjustment for prognostic factors when analysing for treatment differences.

Overemphasis on significance testing

Significance tests and confidence limits

Some fundamental issues in significance testing are illustrated by the reported findings in the Lipid Research Clinics Coronary Prevention Trial.[8] A total of 3806 men with high serum cholesterol concentrations were randomized to treatment with cholestyramine (a drug that lowers cholesterol concentrations) or placebo. The following table presents the results for the prespecified primary endpoint, definite coronary heart disease, after an average follow up of 7.4 years:

	Placebo	*Cholestyramine*
Total number of men	1900	1906
Number with definite coronary heart disease	187 (9.8%)	155 (8.1%)

$\left.\begin{array}{c} \\ \end{array}\right\}$ $p<0.05$ one-sided test

There were fewer coronary events with cholestyramine, but the comparison is statistically significant at the 5% level only if a one-sided test is adopted. This borderline significance should convey the message that uncertainty remains whether cholestyramine reduces the risk of coronary heart disease. Unfortunately, in an aspect of the epidemiology of heart disease that provokes some strongly committed views, the study findings have been interpreted in a more dogmatic fashion, particularly by the press. For instance, the *Daily Telegraph* (January 1984) carried an article headed 'Heart disease study points finger at cholesterol,' which went on to state, 'the study ... proved that lowering cholesterol in the blood reduced both the signs of heart disease and fatal heart attacks.'

This example illustrates that the accept/reject philosophy of significance testing based on the 'magical' $p = 0.05$ barrier remains dominant in the minds of many non-statisticians. Indeed, the statistical profession itself has not always been effective enough in overcoming this misconception. We need continually to assert that p-values are only a guideline to the strength of evidence contradicting the null hypothesis of no treatment difference and that they should not be regarded as indicating proof of treatment efficacy. It may be more productive to shift the emphasis towards estimation methods such as confidence limits.

In this trial the observed percentage reduction in risk in the group given cholestyramine was $(9.8 - 8.1) \times 100/9.8 = 17\%$, which is adjusted to 19% after a stratified analysis. The authors reported 90% confidence limits for this percentage reduction of +3% and +32%. One might argue in favour of the more conventional 95% confidence interval, which would have included zero reduction and helped to emphasize the lack of conclusive proof for treatment benefit.

It has become fashionable to use such percentage reductions in risk, but for potential patients the difference in risk may be more meaningful. In this trial the observed difference in favour of cholestyramine was $9.8\% - 8.1\% = 1.7\%$, with 95% confidence limits of -0.1% and $+3.5\%$. Either way, the use of confidence limits readily conveys the considerable uncertainty about the effect of cholestyramine on coronary risk.

One issue highlighted by this trial is the use of one-sided testing. Ideally the distinction between one and two-sided tests should be unimportant if p-values are interpreted as informal guidelines where there is no radical distinction drawn between $p = 0.06$ and $p = 0.04$. Even so it would make sense always to use two-sided tests, as one-sided testing rests on a subjective judgement that an observed difference in the opposite direction (for example, against cholestyramine) would be of no interest whatsoever. In particular, the use of a two-sided test in this trial would have resulted in $0.05 < p < 0.1$, which might have helped to tone down some of the more exaggerated claims derived from this well-conducted and valuable but inconclusive trial.

The problem with significance testing would not be so bad if there was only one test per trial. Many trials, however, generate a multiplicity of data, which may provoke a plethora of significance tests. It is worth focusing on three issues: interim analyses, subgroup analyses, and multiple endpoints.

Interim analyses and stopping rules

Many trials continue without formalized stopping rules, with the consequent risk of exaggerating both the significance and the magnitude of treatment effects. Our experience at the Royal Free Hospital with a trial comparing D-penicillamine and placebo in treating primary biliary cirrhosis illustrates some of the problems associated with interim analyses.[9] The trial began in 1975 with survival as the main endpoint. In line with the arguments above, the randomization was unbalanced with three-fifths of patients assigned to D-penicillamine.

The changing pattern of survival was as follows:

	Number of deaths/Number of patients			
	Placebo	*D-penicillamine*	χ^2	*p*
First analysis, summer 1980	8/32	2/55	9.1	0.003
Publication, 1981	10/32	5/55	7.2 (logrank)	0.01
Most recent analysis, 1984	16/37	18/61	3.0 (logrank)	0.08

In the summer of 1980 the results looked interesting and so the investigators were encouraged to seek a first analysis of the data despite the few deaths overall. This showed a highly significant result which suggested that, even though no formal stopping rule had been planned, patient entry should be stopped and the results published. The published findings in 1981 indicated that the logrank χ^2 had been reduced in the few extra months of follow-up but that the treatment difference was still significant at the 1% level.[9]

Three years further on, the latest analysis of patient survival in January 1984 still showed a lower death rate with D-penicillamine, but the difference was only marginally significant ($p = 0.08$). These updated findings leave greater uncertainty regarding the value of D-penicillamine, a toxic drug that needs to show clear survival benefit before its general use could be recommended. One possibility worth considering is that there is a genuine decline in the treatment difference over time – that is, does D-penicillamine delay some deaths that would otherwise occur in the first year or two of follow-up? Inspection of the current life table plots, however, gives no indication of such a 'treatment-time interaction', and indeed trials in this disease need more patients to establish the true answer.

This trial illustrates a couple of general messages that need wider recognition:

(a) Interim trial publications claiming significant treatment differences will tend to exaggerate the true magnitude of the treatment effect.

(b) Subsequent analyses (if possible) are likely to show a reduction in both the significance and magnitude of treatment differences.

Both these phenomena may be explained by the fact that interim publications are often timed (either deliberately or unwittingly) to reflect a 'random high' in the treatment comparison. Unfortunately, this potential bias in the timing of publication is widespread as most trials have no formal policy on when to publish.

Subgroup analyses

Clinical trials are sometimes accused of providing only global treatment comparisons, which may not be suited to the needs of individual patients. Hence there is always pressure to try to identify particular subgroups of patients who responded especially well (or badly) to a new treatment. The problems here are:

(a) trials can rarely provide sufficient power to detect such subgroup effects;

(b) medical publications tend erroneously to use separate significance tests for each subgroup rather than the appropriate (but more complex) tests of interaction; and

(c) there are often many possible prognostic factors from which to form subgroups, so that one has to guard against 'data dredging'.

To illustrate the problems of subgroup analysis I will refer to the Multiple Risk Factor Intervention Trial.[10] This randomized trial of 12,866 men at high risk of coronary heart disease compared special intervention aimed at affecting major risk factors (for example, hypertension, smoking, diet) and usual care in the community. The overall rates of coronary mortality after an average seven year follow-up (1.79% with special intervention and 1.93% with usual care) are not significantly different. The trial report contains several subgroup analyses, the most striking of which is the following:

		Number of coronary deaths/Number of men (%)	
Hypertension	Electrocardiographic abnormality	Special intervention	Usual care
No	No	24/1817 (1.3)	30/1882 (1.6)
No	Yes	11/592 (1.9)	15/583 (2.6)
Yes	No	44/2785 (1.6)	58/2808 (2.1)
Yes	Yes	36/1233 (2.9)	21/1185 (1.8)

For those with hypertension and electrocardiographic abnormalities at initial screening, it appears that the coronary death rate is higher in the special intervention group, whereas the three other subgroups show a difference in the opposite direction. At face value such a subgroup effect looks impressive and worthy of clinical interpretation. Nevertheless, a formal test for interaction[11] shows no significant departure from the null hypothesis that the logical difference in coronary death rates for the special intervention and usual care groups is the same in all four subgroups ($p = 0.1$). Given that this was not the only subgroup analysis performed, we should assert that there are inadequate grounds for supposing that the special intervention harmed those with hypertension and electrocardiographic abnormalities.

The message is that we should be wary of overinterpreting subgroup analyses. It would be too extreme to suggest that they should be avoided altogether – rather that they should be used cautiously in a spirit of exploratory data analysis, provoking ideas to be confirmed (or refuted) in future studies.

Multiple endpoints

In many trials it is appropriate to record and analyse several different aspects of each patient's response to treatment. Descriptive statistics on such multiple endpoints may provide valuable insight into the pattern of progress of the disease with each treatment. Nevertheless, the corresponding use of multiple significance tests carries an increased risk of a type I error – that is, false claims of treatment benefit. Accordingly, at the planning stage it has become standard practice to designate one primary endpoint whose significance test will be the main criterion for assessing treatment differences.

As an illustration, consider the report of a trial of 1232 men in Oslo, Norway, at high risk of coronary heart disease who were randomly assigned to the intervention or control group.[12] The intervention was recommendation to change diet and stop smoking. After five years the mortality and cardiovascular events in each group were as follows:

	Intervention group (604 men)	*Control group (628 men)*	*p*
Sudden death	3	12	0.02
Fatal myocardial infarction (MI)	3	2	
Fatal MI + sudden death	6	14	0.09
Non-fatal MI	13	22	0.15
Total coronary events	19	36	0.03
Fatal stroke	2	1	
Non-fatal stroke	1	2	
Total cardiovascular events	22	39	0.04
Total cardiovascular deaths	8	15	0.17
Total mortality	16	24	0.25

The above seven significance tests would pose considerable problems if all were presented on equal terms. In fact, the authors prespecified total coronary events as the primary endpoint, in which case they interpreted this single test at $p = 0.03$ as evidence for intervention being beneficial.

Interestingly, one sudden death in the control group was 'unexplained', in that confirmatory evidence of a coronary cause could not be obtained. If this death was not related to coronary disease it might be considered to have been unrelated to intervention. Let us suppose that this man had been randomized to the intervention group instead – then if this one sudden death had still occurred the significance tests for sudden death, total coronary events, and total cardiovascular events would all have become non-significant at the 5% level. Thus the statistical significance of this trial depends on one possibly unavoidable death being in the control group. This illustrates how fickle statistical significance may be, particularly if one were to rely too heavily on specific cut-off points such as $p < 0.05$.

Size of trials

All too frequently statisticians claim that most trials do not have enough patients to provide a reliable comparison of treatments. It would help to emphasize this fact if trial publications had to indicate the uncertainty of therapeutic differences by using interval estimation methods such as confidence intervals. Nevertheless, once the results of a trial are analysed and published it is too late to improve things.

Hence greater emphasis should be given at the planning stage, where power calculations should be used realistically. Unfortunately power calculations have the habit of producing unduly large sample sizes which are incompatible with the number of patients available. It is tempting to 'improve the situation' by modifying the arbitrary levels of power and treatment difference to be detected, but this may lead to overoptimistic specifications.

For instance, the Oslo trial specified a 60% chance of detecting a 50% reduction in coronary events in the intervention group at the 5% level of significance, which required a trial size of 1230 men.[12] Such a dramatic reduction in coronary heart disease by diet and smoking intervention is highly desirable, but is it realistic to expect such a large effect? A 30% risk reduction would also be important to detect, but a trial size of 1230 men has only about 30% power of picking up such an effect as being significant at the 5% level – that is, if a true 30% risk reduction were to exist, this would be detected as significant only if the observed difference happened by chance to be somewhat greater. Thus, although recruitment of 1230 patients is a substantial undertaking, in the context of primary prevention trials for coronary heart disease such a sample size is inadequate.

Other trials on this question, such as the multiple risk factor intervention trial, have not shown such large benefits of intervention, so that it seems that this Oslo trial, though well executed in all other respects, may have achieved an inflated point estimate of risk reduction (47%)

because of the random error inherent in having only 55 coronary events overall.

Evidently prevention trials in heart disease require particularly large numbers of patients compared with therapeutic trials for other diseases. Nevertheless, the deficiency in patient numbers in clinical trials is a general phenomenon whose full implications for restricting therapeutic progress are not widely appreciated. The fact is that trials with truly modest treatment effects will achieve statistical significance only if random variation conveniently exaggerates these effects. The chances of publication and reader interest are much greater if the results of the trial are statistically significant. Hence the current obsession with significance testing combined with the inadequate size of many trials means that publications on clinical trials for many treatments are likely to be biased towards an exaggeration of therapeutic effect, even if trials are unbiased in all other respects. Such 'publication bias' and its liability to produce an excess of false positive findings has been reported elsewhere.[4,13,14]

In a short chapter it is not possible to explore fully these fundamental statistical problems affecting clinical trials. Nevertheless, I hope that airing such issues will prove thought-provoking and may encourage colleagues, both clinical and statistical, to an increased awareness of the subtle biases that may arise in published reports of clinical trials.

References

[1] Smithells, R. W., Shepperd, S., Schorah, C. J., *et al.* Possible prevention of neural tube defects by periconceptional vitamin supplementation. *Lancet* 1981; **i**: 339–40.

[2] Smithells, R. W., Shepperd, S., Schorah, C. J., *et al.* Vitamin supplementation and neural tube defects. *Lancet* 1981; **ii**: 1425.

[3] Medical Research Council. Vitamin study. *Lancet* 1984; **i**: 1308.

[4] Pocock, S. J. *Clinical Trials: A Practical Approach.* Chichester: Wiley, 1983.

[5] Simon, R. Restricted randomization designs in clinical trials. *Biometrics* 1979; **35**: 503–12.

[6] Pocock, S. J., Lagakos, S. W. Practical experience of randomization in cancer trials: an international survey. *Br J Cancer* 1982; **46**: 368–75.

[7] White, S. J., Freedman, L. S. Allocation of patients to treatment groups in a controlled clinical study. *Br J Cancer* 1978; **37**: 849–57.

[8] Lipid Research Clinics Program. The lipid research clinics coronary prevention trial results. *JAMA* 1984; **251**: 351–74.

[9] Epstein, O., Lee, R. G., Bass, A. M., *et al.* D-penicillamine treatment improves survival in primary biliary cirrhosis. *Lancet* 1981; **i**: 1275–7 .

[10] Multiple Risk Factor Intervention Trial Research Group. Multiple risk factor intervention trial: risk factor changes and mortality results. *JAMA* 1982; **248**: 1465–77.

[11] Halperin, M., Ware, J. H., Byar, D. P., *et al.* Testing for interaction in an I × J × K contingency table. *Biometrika* 1977; **64**: 271–5.

[12] Hjermann, I., Holme, I., Velve Byre, K., Laren, P. Effects of diet and smoking intervention on the incidence of coronary heart disease. *Lancet* 1981; **ii**: 1303–10.

[13] Peto, R., Pike, M. C., Armitage, P., *et al.* Design and analysis of randomized clinical trials requiring prolonged observation of each patient. 1. Introduction and design. *Br J Cancer* 1976; **34**: 585–612.

[14] Zelen, M. Guidelines for publishing papers on cancer clinical trials: responsibilities of editors and authors. *J Clin Oncol* 1983; **1**: 164–9.

3 Error and bias in single group and controlled data trials

Stuart J. Pocock

Summary

The randomized controlled trial, performed double blind, is the gold standard for studies aiming to prove that therapy is effective. This type of rigorous plan has evolved to exclude error and bias, as far as this is possible, and to estimate the probability that chance alone could have caused the observed effects of therapy. This chapter examines the various elements contributing to this rigour and shows that the same principles must be considered in planning any clinical research.

Introduction

As a medical statistician, I shall focus this chapter on randomized controlled clinical trials, partly for their own sake and partly because the principles governing randomized controlled clinical trials are also relevant to other forms of clinical research that you may wish to undertake. Clinical trials are scientific experiments. They are about the evaluation of treatment, getting an unbiased assessment of the efficacy and safety of one or more treatments, with the complication that they require continuous consideration of medical ethics. We are faced with the dilemma that good science (i.e. the advancement of knowledge about treatment) has to be undertaken in the context of what is good ethical practice, and basically a lot of common sense is needed in balancing good science with good ethics.

A key issue in the planning of trials is the careful development of the study protocol, the documentation of what it is intended to do. It is essential to document all aspects of the scientific design, the practical organization, the data collection and the intended evaluation of the study. There are three key issues in the conceptualization of the clinical trial: the first is what *patients* you are going to study, the second is what *treatments* you are trying to compare or study, and the third is what *methods of evaluation* you are going to apply.

1 Patients to be studied

Definition of patients might seem very obvious on many occasions, but precise definition is necessary to avoid trouble. You need to specify the criteria for inclusion and the exclusions, those patients that you deem unsuitable, limitations based on age and other criteria. It is a good idea to keep a register of all the patients coming through who might be considered for the trial but for various reasons are excluded, so that you can see whether they are a representative group capable of giving results that are applicable to a wider variety of patients.

2   Treatments

The next issue is treatments. You need to define precisely what your treatment package is going to be, specifying any dose schedules that are involved and any modification required in response to a patient's circumstances. There is a philosophical distinction I am becoming aware of in complementary medicine. There are *pragmatic* trials, in which the intention is to study the whole policy of a particular approach to therapy; for instance, the approach of one particular type of complementary medicine. There are also *explanatory* trials, which are trying to subdivide that policy to see which bits of it actually work, separating out the various components of the therapy to see whether it is one component or the whole approach that is effective. This distinction between pragmatic and explanatory is an important concept and you should be clear which type of trial you are actually aiming to carry out. In a given area of study you may require a pragmatic trial first to examine whether the whole package of a particular form of complementary medicine produces good effects, and then home in later with an explanatory trial to look at which components of the therapy are being effective.

Assuming that the treatment has been defined, how many different kinds of treatment should you have in a trial? If you are an enthusiast you will probably want to have lots of alternative treatments, but if you are realistic you will have more limited objectives. The essence of most clinical trials is that they compare one new treatment group, the experimental treatment group (which may be a complementary therapy) with a control group on standard therapy or none. The simplicity of a structure that has one new treatment group versus one control group is an important principle to try and maintain when you are planning a clinical trial.

3   The need for a control group

Why do you need a *control group*? Time and time again in therapeutic research you follow a group of patients and do nothing exceptional to them and they tend to get better over the course of time. One reason for this is that patients tend to enter a study when their disease is particularly bad, otherwise they wouldn't be there, and the decision to enter a study or to become available for a study is related to the severity of the disease. The disease has an ebb and flow, so naturally you tend to see an improvement in the disease over time in most groups of patients that are studied, regardless of what the treatment is. That is why it is essential to have a control group so that you can then assess whether there was any additional benefit associated with what you actually did. If you do not have controls you cannot establish this. So uncontrolled studies are inevitably inconclusive. That is not to say that they have no value. They may be valuable pilot studies in setting the tone of how you are going to tackle a whole therapeutic area, but it is important not to fool yourself that they have the definitive answer to whether or not a certain form of therapy works. Another point is that the same treatment carried out on a number of different groups of patients tends to show quite wide differences in the degree of response. So the selection of patients may be the key to the response that is noted; without the control group you cannot possibly say how much the treatment was adding.

4 The role of the control group

What is the precise role of the control group? Suppose that you are comparing a standard treatment group with a control group and at the end of the trial you have a difference of response; one treatment group did better than the other. What does it mean? There are three possibilities. The response may be due to a genuine difference between the *treatments*, it may be due to *chance*, or it could be due to *bias*. You can get chance out of the way by using statistical techniques, such as significance tests, to assess (providing you have a large enough study) whether the difference could realistically occur by chance alone. With regard to bias, you need to consider whether there are aspects of the comparison which made it unfair; whether, for instance, you put better quality patients in the new treatment group than in the control group. Was patient selection biased, or was there some aspect of the way you evaluated patient care over time which led to a bias in evaluation, or is the whole experimental environment different between the two groups? Were enthusiasm or record-keeping or observer variations somehow interfering with the comparison?

5 Randomization

The only way round this problem that has any credibility in the research world is *randomization*. For each patient you must reach a point in time when the patient is available to enter the study, and is then randomly allocated either to the new treatment group or to the control group. The time sequence of doing this is important: 1) you recognize that the patient needs treatment; 2) you recognize that the patient is actually suitable for the trial that you are carrying out; 3) you establish that the practitioner is willing to accept the principle of randomization; 4) you obtain the patient's consent to participate in the trial; 5) only then is the patient formally recognized as in the trial for good; 6) the patient is randomly assigned to one treatment or another; 7) you document the base line observation; and, 8) treatment gets under way. This is usually a very rapid process, often taking place within an hour or so, but it is essential that the decisions are made in this order. If, for instance, you assign treatment from a randomization list and then find that either the investigator or the patient is unwilling, the patient is withdrawn and it messes up your study and may make the comparison invalid; getting the right sequence of events surrounding randomization is important for the validity of the study. There are various methods of implementing randomization. The sealed envelope technique is a simple technique that is widely used but requires careful supervision to avoid error. Tables of random numbers should be used to set up your randomization in advance.

6 Blinding

The next key component in a randomized trial is *blinding*. The gold standard of trials is to achieve a double blind design, where neither the patient nor those who are concerned with the treatment or evaluation are aware of which treatment he is receiving. In some areas of complementary practice that may be feasible (for instance in homoeopathic medicine), but in other areas it may be extremely difficult even to contemplate this sort of a double blind trial, because the patient or investigator has to know what is going on. In such circumstances, you think of other ways of reducing the risk of bias, for instance *blinded evaluation*; you get someone else who does not know which treatment the patient has been having to evaluate how well he has done. The role of a placebo in preserving blindness needs to be carefully considered and in each trial the question arises as to what is meant by placebo and whether there is an acceptable placebo that can be used.

7 Evaluation of outcome

The key to the evaluation of patient response is objectivity. Evaluation concerns three areas: the condition of the patient before treatment (which needs to be fully documented); the disease outcome (that is, the progress of their disease state in terms of both the objective observation you can make, and the patient's own assessment of how they are doing); and any adverse effects that may have occurred. Objective assessment is trying to improve on clinical opinion, by achieving standardization of technique. For instance, the assessment of depression is better done by structured interview techniques, such as the Hamilton Rating Scale, than by just asking the patient how he feels. If possible, use good quality standard techniques that have been tested. This helps to reduce observer variation. If it is a large study and you need a number of observers, you need to train the observers to get consistency between them. The period over which you will be assessing the response also needs to be defined.

8 Design of forms

The design of forms is an important aspect of any trial. It is often the most tedious and long drawn out part of the preparation. It has been said that clinical trials are 5% inspiration and 95% sheer slog, and the worst part of that slog is often designing the forms on which you are going to record your data. Systemization of data collection is crucial in undertaking clinical studies. In any area where you want to get grading of response to therapy you must come up with standardized questions, because for analysis all the data should usually end up in numerical form. Free recording and open-ended questions simply do not work in organized clinical research, whether it is part of a clinical trial or not. Forms with a good, tightly packaged structure, with well-formulated questions, are extremely important. So before you start the trial go out and test your forms on patients who are not in the trial and see whether they work or not.

9 Principles of analysis

At the end of the trial you will be analysing the data to see if you can establish whether there is any difference between the effects of the two treatments. In this chapter I shall only outline briefly the principles underlying the *statistical analysis*, which are also important in understanding the planning of trials. Significance tests compare the patient response in the two treatment groups and arrive at a *p* value which is a probability, the probability of the observed difference occurring by chance even when the active treatment was totally ineffective. There are different ways of applying the significance test, applicable to different circumstances; if the probability of the difference occurring by chance alone is sufficiently small, the study is said to be statistically significant. In every clinical trial, you perversely put forward a null hypothesis which says, 'Suppose that what I was hoping was my good treatment is no good at all'. You then see to what extent the data contradicts that negative declaration, in order to produce evidence that the new treatment really does work. Statistical analyses are often abused in the medical literature with people working on the assumption that if they can only get their *p* value down to less than 0.05 they have proved it worked. Although the smaller the *p* value the stronger the evidence that there is a difference between the two groups, dogmatic claims of proof are unjustified.

You also want to know how well the treatment works, i.e. to quantify the magnitude of the treatment effect by calculating a point estimate of the treatment difference. But as this is based on a finite number of patients, you need to estimate the error involved in this point estimate (taking account of the number of patients). This is often done using a statistical technique called the *95% confidence interval*; the result roughly means that you are 95% sure that the true effect will lie within the limits which you calculate.

The size of a clinical trial is important and affects statistical significance greatly; the more patients you have the more chance you have of showing a genuine difference if it exists. The worst thing about doing small trials is that you might fail to show a difference when it is there; that is called a type II error. So to achieve significance you need to think about two things; the magnitude of the real effect that it would be important to detect and hence, the number of patients needed to demonstrate it. If you economize on the number of patients you may be disappointed in the result because you had too few patients to show the effect. There are statistical techniques called power calculations which are used to find the numbers needed.

10 Protocol violations

Another problem is that of *patient withdrawals*; this affects single group studies as well as controlled trials. You can easily delude yourself that your therapies are wonderful if you only document those patients who stay on them. Your drop-outs (those patients who disappear during the course of therapy) must be accounted for in the results you produce at the end of the study. This is just as important in a single group study as in a controlled study. If some patients have to fall out of a trial because of toxic effects or other unacceptable effects of the treatment and are not accounted for, the trial will give a falsely optimistic view of what that treatment was achieving. So accounting for all the patients is an extremely important part of the follow-up and analysis and publication of all studies.

Conclusion

The double blind randomized controlled trial is not the strategy to choose for a first essay into research, but it is the plan to aim for if the therapy you are concerned with can be tested in this way; other strategies can be used to reduce the possibility of observer error if your therapy cannot be given blind. In complementary medicine it is often appropriate to consider a pragmatic trial in which the whole policy of a particular approach to therapy is tested, before going on to an explanatory trial, testing which parts of that policy actually work.

If you are aiming to do a clinical trial you must write a detailed protocol, first focusing on the definition of patients, treatments, and outcome measures. You must think carefully about the design of your study, considering such issues as: 1) should it be a single group or a controlled trial?, 2) the principle of randomization, 3) the size of trial, 4) the degree of blinding, 5) forms and data management, 6) statistical analysis, 7) patient withdrawals and other possible violations. If the study is to be worthwhile, at the end of the day it should produce findings which can be published and generalized to other patients, giving it a wider clinical relevance. Hopefully, by taking all these things into consideration you will not only come up with the relevant answer but also one which is truthful.

Reference

Pocock, S. J. *Clinical Trials: A Practical Approach.* Chichester: Wiley, 1983.

4 Every doctor a walking placebo

George T. Lewith

Summary

The evolution of the concept of placebos is summarized, and the pharmacological, physiological and psychological aspects of placebo response and placebo responders discussed. Emphasis is placed on the ability of the health care provider to elicit an effective placebo response and possible mechanisms through which this can be maximized in each consultation. Placebo response in the context of controlled clinical trials is also discussed.

Introduction

The medical scientist seems to view the placebo response as a problem that must be rigorously controlled in the context of scientific clinical trials, so that the objective value of specific treatment can be assessed. While this may be overstating the view of many clinicians, such an approach has some validity; we must have criteria for evaluating the effects of treatment, but should we place the placebo in such a negative context? All too often, both in self-limiting illness and in many chronic complaints such as intractable pain, we have little to offer the patient in the form of proven specific treatment. It therefore seems wise for us to re-examine the idea of the placebo effect so that we can understand it more completely. Perhaps through this understanding we may be able to develop a better method of maximizing the placebo response, thereby providing help, symptom relief and possibly even cure for more of our patients.

Defining the placebo presents us with problems. Laurence implies that the placebo response is 'a subjective improvement in the patient's condition that is not directly attributable to the pharmacological or physiological effects of treatment',[1] while Wolf suggests that the placebo effect is 'any effect attributable to a pill, potion or procedure, but not to its pharmacodynamic or specific properties'.[2]

These definitions allow us to analyse the effect of placebos in the context of clinical trials evaluating both pharmacological preparations and surgical procedures. However, they tell us nothing about the possible placebo effect of the quality and quantity of personal contact between the doctor and the patient. Furthermore, because our current concept of the placebo tends to be reductionist and materialistic, the definitions available are formulated in order to explain the observed placebo response encountered during controlled clinical trials. The argument is tautological; patients get better naturally even when suffering from severe chronic complaints; therefore we must invoke some explanation for this phenomenon. The model used does not adequately analyse the possible reasons for improvement, but simply uses a jargon word (placebo) to reinforce, and consequently make respectable, our empiricism.

The placebo response

Placebos have undoubtedly been a vital part of the physician's toolkit since time immemorial, but before the 1950s very little had been written about them. Beecher was one of the first to look at the placebo response in the context of both medication and surgical procedures.[3,4] His conclusions are based on a variety of studies which include conditions such as post-operative pain, angina, headache, cough, anxiety and even the common cold. These studies provide conclusive evidence that the placebo is effective in a wide range of conditions.[5]

Furthermore, the placebo response is consistent (35.2% ± 2.2%). The main method of defining this response had been based on the patient's subjective evaluation of response to treatment. It is impossible to measure many symptoms, such as pain, objectively and so most clinical studies, however carefully constructed, are necessarily subjective when it comes to measuring important endpoints such as treatment efficacy.[6]

Surgery is also a powerful placebo, and undoubtedly the surgeon's enthusiasm has a significant effect on outcome. This observation is supported by detailed investigation into two surgical procedures: ligation of the internal mammary arteries for angina and the treatment of duodenal ulcer by gastroenterostomy.

Enthusiasts supporting the operation of internal mammary ligation for the treatment of intractable angina began to report excellent results during the late 1950s. Complete or significant pain relief associated with subjective reports of good improvement in function occurred very shortly after the operation in a large number of patients. An early study by Kitchell *et al.*[7] suggested that 68% showed significant subjective clinical improvement, but only 42% showed an objective improvement on investigations such as ECG and exercise tolerance. Sceptics such as Cobb,[8] using exactly the same procedure, reported only a 6% success rate.

In a sense the debate about coronary artery ligation was answered in a paper by Dimond *et al.*[9]; they carried out a double blind study of internal mammary ligation in 18 patients. Skin incisions were made in all 18, but only 13 had ligation. The cardiologist assessing the patient's response to the operation was unaware as to which procedure they had undergone. A marked improvement in clinical state and anginal pain occurred in ten of the 13 ligated patients. All five who had the sham operation also described a marked clinical improvement.[10]

A similarly dramatic difference in clinical response can be elicited when evaluating the effect of gastroenterostomy as a long-term treatment for duodenal ulcers. Enthusiasts like Douglas claimed an 82% five-year cure with almost no unpleasant or adverse reactions, whereas sceptics such as Lewishon claimed only a 47% five-year cure rate with a much higher proportion of adverse reactions.[4] Surgery therefore is a powerful placebo, and illustrates very dramatically how the enthusiasm of the operator can have a major effect on treatment outcome over a prolonged follow-up period.

Patients respond to placebos in a variable manner; Lasagna *et al.* report a double blind placebo-controlled study on post-operative pain which suggests that 14% of patients were consistent placebo responders and 21% were non-consistent placebo responders. The remaining 65% varied in their degree of placebo response in no obvious or predictable manner.[11] Placebos have their own pharmacology; the dose response curve to placebo treatment is similar to that of many real medications. Patients experience adverse reactions to placebos and on occasion can become quite ill in response to placebo medication. Cumulative or 'carry-over' effects can also occur if the placebo medication is given repeatedly; patients may complain of feeling overmedicated or even addicted to the drug.[12]

We have therefore made some attempt to quantify the placebo response. We must be aware that a placebo effect will occur in response to almost any procedure in approximately 35% of patients. The effect is variable although there is a small group of consistent placebo responders. Furthermore, placebos have a discrete pharmacology which includes both a dose response curve and the potential for adverse reactions.

The psychology of the placebo response

What are the psychological parameters governing the placebo response? Beecher has shown that the more anxious the patient, or the more anxiety-provoking the procedure – for instance, heart surgery – the more likely a placebo response will be elicited.[5] Therefore procedures such as open-heart surgery which are dangerous and life-threatening, and which also involve prolonged periods of recuperation in stressful, high-technology environments such as chronic coronary care units, must be successful at invoking a significant placebo response.

Sex, educational background, attitudes towards drugs, doctors, nurses, hospitals and church membership are *not* important predictors of placebo response.[13] However, it does appear that placebo reactors have a tendency to be more emotional, gushing and neurotic. They are more grateful for, and impressed by, hospital care and ask less frequently for medication. In one study the nursing staff noted that placebo responders tended to be more cooperative and talkative than non-responders. Furthermore, the placebo responders more commonly gave a history of psychosomatic symptoms and had a higher chance than a control population of being addicted to purgatives or analgesics. Female placebo responders tended to be more prone to dysmenorrhoea, and psychological testing suggested that placebo responders were more inward-looking and preoccupied with their own internal body processes.[14] This psychological picture does not provide enough information to predict which patients will (or will not) respond to a given placebo. It does, however, suggest that placebo responders may have a tendency to be more sensitive and neurotic.

The doctor/patient relationship is often an essential factor in eliciting the placebo response. Wolf reports the case of a patient with achlorhydria in whom a gastric cancer was suspected. She was saved from laparotomy when the surgeon who had enquired into her background asked: 'Why did you not take your husband back when he returned from overseas?'. She promptly produced gastric acid without a histamine stimulus.[2] Further support for the importance of the therapeutic relationship as one of the possible initiators for the placebo response can be found from Hankoff *et al.* They treated schizophrenic patients first with a placebo and then with an active medication. Of the patients who failed to respond to a placebo, 87% also failed to respond to the active medication. The common factor in deciding upon patient response seems to be the relationship between the patient and the doctor. Hankoff *et al.* regard the placebo response as a non-verbal communication between patient and doctor.[14]

Gliedman *et al.* have suggested that the placebo response is in some ways similar to a conditioned reflex.[15] It is quite clear that patients' responses can to a certain extent be conditioned by the expectation of the doctor or therapist dealing with them. Such conditioning is enhanced by central excitatory states, such as those frequently seen in doctor/patient consultations. Therefore the expectation of help when the patient consults a doctor may be part of a 'conditioned placebo response', of a nature that we have come to expect from almost any therapy.

The mechanism of the placebo response

Levine *et al.* have suggested that the placebo response is endorphin mediated, as it can, in some instances, be naloxone reversed.[16] This implies that an unknown trigger may be stimulating a response within the central nervous system that is at least partially mediated through known neurotransmitters. In spite of the fact that endorphins have been invoked as an explanation for many poorly understood treatments such as acupuncture,[17] this does not negate the validity of such therapies. Conversely, it suggests there is a coherent quantifiable pathway through which their activity can be assessed, and the treatment better understood and evaluated.

It is possible that the trigger stimulating endorphin release may be variable; a stressful situation may stimulate the same neurohumoral pathway as the warmth and sympathy of a good doctor/patient relationship or the effect of a trained healer. Perhaps the healer's art may be to maximize the placebo response by stimulating the body's own natural powers of homoeostasis and recuperation through neurohumoral mechanisms such as endorphin release.

The emerging field of psychoneuroimmunology was predicted by Wolf in 1959. He suggested that 'strong experimental evidence indicates that many of the component changes in disease process, including fever, leucocytosis, headache and nausea, are capable of being set in motion by impulses arising in the cerebral cortex'. By suggesting this he did not mean that all illnesses are psychosomatic or neurotic, but rather that the psyche has a significant influence on the progress and outcome of somatic disease.[2]

Solomon's more recent review provides some 14 hypotheses through which psychological events may affect the immune system of both man and experimental mammals.[18] For instance, the hypothesis that 'severe emotional disturbance should be accompanied by immunological abnormalities' is supported by data demonstrating that clinical depression causes immune suppression[19] and that schizophrenics display abnormal lymphocytes both functionally and morphologically.[20] The detailed information presented by Solomon is overwhelming; how we feel obviously affects how we deal with illness at a physical as well as a psychological level.

We now know that certain stressful environments, if they are controlled by the individual or animal under stress, can be used in a positive and constructive manner and appear to potentiate our immune response, while feeling out of control or overwhelmed by any stress causes a significant depression of immune response.[21] Psychoneuroimmunology has vindicated Wolf's original suggestion 25 years ago; the mind does affect how we deal with illness. How we feel must to some extent be affected by our relationships with others and therefore our relationships with others must in turn affect how we deal with illness. This must necessarily include the doctor/patient relationship as well as all the other personal interactions we experience on a day-to-day basis.

All too often treatments are illogically promoted because the researcher has failed to understand that the illness may improve spontaneously. For instance, post-herpetic neuralgia shows a 50% spontaneous resolution rate in the first three months after the last evidence of acute shingles has disappeared.[22] Studies evaluating potential treatments must either be an improvement on the expected natural history, or be instituted after the pain has been established for three months, when the rate of spontaneous improvement diminishes significantly.[22,23] The fact that many chronic illnesses tend eventually to improve, or at least show relapses and remissions, must not be confused with the distinct concept of the placebo response. The placebo response implies a natural healing process that is *triggered* by events as yet unclearly defined.

The controlled clinical trial

Heron has written extensively about the contextual and philosophical validity of clinical trial methodology.[24] His criticisms of controlled clinical trials are many, but can be best summarized by the statement 'What is the treatment of choice for this individual and idiosyncratic patient?'. His question suggests to us that the normal clinical practice of diagnosing a constellation of signs, symptoms and investigations, with a particular label, and then using a standard treatment for that disease, is a gross oversimplification. This rather rigid view is necessary in the context of conventional controlled clinical trials. However, it is not used in day-to-day clinical practice, which is far more flexible both in terms of diagnosis and therapy. Our evaluation and treatment of illness should, therefore, be based on similar criteria to that of normal clinical practice and not on the artificial situation encountered in a controlled clinical trial.

If we think of a complex illness such as migraine, then the validity of Heron's ideas may appear more convincing. We know migraine headaches may respond to medication, acupuncture, manipulation, dietary avoidance and relaxation techniques such as biofeedback.[25,26,27] If we were to suggest a controlled study that involved assessing the value of acupuncture in migraine headaches, then the assessment and treatment protocol would involve elements of constructive and supportive consultation techniques along with a period of enforced stillness every week (lying down for 20 minutes while acupuncture needles were inserted and removed).

We are, in effect, providing three simultaneous treatments. We cannot in reality assess acupuncture without deciding on the best acupuncture treatment (talking to and examining the patients) and then treating them (lying them down and inserting needles). Perhaps the patients entered into the migraine study have overwhelming food sensitivities and may not respond to acupuncture. However, they still do have the diagnostic label of migraine. How can we realistically assess treatment in this situation, when our diagnostic entities are so poorly differentiated and our treatments so crude and impossible to analyse in an independent and objective manner? The purely objective controlled clinical trial must therefore be an unattainable goal.

Heron suggests an approach based on contextual validity. This allows for the assessment of treatment based on a case-by-case analysis and does not assume that all patients with migraine have an essential homogeneity, and by inference a single causal mechanism and therefore a single therapy. Such an approach leaves us with less of a need to explain away placebos as the control or untreated group within a clinical trial. This approach is similar to 'the single patient' controlled trial.[28] It implies that the placebo response may have much to do with factors such as the patient's belief system, the doctor/patient relationship and the use of touch, healing and other psychodynamic mechanisms. Heron's opinion would appear to be supported by the evidence available from psychoneuroimmunology and by studies such as those of Hankoff *et al.*

While it would be foolish to reject the controlled clinical trial completely, it would also be most unwise to look upon it as the final arbiter of treatment efficacy in the vast majority of clinical conditions that we see on a day-to-day basis. Results from clinical trials, both for specific treatment and placebo groups, must therefore be interpreted with caution.

Conclusions

The placebo response is a definite clinical entity with its own pharmacology and pharmacodynamics. While it is important to assess therapy, the controlled clinical trial must be seen in its proper context and understood as an artificial and often clumsy method of assessing the actual effects of treatment.

The placebo response itself means different things to different people; to the pharmacologist it's the 'control group', while to the general practitioner it may be the only treatment available. The general practitioner may therefore wish to employ all his or her knowledge, enthusiasm, consultation technique and sympathy to create the best possible atmosphere in which to elicit a placebo response from the patient.

Perhaps in reality what we are debating is simply terminology. Patients have always improved spontaneously; some cultures have amplified this homoeostatic process by a variety of magical and mystical procedures. Our current technological magic involves us in invoking the clinical trial and the placebo response. After all, we can hardly claim, as conventional medical scientists, to be simply 'healers'. We need more objective evidence, or do we? The arguments presented take us full circle in an objective and scientific manner. What you say and how you say it almost certainly matters; perhaps a placebo response is as far as the medical scientists will go towards evaluating this healing ability in the context of a controlled clinical trial.

References

1 Laurence, D. R. *Clinical Pharmacology*. Edinburgh and London: Churchill Livingstone, 1980.

2 Wolf, S. The pharmacology of placebos. *Pharmacology Review* 1959; **11**: 689–704.

3 Beecher, H. K. The powerful placebo. *JAMA* 1955; **159**: 1602–6.

4 Beecher, H. K. Surgery as placebo. *JAMA* 1961; **176**: 1102–7.

5 Beecher, H. K. Evidence for increased effectiveness of placebos with increased stress. *Am J Physiol* 1956; **187**: 163–9.

6 Huskisson, E. C. Measurement of pain. *Lancet* 1974; **2**: 1127–31.

7 Kitchell, J. R., Glover, R. P., Kyle, R. H. Bilateral internal mammary artery ligation for angina pectoris; preliminary clinical considerations. *Am J Cardiol* 1956; **1**: 46–50.

8 Cobb, L. A. Evaluation of internal mammary artery ligation by double blind technique. *N Eng J Med* 1959; **260**: 1115–18.

9 Dimond, E. G., Kittle, C. F., Crockett, J. E. Evaluation of internal mammary artery ligation and sham procedure in angina pectoris. *Circulation* 1958; **18**: 712–13.

10 Dimond, E. G., Kittle, C. F., Crockett, J. E. Comparison of internal mammary artery ligation and sham operation for angina pectoris. *Am J Cardiol* 1960; **5**: 484–6.

11 Lasagna, L., Mosteller, F., von Flesinger, J. M., Beecher, H. K. A study of placebo response. *Am J Med* 1954; **16**: 770–81.

12 Lasagna, L., Laties, V. G., Dohan, J. L. Further studies on the pharmacology of placebo administration. *J Clin Invest* 1958; **37**: 533–7.

13 Lasagna, L. Psychological effects of medication. *Proc Roy Soc Med* 1955; 773–6. *Br Med J* 1961; **1**: 43–4.

14 Hankoff, L. D., Engelhart, D. M., Freedman, N., Mann, D., Margolis, R. The doctor–patient relationship via psychopharmacological treatment setting. *J Nerv Ment Dis* 1960; **131**: 540–6.

15 Gliedman, L. M., Horsley-Gantt, W., Teilelbaum, H. A. Some implications of conditional reflex studies for research. *Am J Psychiat* 1953; **113**: 1103–7.

16 Levine, J. D., Gordon, N. C., Fields, H. L. The mechanism of placebo analgesia. *Lancet* 1978; **2**: 654–7.

17 Lewith, G. T., Kenyon, J. N. Physiological and psychological explanations for the mechanism of acupuncture as a treatment for chronic pain. *Soc Sci Med* 1984; **19**: 1367–78.

18 Solomon, G. F. The emerging field of psychoneuroimmunology. *Advances* 1985; **2**: 6–19.

19 Kronfol, Z., Silva, J., Greden, J., Dembiski, S., Carroll, B. J. Cell-mediated immunity in melancholia. *Psychosom Med* 1982; **44**: 304.

20 Fessel, W. J., Hirata-Hibi, M. Abnormal leukocytes in schizophrenia. *Arch Gen Psychiat* 1963; **9**: 601–13.

21 De Vries, M. Research into restoration of health: models, method makers and measurements. Conference held at Charing Cross Hospital Medical School, 1986.

22 Hope-Simpson, R. E. Post-herpetic neuralgia. *J Roy Coll Gen Pract* 1975; **25**: 571–5.

23 Lewith, G. T., Field, J., Machin, D. Acupuncture compared with placebo in post-herpetic pain. *Pain* 1983; **17**: 361–8.

24 Heron, J. Critique of conventional research methodology. *Comp Med Res* 1986; **1**: 12–22.

25 Lewith, G. T. Headache and its management: A personal review. *Ann Swiss Chiro Ass* 1985; **8**: 7–16.

26 Dowson, D. I., Lewith, G. T., Machin, D. The effects of acupuncture versus placebo in the treatment of headache. *Pain* 1985; **21**: 35–42.

27 Marcer, D. Biofeedback and meditation. In: Lewith, G. T. (ed.) *Alternative Therapies*. London: Heinemann, 1985; 109–49.

28 McLeod, R. S., Cohen, Z., Taylor, D. W., Cullen, J. B. Single patient randomised clinical trial. *Lancet* 1986; **1**: 726–8.

5 Why measure outcomes?

Honor M. Anthony and Frank M. Parsons

Summary

Assessing outcome is an essential part of the work of all therapists if they are to learn from their experience. There are ethical, moral, social, economic and political reasons for instituting more formalized attempts to measure the outcome of therapy in a holistic way, both in orthodox and in complementary medicine. These are particularly insistent in relation to complementary medicine if the aim of bringing effective therapies of this type into the mainstream of modern medical practice is to be met.

Introduction

Measurement of the outcome of therapy takes many different forms. At its simplest it consists of assessing the effect of each treatment, or each part of treatment, to determine the next appropriate action and to gain experience to draw on in the future. Both parts are essential activities for any therapist of any discipline.

Everyday assessments may be made according to a pre-arranged plan, and at pre-arranged times, or spontaneously when the occasion arises. They may be limited to the effect of the treatment on the condition or symptom that led to the consultation, or include other aspects of the patient's health. Whatever their form or pattern, they are an essential element of the treatment of the patient and of the professional development of practitioners. It would be true to say that no patient would willingly trust himself to any practitioner whose ability to learn from experience was suspect.[1]

Perhaps the title of this chapter might then be rephrased to ask why we should try to find, validate, and apply methods of measuring outcome that can be used by different therapists, and applied under different conditions: why organized efforts to assess outcome are important.

The first part of the question concerns the formality. In repeated consultations between an individual therapist and a patient, spontaneous and intuitive assessments play an important role, not easily mimicked by any formal system involving different therapists. Why is the spontaneous, intuitive assessment insufficient? Assessments need to be formalized to discipline the memory, to promote communication between therapists, to help in the recognition of patterns, to ensure that other effects of treatment on the patient are looked for (for instance, effects on other systems or delayed effects), and to examine problems too complex or too rare to be evident to individual practitioners.

Formal assessment systems range from the restriction of the use of certain words within a discipline to describe specific features, through the designation of certain descriptive categories (nominal categories), and of ordered categories (ordinal categories: e.g., slight pain/moderate pain/severe pain) through numerical measurements which are merely ordinal in character, to numerical measurements directly related to the property in question. All of these can be thought of as 'measurements': all can be validated as measures of outcome. Indeed, although results in numerical form are convenient and give an impression of accuracy, this may be illusory unless the numbers are related to the property throughout their range; if there are doubts about this a nominal or ordinal category scheme that accurately reflects the property may be a more satisfactory outcome measure. Each measure must be able to be applied consistently by different individuals, and be examined to see how validly it is able to reflect changes in the condition under consideration.

Accepting the need for formalization, the other part of the question is concerned with the value of the extra information that may be obtained by the use of formalized measures. The nature, and therefore the significance, of this information is determined by who does the assessing, the type and range of measures used, and the time-scales: these also determine the character and quality of the professional insights which result.

However, our task is to examine the ethical, moral, social, economic and political reasons for a disciplined approach to the measurement of outcomes of therapy.

What is a successful outcome?

The determination of what is, and what is not, a successful outcome lies at the heart of the social, economic and political aspects of this question. It is not a simple matter; and simplifications that lose the essence may have serious consequences. Because outcomes are difficult to assess, there are tendencies for other measures to be used in their place, for instance in the decision of government to use information derived from routine statistics in evaluating the cost-effectiveness of the NHS:[3] according to the performance indicators in use, a short stay in hospital is evidence of greater efficiency than a longer stay. This sounds innocuous until you realize that hospital statistics are based on admissions, not people. The patient who is discharged too soon and has a relapse and has to be re-admitted is therefore viewed by the statistics (though not by anybody else) as evidence of greater efficiency than the case who stays in another day or two and progresses favourably. It is of course an absurdity, carried to even more farcical extremes if the calculation does not take notice of whether the patient lived or died, information which is available in the hospital statistics. Rathwell and Barnard[3] have summarized other criticisms of these performance indicators – that they are based on data which is itself suspect, that the system is institution-based and therefore not a true measure of performance, that it concerns the *process* of health care and not its effect on people, and that it is a measure of effort rather than the results of effort. The situation has arisen because it has been deemed to be too costly or too difficult to get any real assessment of the outcome of treatment. This may be seen as a failure of government, or of health administrators, but perhaps we practitioners should ask ourselves whether the failure to develop and validate good measures of outcome should not be laid at our door. We would not appreciate the imposition by non-practitioners of criteria to be used to evaluate the success of our treatment (though we might value their collaboration) so it behoves us to make the running ourselves.

Traditionally the doctor has seen himself as the sole arbiter of what constitutes successful treatment (except where negligence is concerned): in the consulting room doctors have relied largely on observation, intuition and on what the patient says: in contrast, organized studies of outcome have concentrated on objective measurements and subjective data has been regarded as suspect. Objective measures, provided they are appropriate, valid and significant, give a definition to the measurement of outcome difficult to achieve in any other way. Other measures are always at risk from the optimistic self-deception (or sometimes its obverse) which is common and natural in both therapists and patients, since both are hoping for justification of the time, effort and cost involved in the therapy. Objective measures of outcome help to avoid these pitfalls; these may involve measures of *time* – length of time to complete recovery, length of survival – or objective measures of *condition* at certain points in time, derived either from direct examination of the patient or from investigations, or from records of the patients' need for other medication.

Objectivity is desirable, but appropriateness is essential. Take the inoperable cancer patient as an example. The easiest and most objective measure of treatment outcome is the length of survival: but is it appropriate? If the quality of life is good, strain on the family minimal, or the patient has some personal reason for wishing to live a little longer, it may be. Under other circumstances it may be an extension of a misery which is almost unendurable, and therefore prolongation may be far from being an appropriate measure of the 'success' of treatment.

The assumption that decisions about the success of outcomes are professional decisions to be made only by practitioners has been increasingly challenged recently. On the one hand the wide range of 'user' groups which have been set up signifies that various kinds of patients have not received all the help they were aware of needing, or that what seemed a satisfactory outcome to practitioners did not seem so to the patient (or to his relatives). One example is the movement to provide for mothers to accompany small children into hospital. In the past, many hospitals admitting young children not only took them in without their mothers, but actually imposed very severe limitations on visits, because the children cried when their mothers left. Estimating 'success' of management in terms of quiet children in hospital, this strategy was fairly effective, but mothers saw the other side, the months or years that many of the children took to recover, not from the illness but from the separation imposed during treatment. Another example is the groups formed to draw together patients with certain chronic diseases and their families, and patients disabled by illness or its treatment, so that they can support each other and pass on useful information. The existence of these associations is saying to practitioners: 'We have to learn to live with these conditions. You may assess whether your surgical intervention, or medical management, or other interventions were appropriate and effective, but only if we have access to adequate information and help can we make the appropriate adjustments; these adjustments are a significant item in the long-term outcome.' Assessment of the outcome in these types of condition is incomplete unless the patients' contribution is included.

Just as the choice of treatment must take into account the characteristics of the individual,[4] so successful treatment will not return all patients to the same level of activity and/or interest. Many elderly people may be delighted to recover sufficiently to potter down to the shops because they have not been more energetic than that for years, but this might represent a severe handicap to the unusual individual who still regularly climbs mountains or plays 18 holes of golf. A limitation of pronation of the wrist may be relatively unimportant for many, but a disaster for a pianist. This complicates the concept of outcome assessment by stressing the need for it to be appropriate for individuals, and indicates that blanket values, even when they are developed in collaboration with patients, may not be a valid measure for all the patients. For some therapy situations, particularly perhaps where attempts to change addictive behaviours or unhealthy habits are concerned, or in studies in mental illness, there may be such a large individual element that it is unrealistic to try to find common outcome measures, and individual goals may need to be set with each patient. Whatever strategy is employed, respecting individuality in this way imposes additional problems in devising assessments.

But the patient's impression of progress cannot always be relied upon. In addition to the optimistic self-deception referred to previously, there are some therapeutic situations where the patient is *expected* to get worse before he gets better, and others where the untreated outcome would have been so bad that even recovery with a substantial degree of disability represents a genuine success, which the patient may not be in a position to realize. The decisions on outcome must be a cooperative exercise in which patient and therapist both take part: in organized studies which rely on subjective assessments an independent observer should also be involved wherever possible.

The ethical viewpoint

The question of who should decide on what constitutes a 'successful' outcome is linked to the philosophy and ethics of practice. There is still evidence of the paternalistic model, that sees treatment as something done to, or prescribed for, the patient by the doctor, for instance in the status accorded to the general practitioner in the UK as the sole arbiter of what other medical personnel the patient should (or may) consult (except in an emergency), in the autocratic way in which some consultations are conducted, and in the acceptance of a system which allows only brief consultations, inadequate for much discussion or training. This model vests the decisions about both treatment and outcome primarily in the practitioner, with the patient playing a largely passive role of concurrence or changing to another doctor. It is gradually being replaced by a more collaborative model in which the patient takes more responsibility for his own health – a patient-directed or partnership approach – but much of the impetus for this is coming from the patients. As patients understand more about their own health and play a larger role in deciding how successful treatment has been, the emphasis may change; they may increasingly accept as 'success' those strategies which *prevent* the occurrence of illness rather than those which relieve it, a view to which lip-service has been paid[5] but inadequate investment made.

Any model of practice implies responsibility both for reaching the highest attainable standards of practice, and for refraining from doing harm, which is another face of the assessment of outcomes. It is rarely possible to be certain that adverse effects not previously reported were caused (or not caused) by treatment from the experience of a single practitioner, except when the effects are bizarre or frequent in a much-used treatment. Correct attribution depends on awareness, organization and cooperation between practitioners, as in the Yellow Card scheme for drug reactions in the UK. This is another form of measuring outcome, and has had some effect in minimizing severe and sometimes tragic side effects, but might have had even greater success if *all* practitioners had reported *all* patients who showed unexpected reactions. Ill effects occurring after months or years sometimes feature in these reports, but often do not because of the increasing difficulty with time in seeing the association between treatment and effect. It is sobering to reflect that the ill effect of stilboestrol treatment given to pregnant women on their unborn daughters[6] was only recognized because it caused a rare tumour at an unusual age; it is unlikely that induction of a common tumour or an effect on health in general would have been detected.

Complementary practitioners have the advantage over orthodox doctors in this respect because many of their therapeutic measures do not involve potentially toxic substances, but some do, and the recent moves to insist that natural medicines also are properly tested are to be welcomed, provided that they are applied with discretion. The fact that a medicine has an impressive historical record makes it unlikely that acute side effects have passed unnoticed (provided that production methods are unchanged), but it is no guarantee of efficacy or of freedom from unwanted long-term or delayed effects. The same is true of some of the older allopathic remedies. However, if a treatment used repeatedly by several generations of patients is discredited by the results of a randomized trial, it is reasonable to look for the source of the discrepancy perhaps in the conduct of the trial or in the criteria used, rather than pinning unquestioning faith in the results, just because they came from a randomized controlled trial.

Social and economic factors

Complementary medicine contrasts with the bulk of orthodox medicine in this country in having a direct commercial aspect: patients *pay* for treatment. This may mean that the patients are more active in the evaluation of the short-term effects of treatment, since a patient who is not convinced it is helping will be less likely to spend substantial sums of money as well as time in coming back for more. But it may also make it more difficult to get compliance and perseverance with treatments whose benefits are delayed, and mean that long-term treatments may be curtailed for financial reasons alone.

Both these possibilities provide strong arguments for *organized* studies of outcome in complementary medicine. On the one hand encouraging results from a well-planned, competently executed study of patients with similar problems provides encouragement to persevere. On the other hand financial support for complementary therapies on the NHS is only likely when there is consistent, significant evidence of effectiveness in rigorous studies. It may be that as the holistic nature of illness and of the response to therapy is recognized, changes will come about in the sort of study that is accepted[7,8] but the same degree of rigour will be demanded. In fact *greater* rigour is likely to be required than that for treatments already financed by the NHS, even though some of the latter do not have such support.

There is another sense in which economic and social factors call for more realistic and holistic assessment of outcomes, this time initially in orthodox medicine. It is generally agreed[9,10] that irrespective of how the bills for treatment are met, whether privately, through some sort of insurance, or through state provision, there is a limit to the amount of money that any community can afford to spend on health care, quite apart from the present political pressures to reduce public spending. Even if the government were being generous to the health service, choice would still be required over what could be afforded and what not: the problems will get worse as the sophistication and expense of treatments continue to increase. The important question concerns the grounds on which such choices are made. One would expect choices of this importance to be made on explicit grounds of value to the community as a whole and compassion for the sick, based on a rigorous assessment in the widest possible terms of the need for, the success of, and the cost-effectiveness of various types of provision.

To an extent priorities have been set, but there is no evidence that they have been based on this kind of data, because with few exceptions the data is not available; indeed, in 1982, in his critique of the bases of decision-making in health care, Maynard[9] went so far as to say that 'there are no good health status measures in use today'. The priorities set seem to be acute illness, children, childbirth and cancer, largely on pragmatic and compassionate grounds with the precise pattern of support influenced by the news-worthiness of the patients' dilemmas, the vociferousness of pressure groups and locally by the political acumen of rival hospital consultants. Adequate study of the medical, personal and social consequences of various types of management and treatment might come up with quite different priorities. In some therapy situations, such as cancer, detailed studies of outcome which pay attention to quality of life, strain on the family and on family relationships and the summation of suffering over time might well tilt the scales away from 'high-tech' interventions and cytotoxic drugs except where the chances of 'cure' were substantial: heart transplants in babies and the resuscitation of patients whose lives are already severely restricted by ill health might well be other examples.

I suspect that an exercise of this sort would still put acute illness in fairly healthy individuals, childbirth and 'curable' cancer towards the top of the list, but that those treatments which restore the ability to live a full life (like hip replacements, and the repair of hernias, prolapses and haemorrhoids, all low in priority at present), and treatments aimed at achieving a greater degree of wellness would make dramatic upward moves. The difficulty lies in the fact that there is limited room at the top of the priorities list, and the only genuine way out of the dilemma is to prevent illness or to find less 'high-tech' managements which are actually preferable for some of the emotive conditions. An example of this is the management of dying cancer patients in hospices or with support at home; but establishing that such alternatives *are* preferable is difficult without good measures of quality of life that are applicable to the particular situation.

Getting studies of outcome to meet these requirements would involve the cooperation of doctors, adequate personnel – epidemiologists, statisticians and data processors – and the necessary finance. Obtaining the cooperation of doctors is likely to prove to be the greatest difficulty because of the importance given to the freedom of the individual doctor to act as he or she thinks best. This is important, but it is equally important that decisions about priorities in the allocation of money to treatment, and to equipment and facilities for treatment, are *not* based on inadequate data. Practitioners must press for the collection of data from indepth holistic studies of outcome which will allow the replacement of the present haphazard system of priorities with a modern compassionate and intelligent approach, before it is too late: this must be based on providing the care, advice or management most appropriate to the person with the illness, not merely to the illness. We might perhaps consider insisting that the public purse (our purse) should pick up the bill only for the more expensive treatments of all sorts where there was full cooperation with outcome measurements in the widest sense, and agree to similar short-term restrictions on the use of specific drugs or groups of drugs from time to time, to allow their effectiveness to be assessed. The only apparent alternative, of administrative decisions made without adequate data being imposed by financial stringency, is quite unacceptable. The freedom of the individual doctor to act as he or she thinks best in respect of each individual patient becomes hollow when faced with a patient desperately needing facilities which are not available.

Renal physicians and surgeons throughout Europe have kept a register of patients treated by dialysis and/or transplantation for the last 21 years, and have recorded survival and made many attempts to assess the effects of their treatments on the quality of life achieved. The inherent problems have been compounded by the differences in language, customs and habits in the 29 countries involved, and the only measure which has been interpreted successfully has been length of survival. Without dialysis, patients with renal failure died with a few weeks; with dialysis, 70% of young adults lived more than five years.[11] The UK was next to bottom among the 17 Western European countries in the numbers of new cases accepted for treatment (per million population),[12] but accepted equal numbers under 40 years of age: presumably the older age groups were left to die. This was partly because of a shortage of central DHSS funds and partly because of switching as far as possible to home dialysis as a means of limiting the danger from hepatitis B infection to patients and staff; older patients found home dialysis more difficult to learn. In this situation outcome measures needed to consider the health of the staff as well as the patients: continuous audit of progress led progressively to home dialysis and continuous peritoneal dialysis and to the testing of all donor blood, which improved the uptake of older patients in the UK.[13] With dialysis, most patients return to leading a near-normal life, in contrast to many other treatments for similarly life-threatening conditions, for instance chemotherapy for advanced cancer. The difficulty in designing quality of life measures applicable equally to all this very disparate group of patients, whose only common factor is failed kidneys, means that, in spite of all their efforts, the European Dialysis and Transplant Association has failed to produce the sort of evidence which might give it precedence for funding over, for instance, cancer chemotherapy on the basis of the relative benefits, in terms of quality of life, that are achieved. This illustrates both the difficulties experienced and the importance and urgency of developing reliable measures.

Complementary therapists would be wise to participate in these developments and to set up rigorous and wide-ranging studies of the effectiveness of their therapies, to be in a position to bid to fill appropriate roles, particularly in manipulation, and in the preventive, supportive and retraining areas whose importance is likely to become more apparent if a sizeable exercise of this sort were to get under way.

The political aspect

We have looked briefly at the professional, ethical, moral, social and economic reasons for more thorough measurement of treatment outcomes in a holistic setting. But the last topic discussed was as strongly political as economic or social. In addition to wishing to be seen as genuinely complementary to orthodox medicine (i.e., in having a role as a complement to orthodox treatment and functions they can fulfil as well as, or better than, orthodox medicine), complementary therapists, like their orthodox counterparts, are also citizens and, either at present or almost certainly sometime in the future, patients. We all have a vested interest in the way in which our money is spent and the provisions for health concern us all as clients as well as providers. We have a political right and duty to demand that expensive therapies are evaluated using measures of outcome that register the human costs and gains in terms of suffering, personal and family distress, quality of life both now and in the future, and the chance of the long-term 'success' of the treatment. Inappropriate short-term kindness can cause longer term misery and we need to find ways of reducing the compulsion to use a treatment just because it is available. According to Maynard: 'Clinical freedom and professional power have led to a failure to create mechanisms which ensure that practitioners evaluate clinical outcomes and their cost implications. Such behaviour is not only inefficient but is unethical: resources used inefficiently are not available to treat those who are in the queue and who could potentially gain more, in terms of health status, if they were treated.'[9]

Complementary therapists might challenge orthodox doctors to a dialogue about, and subsequent studies of, the appropriate measures to evaluate outcome in the sorts of conditions they treat most often; they must produce good evidence of efficacy if they wish their treatments to be available to patients who need them, regardless of ability to pay. The same is true of some of the neglected developments in orthodox medicine, particularly in the field of allergy to food and chemicals and its bizarre manifestations[14] largely ignored by the establishment; good management of food allergy is capable of bringing about dramatic health improvements, in migraine,[15] irritable colon[16] and asthma[17] for instance. Undervalued disciplines, both orthodox and complementary, need initially to demonstrate efficacy, producing the sort of evidence that will encourage GPs to refer patients; but the eventual aim must be that of forcing the NHS to make all effective therapies available through the health service. This is the political impetus for the measurement of outcomes. Rival bids for financial support from preventive and therapeutic medicine, from primary care and the hospitals, from different specialities and different individual consultants, and in the future from orthodox and complementary medicine must be settled on the basis of the findings of rigorous, wide-ranging studies of efficacy, not on the basis of who has the most 'clout'.

Future generations may well see the monitoring of health and wellbeing in relation to the effects of other social policy as an even more important political function at this time; not only in monitoring the obvious effects of unemployment and destructive habits such as smoking and drugtaking, but also the effects on health of reducing chemical pollution, of reducing continual pressures to acquire material goods, of increasing cooperation in the work-place, and of re-invigorating communities. Contrary to popular belief, the battle against tuberculosis was largely won before the advent of chemotherapy and vaccination, by the virtual elimination of gross malnutrition and the reduction of overcrowding.[18] In much the same way, changes in social policy might make a more important contribution to health in our age[19] than discovering the best ways – orthodox and complementary – of picking up the pieces. If so, monitoring the health consequences associated with such changes, or with localized differences, with the aim of producing data to support claims for further change, might be of more lasting significance than studies of the effects of therapy. This possibility presents a challenge to all who regard themselves as health professionals; it cannot safely be left to other people. There is a further twist to this, increasing our responsibility, since McKnight[20] points out that 'publicly financed medical insurance systematically misdirects public wealth from income to the poor to income to medical professionals': he holds that this may actually be increasing illness, since the most potent factor for health is the absence of poverty. Stressing the need for measurement of the effect of social changes on health and wellbeing is appropriate in this book since complementary therapists show more concern about positive aspects of health than most orthodox doctors.

Conclusion

There are strong and interrelated professional, ethical, social and economic reasons for measuring outcome of therapy in a holistic way, insistent both for orthodox and complementary medicine if the most appropriate help is to be available to patients. But a case can also be made for extending the debate into the area of health promotion and of measuring the beneficial effects of moderating destructive health habits and environmental influences of all kinds. In each case a political dimension is involved since measurements taking account of all the physical, personal, family and financial costs are likely to result in findings which call for corporate action. Health professionals need to be in the forefront of these developments if health decisions are to be made on rational grounds.

References

1 Marmot, M. Chairman's summing-up. *Comp Med Res* 1987; **2**: 117–21.

2 Department of Health and Social Security. *Health Care and Its Costs.* London: HMSO, 1983.

3 Rathwell, T., Barnard, K. Health services performance in Great Britain. In: Long, A. F. and Harrison, S. (eds.) *Health Services Performance; Effectiveness and Efficiency.* London: Croom Helm, 1985; 126–62.

4 Anthony, H. M. (ed.) The patient as individual and statistic. Proceedings of the Second Conference on Research Methodology for Complementary Medicine. *Comp Med Res* 1987; **2**: 48–121.

5 Department of Health and Social Security *Prevention and Health: Everybody's Business.* London: HMSO, 1976.

6 Scully, R. E. Vaginal and cervical abnormalities, including clear-cell adenocarcinoma related to prenatal exposure to stilboestrol. *Ann Clin Lab Sci* 1974; **4**: 222–33.

7 Canter, D. A research agenda for holistic therapy studies. *Comp Med Res* 1987; **2**: 104–16.

8 Anthony, H. M. Some methodological problems in the assessment of complementary therapy. *Stat Med* 1987; **6**: 761–71.

9 Maynard, A. The regulation of public and private health care markets. In: McLachlan, G. and Maynard, A. (eds.) *The Public/Private Mix for*

Health. London: Nuffield Provincial Hospitals Trust, 1982; 471–511.

[10] Long, A. F., Harrison, S. Health services performance: an overview. In: Long, A. F. and Harrison, S. (eds.) *Health Services Performance; Effectiveness and Efficiency*. London: Croom Helm, 1985; 1–9.

[11] Parsons, F. M., Brunner, F. P., Burck, H. C. *et al*. Combined report on regular dialysis and transplantation in Europe, IV, 1973. *Proc Eur Dial Transpl* 1973; **11**: 3–67.

[12] Parsons, F. M., Ogg, C. S. (eds.) *Renal Failure – Who Cares?* Lancaster: MTP Press, 1983.

[13] Wood, I. T., Mallick, N. P., Wing, A. J. Prediction of resources needed to achieve the national target for treatment of renal failure. *Br Med J* 1987; **294**: 1467.

[14] Brostoff, J., Challacombe, S. J. (eds.) *Food Allergy and Intolerance*. London: Baillière Tindall, 1987.

[15] Munro, J., Carini, C., Brostoff, J. Migraine is a food-allergic disease. *Lancet* 1984; **2**: 719–21.

[16] Alun Jones, V., McLaughlin, P., Shorthouse, M. *et al*. Food intolerance, a major factor in the pathogenesis of irritable bowel syndrome. *Lancet* 1982; **2**: 1115–17.

[17] Rowe, A. H. Bronchial asthma because of food and inhalant allergy and less frequently drug and chemical allergy. In: Rowe, A. H. (ed.) *Food Allergy*. Springfield: Charles C. Thomas, 1972; 169–77.

[18] Cochrane, A. *Effectiveness and Efficiency: Random Reflections on Health Services*. Nuffield Provincial Hospitals Trust.

[19] Draper, P. Nancy Milio's work and its importance for the development of health promotion. *Health Promotion* 1986; **1**: 101–6.

[20] McKnight, J. L. Well-being: the new threshold to the old medicine. *Health Promotion* 1986; **1**: 77–80.

6 Choice of health indicator: the problem of measuring outcome

Ann Bowling

Summary

Research on outcomes of care goes beyond descriptions to look for causal relationships. The problem under study should be carefully defined and appropriate procedures chosen for measuring outcome. To do this one should:

1 Specify the purpose of the measurement (is the study descriptive or evaluative?).

2 Specify the population under study. If the sample is one of the normal population, a measure is needed that discriminates in terms of positive and negative health. Samples with a specific diagnosis will need measures which identify and discriminate between the problems caused by the particular disease. This is particularly relevant when choosing a disability measure.

3 Specify what resources are available for preparation for the study, administration of the instrument, etc.

This chapter considers the choosing of appropriate instruments for measuring outcome with special reference to the measurement of functional ability and perceived health status.

Introduction

There is now general agreement among health service planners and care providers that when setting objectives to reduce ill health and promote good health, one must define needs and evaluate the extent to which these are met. This involves a separate but equally important question for evaluative research: are some types of care and treatment more effective than others? Such questions focus attention on the health outcomes or consequences of care. However, the methods of evaluation and the measurement of outcomes remain controversial.

Almost as soon as the first potent medical therapies became available in the 1940s and 1950s the medical profession realized the importance of evaluating their effectiveness. This led to the introduction of the so-called 'clinical trial' to assess the efficacy of new medicines, and later, new operations, developing into the randomized controlled trial which compares the new treatment under study with a placebo or with the previous standard treatment. If possible, this is done on a double blind basis, where neither doctor nor patient knows whether the test or control treatment is being administered.

This type of trial provided no information on financial costs or economic benefits. Thus the 1950s and 1960s saw the development of cost-benefit analyses – for example, it was shown that the cost of modern drugs to treat TB was far outweighed by savings in hospital costs and reduced sick leave costs, and premature mortality. This then led to cost-effectiveness analyses in the 1960s and 1970s as it came to be realized that modern medicines increased longevity and extended the scope of therapy – so leading to *increases* in overall costs out of all proportion to the initial economic benefits. Cost–benefit analyses set out to answer the questions: 'Does this treatment bring a greater or smaller economic benefit than its predecessor?' and, 'Which treatment, assuming outcomes are the same, provides better value for money?'. Neither of these answers the broader question of how much overall benefit a service is yielding. In the 1970s economists applied cost–utility analysis to the question: 'How does the treatment affect the length and quality of life?' The principle of utility has become increasingly important in health care as few treatments now yield actual financial savings.

Cost–utility analysis thus attempts to measure the degree of wellbeing achieved in relation to its cost. However, measures of outcome are needed for reasons other than justification of cost: they are needed to justify the risks involved in medical intervention. Professionals are increasingly sensitive to patients' perspectives and assessments of need.

The problem of measuring outcome

Research on outcomes of care goes beyond descriptions to look for causal relationships. The problem under study should be carefully defined to ensure that it can be identified and clearly distinguished from other problems.

In order to choose an appropriate procedure for assessing outcome, in terms of study design and method of measurement, one should:

1 Specify the purpose of the measurement (is the study descriptive or evaluative?).

2 Specify the population under study. If the sample is one of the normal population, a measure is needed that discriminates in terms of positive and negative health. Samples with a specific diagnosis will need measures which identify and discriminate between the problems caused by the particular disease. This is particularly relevant when choosing a disability measure.

3 Specify what resources are available for preparation for the study, administration of the instrument and data analysis.

The researcher will also need to be aware of the strengths and weaknesses of existing measures of symptom severity, functional dependency, health status, etc., some of which are discussed later in this chapter. Evidence of validity and reliability should constitute essential criteria for the choice of instruments.

Finally, the choice of the research design (although hopefully not the method of measurement) will usually be a compromise between the ideal and what is practicable. The classic double blind randomized controlled trial is often not feasible. It will often be necessary simply to compare populations exposed and not exposed to defined inputs and those with and without desired outcomes.[1]

In order to measure health outcome a measure of health status is required. This, in turn, must be founded on some concept of what constitutes health. The limitations of the widely used negative definition of health as the absence of disease and the World Health Organization's definition of health as social, psychological and physical wellbeing have long been recognized. In the absence of satisfactory definitions of health, how should health outcome be defined?

Measures of health outcome

Mortality rates

As a measure of health outcome, mortality rates have the advantages of being collected routinely and being easily available, but in more affluent societies they are less useful as health indicators. As life expectancy increases, it becomes more difficult to diagnose cause of death unequivocally because of the increase in chronic multicausal disease and disability; for some conditions the death rate may be low and therefore subject to artificial fluctuations. Moreover, improved mortality rates are not necessarily associated with a generally improved health status.

Morbidity rates

Morbidity rates are less widely available and are subject to variations in quality. Attempts to improve them have developed in the following ways:

1 Refined indices, such as incidence and prevalence rates for specific conditions; absence from work; episodes of illness and type; and duration of disability.

2 Disability measures, which assess the degree to which people are able to perform the essential tasks of daily life. These should also include effects on social and occupational roles.

3 Health status and symptom indices, which focus on clinical and perceived health status and symptoms.

These techniques are collectively referred to as 'health indicators'.

Health indicators

All developed measures suffer from one major limitation: they measure deviations away from a state of health, health being the baseline. They are, in effect, indicators of 'ill health'. It is easier to measure departures from health than to find indices of health itself.

Each type of indicator is one method of measuring health status: there are multiple influences upon patient outcome, and these require a broader model of health than can be derived from any one type of indicator. Outcome is also influenced by non-biological inputs which include patient psychology, motivation and adherence to therapy, socio-economic status, availability of health care, social support networks and individual and cultural beliefs and behaviours.

Measurement problems

Measurement problems are rife when attempting measures of health outcomes.

Taking functional disability as an example, there is no 'hard' method of measuring abstract attributes such as disability. We rely on indicators for this purpose; for example, we may watch to assess whether someone is able to wash and dress. Often, several combined indicators are used for one concept. The combination is then called an 'index' or 'scale'.

Indicators may work well or badly, and are usually assessed by tests of reliability and validity. Validity is concerned with whether the indicator actually does measure the underlying attribute or not. Criteria of validity must be met, in particular:

Face validity: Is the indicator, on the face of it, a reasonable one? Is it a credible variable?
Content validity: Do the components of the scale/item cover all aspects of the attribute to be measured? Does the content of the variable match the name it has been given?
Predictive validity: Does the measure predict future differences? Is it of prognostic importance?
Convergent–discriminant validity: Are the results more highly correlated with an attempt to measure the same attribute by a different technique than with a measure of a different attribute by the same technique? Is it able to discriminate effectively between rival hypotheses?
Criterion validity: Can the variable be measured with accuracy? Is it reproducible between observers? On repeat tests, are similar values obtained (reliability)?
Construct validity: Can the results be correlated with an accepted gold standard?

An instrument will also require testing for reliability. A measure is judged to be reliable when it consistently produces the same results, particularly when applied to the same subjects at different time-periods. Three methods of measuring reliability are commonly used: multiple form, split half and test-retest. In addition, tests of internal consistency based on statistical models are becoming more widespread.

Multiple form reliability: This is used where two instruments, which have been developed in parallel and which measure the same attribute, are administered and the scores on each correlated. A high correlation indicates a reliable test.
Split half reliability: This is a method of assessing internal consistency where items on an instrument are divided into two equivalent parts and correlations between the scores on each part are computed. This requires that the items in the instrument should be homogeneous with respect to the attribute being measured. This is useful when a large pool of items measures one attribute.

Test-retest reliability: The test is administered to the same population on two occasions and the results compared, usually by correlation. The main problem with this is that the first administration may affect responses on the second: there may also be genuine changes between administrations which affect the estimate of reliability.

The achievement of standards of validity and reliability requires time and effort. It is a powerful reason for using existing scales: inventing one's own scale involves a waste of resources and leads to the development of a plethora of unreliable and invalid scales. It is a practice to be discouraged.

Measurement theory

Functional disability states and perceived health are defined by descriptions and thus a nominal (or classification) scale is constructed. This means that words (or numbers or other symbols) have been used simply to classify a characteristic or item. This is measurement at its weakest level. The merits of different classifications or sets of descriptions remain controversial and the choice is partly determined by the application. Hypotheses can be tested regarding the distribution of cases among categories by using the non-parametric test, χ^2 (chi-square), and Fisher's exact probability test. The most common measure of association (correlation) for nominal data is the contingency coefficient.

Descriptions can be placed on ordinal, interval or ratio scales. An ordinal (or ranking) scale is applicable where objects in one category of a scale are not simply different from objects in other categories of that scale, but they stand in some kind of relation to them: typical relations may be higher than, more preferred, more difficult (in effect, greater than). This is an ordinal scale. Socio-economic status is one example. Many disability and health status measures are strictly of this type. The most appropriate statistic for describing the central tendency of scores in an ordinal scale is the median, since the median is not affected by the numerical value of any scores above or below it as long as the number of scores above and below remain the same. Hypotheses can be tested using non-parametric statistics such as correlation coefficients based on rankings (e.g. Spearman rs or the Kendal r).

An interval scale is obtained when a scale has all the characteristics of an ordinal scale, and when in addition the distances between any two numbers on the scale are of known size. Measurement considerably stronger than ordinality has thus been achieved, characterized by a common and constant unit of measurement which assigns a real number, but the zero point and the unit of measurement are arbitrary. Temperature is one example (two scales are commonly used and the zero point on each is arbitrary – it differs on the two scales). An interval scale is a truly quantitative scale and all the common parametric statistics and tests (means, standard deviations, t-test, F-test, Pearson correlations, etc.) are applicable, provided that the requirements for normal distribution are met. Parametric tests take advantage of all information contained in interval scale data.

The ratio scale exists when a scale has all the characteristics of an interval scale and in addition has a true zero point as its origin. The ratio of any two scale points is independent of the unit of measurement. Weight is one example. Any statistical tests can be used when ratio measurement has been achieved.

Most behavioural scientists aspire to create interval scales but rarely succeed. Measures of functional disability and health status never strictly reach a ratio or interval scale of measurement. This has implications for analysis since statistical tests implying a higher level of measurement are invalid if used on ordinal scale data.

For the purpose of the comparative evaluation of the outcome of intervention A in comparison with the outcome of intervention B, a nominal scale may be sufficient (for example, 'died' or 'survived'). However, an ordinal scale is likely to provide greater statistical efficiency because a smaller sample may answer the question if a more sensitive measure, such as an ordinal scale of severity, is used. When the question is: 'How much more effective is A than B?', at least an interval scale, providing more precisely quantified data, is required. If the question is: 'Proportionately how much better is intervention A than B?', a ratio scale is ideally required, but not always available. In choosing a scale one must take into account the uses which should be made of it, and those which are likely to be made of it.

Functional disability measures

The terms 'impairment', 'disability' and 'handicap' are often erroneously used interchangeably. The increasing use of the concept of functional dependency has recently added to the confusion. The distinctions between these concepts first require clarification. Philip Wood's work for WHO has resulted in the International Classification of Impairments, Disabilities and Handicaps.[2] This provides a clear and consistent terminology and a classification system.

This system defines the terms 'impairment', 'disability' and 'handicap' and links them together conceptually:

$$\text{Disease or Disorder} \rightarrow \text{Impairment} \rightarrow \text{Disability} \rightarrow \text{Handicap}$$

Impairment is defined thus:

> In the context of health experience, an impairment is any loss or abnormality of psychological, physiological, or anatomical structure or function.

It represents deviation from some norm in the individual's biomedical status. While impairment is concerned with biological function, disability is concerned with activities expected of the person or the body.

Disability is defined thus:

> In the context of health experience, a disability is any restriction or lack (resulting from an impairment) of ability to perform an activity in the manner or within the range considered normal for a human being.

Functional handicap represents the social consequences of impairments or disabilities. It is thus a social phenomenon and a relative concept. The attitudes and values of the non-handicapped play a major part in defining a handicap. It is defined thus:

> In the context of health experience, a handicap is a disadvantage for a given individual, resulting from an impairment or a disability, that limits or prevents the fulfilment of a role that is normal (depending on age, sex and social and cultural factors) for that individual.

These constitute working definitions of impairment, disability and handicap. A working definition, as distinct from an operational definition, must be precise enough to suggest the content of the indicators, but must not be so precise that it cannot be generalized to a variety of contexts. Operational definitions, in contrast, are usually specific to a particular measurement instrument and even to a particular type of study. They define the specific behaviours and the ways in which they are to be classified.[1]

Functional dependency is less easily defined. Impairment and disability may lead to dependency in the same way they lead to handicap. However, they cannot be equated with dependency, nor is there a necessary relationship. Like the concept of handicap, dependency is a social consequence, and the attitudes of others decide its definition Working definitions are limited to specific contexts, which, in the case of dependency, means that they tend to deal with particular types of dependency, for example the type of help from others that is necessary for survival.[1]

Operational definitions, on the whole, concentrate on activities of daily living, often subdivided into domestic and self-care activities. Thus the operational definition of disability is failure to perform certain specified activities to a pre-determined standard.[2]

Measuring functional status

On the basis of the previous definitions, functional status can be defined as the degree to which an individual is able to perform socially allocated roles free of physically (or mentally in the case of mental illness) related limitations.

There is a clear distinction from general health status. Functional status is directly related to the ability to perform social roles, which measures of general health need not take into account. Functional status is just one component of health. It is a measure of the *effects* of disease rather than of the disease itself.

There are several advantages in using functional status measures. First, the theoretical framework is well articulated. Such measures reflect the physical ability of the individual to perform expected roles and activities. The behavioural aspects of functional status are of interest when assessing health and wellbeing. Secondly, measures of functional status are probably the component of health most sensitive to change and hence best suited for use as a criterion in intervention studies.[3,4] Thirdly, functional disability measures have more relevance to people's lives than the more objective measures of timed walking, grip strength, etc.

The problem of measuring functional disability is compounded by conceptual difficulties and interactive factors. One of the major problems with using a functional index is that different patients may react differently to apparently similar levels of physical impairment, depending on their expectations, priorities, goals, social support networks and so on. Functional disability, like dependency, is a multidimensional concept which may relate to physical, mental, cognitive, social, economic or environmental factors. By implication, it is an interactive concept – the disability may not be a necessary consequence of impairment but perhaps, for example, of the siting of bathrooms, toilets and other facilities and the necessity of negotiating stairs. In terms of dependency, severity might be a function of the existence of gadgets and equipment or the frequency and timing of help. Perceptions of the severity of both disability and dependency will also be influenced by previous history, and expectations for the future.

Also, there are often differing points of view of how people ought to be performing, for instance, between therapist and patients. The patient may want to walk without aids or a limp while the therapist may regard 'walking with aids and a limp' as indicative of a satisfactory outcome. Choice is generally ignored by most measures of disability and health status. Elderly people may prefer a strip-wash to the risk of slipping while getting into the bath. It is important to include questions about patients' expectations and satisfaction in a study on outcome of care.

Finally, caution is needed when deciding on which measures to use. Measures tend to be developed, administered and validated in one of two types of samples: people living in the community or in institutions. The measures are not necessarily interchangeable between samples: choice must take account of the type of population. Measures also tend to be age-related – many have been developed to be optimally suitable for a particular age group, and may be inappropriate for use with other age groups.

Content of functional status scales

Most measures of functional disability are self-report methods. Respondents are asked to report limitations on their activities. They tend to focus narrowly on a limited range of functions (mobility, domestic and self-care tasks), ignoring financial, emotional and social needs, which may be equally or more important. Measures of physical functioning and limitations to activity do not assess functioning in everyday social roles, or patients' satisfaction with their level of functioning. More relevant aspects of household roles are also largely ignored: for example, the effect of the condition on the *time taken* to perform chores such as cleaning, cooking, shopping, errands, childcare and other caring roles, and people's satisfaction with their functioning in these areas. Thus, most measures will require supplementation.

Selected functional disability scales

Rheumatology, a discipline traditionally concerned with function, has numerous scales of 'Activities of Daily Living'. Few have been adequately tested for reliability and validity. This has led to researchers not knowing which instrument to use and so to the design of more new ones, resulting in the use of measures of questionable validity. The procedure to be recommended is to choose an existing, well-tested scale where one is happy with all the items and then add to it, with care, to supplement any areas where it seems weak.

There are in addition a number of methodological techniques available for measuring function: direct physical tests of function, direct observation of behaviour, and interviews with the person concerned or a third party. Each method has its limitations, as has been indicated. Direct observation is rarely used because it is so time-consuming. Direct tests of functioning, such as range of limb movement, grip strength, walking time, or standards such as joint swelling, morning stiffness, erythrocyte sedimentation rate and joint counts, while objective, may not necessarily give an accurate indication of ability or performance. Grip strength will tell you how much a patient can and will squeeze a bag on a particular day. Patients may be more concerned with subjective feelings and reductions in activities associated with daily living.

Guttman scales

One of the earliest attempts to scale disability was introduced in the 1940s by Guttman.[5] He ranked degrees of patient disability in respect of a number of activities, such as feeding, continence, ambulation, dressing and bathing.

This method assumes that disabilities can be ordered. For example, six disabilities always score worse than five, and a score of six would assume that items 1–5 had been affirmed. This is satisfactory provided that disability progresses steadily from one activity to another (i.e. patients first have difficulty in bathing, then in bathing and dressing, and so on until they are disabled in respect of all the activities). It yields a single rating from one (no disability) to seven (disabled on all six activities). The resulting type of Guttman scale has been widely used since the 1940s.[6] This method, and the many variants, all assess or 'score' function by putting items in a hierarchy of severity based on the notion that patients who can perform a particular task will be able to perform all easier tasks. Conversely, if they cannot perform a particular task, they will be unable to perform tasks rated as higher. The Normative scale relies on the classification of items into major or minor disability, e.g. 'being able to feed oneself' is given twice the weight of 'being able to dress oneself'. Principle Component Scaling relies on the internal evidence of the data being scaled, calculating the relative weights to be given each item in order to construct a linear additive index. Numerous health index questionnaires fall into these categories.

A more recent Guttman scaling instrument has been developed by Williams *et al.*[7] The activities which make up the scale are not comprehensive in terms of describing activities of daily living but it has the advantage of having two scales, one for men and one for women. Work on developing and refining the scale is continuing.

Activities of Daily Living (ADL)

One of the best known and oldest of the disability scales is the Activities of Daily Living (ADL) index developed by Katz *et al.*[8,9] They designed it in order to describe, for clinical purposes, the states of elderly patients. Patients are graded by interviewers on six ordinal scales related to their ability in bathing, dressing, transferring (e.g. to chair), toileting, continence and feeding. Scores on individual scales were summed, all items being treated as equally important, thus yielding a single total score. On the basis of more than 2000 evaluations of the states of patients, the authors observed that these functions decreased in order, and claimed to have a measure of fundamental biological function, a claim questioned by those using Guttman scales.[7] The index of ADL was shown to predict the long-term course and social adaptation of patients with strokes and hip fractures and was used to evaluate outpatient treatment for rheumatoid arthritis.[10–12] This group later developed a survey instrument for obtaining health status data containing questions about the need for and use of health services and attitudes towards medical care. They defined five ranked categories of 'need' – no disability, restricted activity with no chronic conditions, restricted activity with chronic conditions, mobility limitation, and bed disability – chosen to permit comparisons with existing national surveys.[13] The Katz is one of the earliest and most extensively tested of a group of indices for use in evaluating care of elderly and chronically ill patients: it is useful with a restricted range of patients. However the range of disabilities included in the instrument is not comprehensive and so the populations to which it can be administered are limited. The main disadvantage of the use of a single index is that information about variability is lost because different patterns of restriction, with different implications, can be reduced to the same score. In addition, if any of the items added together in this way to create an overall rating are no more than ordinal, the index also will be no more than ordinal, and the statistical techniques used must reflect this. Scoring may also exacerbate the instrument's distortion of the experience of the individuals. These problems may be avoided by treating all aspects of disability and dependency as equal contributors to overall severity, and expressing the results for each item separately.

Finally, concise indices, such as the Katz ADL, tend to be insensitive to small changes in disease severity and to focus on physical performance. More recently developed measures take a broader view of function and include elements of social activity, anxiety and depression.

Other measures

Among the most widely used measures of functional disability are:

Health Assessment Questionnaire (HAQ)[14–16]
Arthritis Impact Measurement Scale (AIMS)[17–19]

McMaster Health Index Questionnaire (MHIQ)[20,21]
Sickness Impact Profile (SIP)[22,23] (adapted for use in GB and
    known as Functional Limitation Profile (FLP))[24]
Cornell Medical Index (CMI)[25]
Older Americans Resources and Services Inventory
    (OARS)[26,27]

Most of these measure disability, impairment and handicap. Apart from
the SIP, adapted as the Functional Limitation Profile by Patrick for
applicability in the UK,[24] most raise the question of cross-cultural
applicability, since they were developed in the USA and Canada.
However, the HAQ has been used in the UK and the results suggest that
it is applicable.[28] Another criticism of these measures is that patients'
wishes and satisfaction are omitted. Most of their designers are satisfied
with their levels of validity, reliability and sensitivity, although these
have been questioned by others.[29] The HAQ and AIMS are perhaps
among the most popular.

The Stanford Arthritis Centre Health Association Questionnaire (HAQ)

In the process of developing this measure, 62 potential questions were
selected from questionnaires in use in the rheumatic diseases and
elsewhere. Testing the measure for reliability and validity with patients
with rheumatoid arthritis reduced the measure to 21 questions, grouped
into nine components, and graded in ordinal fashion from 0 to 3.

The resulting instrument has subsequently been administered in
numerous settings. It has been extensively validated. Correlations of the
HAQ against observed patient performance ranged from fair to high
(0.47 to 0.88).[15,16,30] It assesses dressing and grooming, rising, eating,
walking, reaching, personal hygiene, gripping and grasp, activities and
pain. It is relatively coherent and concise and is self-administered so
does not rely on skilled personnel to administer. It is therefore relatively
cheap. Administration takes five to eight minutes; manual scoring may
be accomplished in one minute. The HAQ is also sensitive to change,
and thus makes possible long-term studies of outcome in arthritis: in
this sense it is probably more useful than the numerous scales of
activities of daily living.[15,16] It is suitable for use in community settings
and has been administered to patients with rheumatoid and osteoarthritis, systemic lupus and ankylosing spondylitis.

The Arthritis Impact Measurement Scale (AIMS)

This is another self-administered questionnaire that has been extensively validated and is also sensitive to change.[17–19,30] It aims to assess
patient outcome in arthritis and other chronic diseases, and is composed
of 49 items. These are summed into nine scales. Each scale is indexed
from 0 to 10 (minimum to maximum disability). It assesses mobility,
physical activity, activities of daily living, dexterity, household activities,
pain, social activity, depression and anxiety. All nine AIMS scales have
been reported to be highly correlated with physician-produced estimates of health status, and the relevant scales correlated highly with
standard measures of physical function. The content of AIMS overlaps

with the HAQ by about 65% but all the actual questionnaire items are different, except that both instruments contain a single horizontal visual analogue scale assessing the patient's perception of arthritis status, providing a 'global health estimate'. A study administering both instruments (HAQ and AIMS) to patients with rheumatoid arthritis demonstrated that they measure similar dimensions of health status in this type of chronic disease. The instruments were highly correlated, providing convergent validation for the existence of three relatively discrete components of health status: pain, physical disability and psychological status.[30]

Both HAQ and AIMS have good measurement properties, have been extensively tested for validity, and explain the majority of the impact of illness as estimated by patients. However, the specificity of these two instruments makes them unsuitable for use with groups other than the chronically ill.

Health profiles

To some extent disability measures cannot be separated from indices of perceived health status and symptoms. The difference is that the former are more specialized and hence narrow, while the latter give a broader picture of perceived health. Some measures fall into both categories (e.g. CMI, OARS, MHIQ, SIP). There are a number of other well-tested scales.[31]

The Cornell Medical Index (CMI)

This is a good example. It is based on self-report and contains 95 yes/no questions divided into 18 sections relating to physiological disturbance, personal habits, frequency of illness, moods and feelings. The number of problems admitted are scored and the total number is taken to indicate the degree of deviation from health: a medically significant emotional disturbance is considered present if the total score is 30 or more.[25] It is less well tested than other measures.

The Older Americans' Resources and Services Inventory (OARS) and the Functional Assessment Inventory (FAI)

This assessment schedule is more appropriate for use with older persons.[26,27] FAI is a shorter version of OARS. Both have questions relating to mental status, socio-demographic information, mental and physical health, activities of daily living and the use of services. Information is obtained by interview. The FAI has 90 items less than the OARS, fewer response categories and two scales measuring life satisfaction and self-esteem. Both instruments appear to have face and content validity, although discriminant and predictive validity have not been tested adequately. The complexity of the inventory makes it time-consuming to complete.

The McMaster Health Index Questionnaire (MHIQ)

This contains 59 items covering physical mobility, self-care, sight and hearing, general wellbeing, social and occupational role performance, family support, self-esteem, critical life events, personal relationships and emotional functioning. This can be self-administered and it is simple, acceptable, cheap and reasonably reliable. Content, criterion and construct validity have been assessed in a wide variety of patients. The validity of the physical function items is robust but the social and emotional indicators are weak.[20,21]

There are a number of other scales which have been extensively tested for reliability and validity and which appear satisfactory for use in clinical trials and in evaluation of therapies. A number have been reviewed by Brooks.[31]

The Quality of Wellbeing Scale (QWB)

This combines assessments of quality of life with mortality risk and includes symptom combinations such as pain and shortness of breath with measures of functional ability, social activities, self-care and activities of daily living.[32,33] However, it must be administered by trained interviewers and is fairly complex, which limits its application.

There have also been a number of attempts to measure psychological wellbeing, although the reliability and validity of most is questionable and, as most have been developed in the USA, their cross-cultural application is limited (notions of feeling good may well vary cross-culturally).

The General Health Questionnaire (GHQ)

GHQ, developed for community screening, is a well-tested and often used instrument in the UK for the detection of purely psychological problems. It is available in a number of versions of varying length (from 140 items to twelve).[34] It has been found to be effective in detecting mental problems, although not their severity. Many items measured perceived health status insofar as this affects mental health. The questionnaire is self-administered and economical and population norms are available for comparison.

Sickness Impact Profile (SIP)

One of the best developments in the USA has been the Sickness Impact Profile.[22,23] This contains 136 items referring to illness-related dysfunction in twelve areas: work, recreation, emotion, affect, home life, sleep, rest, eating, ambulation, mobility, communication and social interaction. Scores can be in the form of an overall total or separate for physical and psychosocial areas. It may be self-administered. It has established good convergent and discriminant validity and test-retest validity is high. It is suitable for use with a wide range of patients with acute or chronic conditions, and has been used successfully in clinical trials. It is sensitive to change and is valuable for assessing the impact of illness on the chronically ill and for measuring the effects of non-curative interventions.[35,36] Its limitations are its length and the fact that it can only be used with people who are regarded, or who regard themselves, as ill. A modified version (based on language changes more suited to our population) has been used at St Thomas's Hospital for a community disability survey.[24] However, the changes are not entirely satisfactory and its appropriateness for use in Britain has yet to be established.[37]

Nottingham Health Profile (NHP)

In Britain the recent development of the Nottingham Health Profile, as a measure of perceived health, was planned to overcome some of the problems outlined.[37] It is based on lay perceptions of health status; it is short and simple, based on British samples, and is suitable for clinical or survey work. It can be used with groups of patients or a general population. It is suitable for people who have not been labelled as unhealthy or ill. However, like others, it focuses on negative rather than positive experiences.

Symptoms are not included in the measure so those who have not been labelled as unhealthy or ill can complete it. It is suitable for a wide range of groups, including the elderly. Pilot work identified key concepts; statements were drawn up which exemplified those concepts; after piloting and much refinement and elimination of ambiguity, statements were finally categorized into six areas: physical mobility, pain, sleep, energy, emotional reactions and social isolation. Respondents are asked to indicate 'yes' or 'no' according to whether the statement applies to them 'in general at the present time'. This comprises Part I of the NHP. Part II asks about any effects of health on seven areas of daily life: work, looking after the home, social life, home life, sex life, interests, hobbies and holidays. It only requires yes/no responses to each of 38 statements in Part I. Part II is simply coded 1 for yes and 0 for no, and then scored. Population norms exist for the instrument, as do scores on individual patient groups, e.g. those recovering from fractures of the hip, heart transplantation surgery and those with osteoarthritis, etc.

The NHP produces scores ranging from 0 (no problems) to 100 (where all problems in a section are affirmed). It has been extensively tested for reliability and validity, and results have been good. It has been tested for face, content and criterion validity and has been found to be a highly satisfactory measure of subjective health status in physical, social and emotional spheres. It was also found to be useful in measuring the extent to which health problems restrict normal physical and social activities, although it is no substitute for a more detailed measure of functional disability, and requires supplementing with a well-validated measure of functional ability (e.g. HAQ) in areas where function is of relevance (as in rheumatology).

Two studies have focused on the reliability of the NHP, using the test-retest technique, one with patients with osteoarthritis and the other with peripheral vascular disease. Both demonstrated a fairly high level of reliability. However, the NHP does not meet the requirements for carrying out split half or multiple form reliability.

In summary, the NHP can provide the following measures:

1 Perceived health status before and after intervention.

2 Comparison of treated patient with population norms.

3 Assessment over a longer period of time after intervention.

It is appropriate for use in the following ways:

1 For evaluation of medical/social interventions, in pre-test/post-test designs.

2 As an outcome measure for group comparisons.

3 As a survey tool with groups such as the elderly and the chronically ill.

4 As an adjunct to clinical interviews.

Some preliminary work has been done with patients suffering from cancer of the breast, genital–urinary cancer, skin and lung cancer. They indicate the NHP has a value in helping to decide on the best treatment for categories of patients, and identifying patients at particular risk.

A main weakness of the NHP is that it is a relatively severe measure and may not pick up minor improvements in perceived health and many forms of treatment may be expected to lead only to small changes.

A problem of concern specifically to the NHP is the distribution of scores obtained which will probably be highly skewed. Careful consideration then needs to be given to the application of statistical tests as parametric tests assume that the results are normally distributed.

Global Health Indices (QUALYs)

Finally, brief reference should be made to the attempts of economists to find single, global health indices which would summarize in a single statistic the health status of populations. Such models typically assign values to days of health, number of illnesses per annum per person, hospital inpatient stays and weightings of the severity of ill health and effects of death, resulting in a comprehensive index in the form of an annual statistic. Chiange produced an index of health which uses the weighted average mean duration of health of a population per annum, the mean duration of health by age groups and includes the effects of illness and mortality.[38] A revised version includes a severity factor.[39] Other single global indices have been developed. There is particular interest in QUALYs – quality-adjusted life years which could be used as units of health benefits and which would be more sensitive than life expectancy, since they take into account interventions to prolong life and activities improving the quality of life which leave longevity unaffected. However, single indices are not heuristic, they lead to a serious loss of information.[40] Global indices also wrongly assume that a healthy lifestyle is of equal value to everyone.

One of the earliest pieces of work attempting to create a single global figure indicating health in the UK was carried out by Rosser and Watts in 1971.[41] They constructed a matrix showing four degrees of distress along one axis and eight degrees of disability along the other. They then allocated each patient to an appropriate box out of the 32 in the matrix. In order to put a value on each box they used a legal textbook which gives the quantum of damages awarded following industrial injury cases.[42] They put about 500 legal cases into appropriate boxes in the matrix, and derived an average value for the compensation given in each of the 32 different conditions, and converted these values into an index. This has led to more sophisticated attempts by Rosser, using the same basic matrix, to get different groups of individuals to put relative degrees of desirability on the different states.[43] In the process of evaluation two survival states were given a score of less than zero – that is, judged worse than death. The use of a one-dimensional scale makes it possible to make a quantitative assessment of relative wellbeing for an individual over time. This has led to the concept of a quality-adjusted life year or QUALY. The principle is that it is no longer simply important to measure life expectancy in unadjusted years because a single year of excellent health may be equivalent in terms of overall utility to more than one year of impaired health. In other words, given the choice, a person would prefer a shorter healthier life to a longer period of survival in a state of severe discomfort and disability.[44] This leads to ratings implying that 18 months confined to a wheelchair and in moderate pain has the same economic utility as one year completely free from disability or distress. The problem with this is that it may be difficult to obtain a universally accepted view of the value (utility) of different states of wellbeing. An elderly person may feel their handicapped and painful existence is just as valuable to them as someone else's apparently healthier existence. A more obvious limitation of such measures is that they discount other factors (e.g. work) which affect a person's quality of life.[45]

Choice of indicator

Before deciding on an instrument, several issues require clarification:

1 What is the research question? What is to be measured? Hypotheses must be formulated clearly.

2 What is it that the suggested instrument measures? Is it functional disability, emotional problems or physical health problems? Is that what requires measuring?

3 For what populations is the instrument to be used? In a sample of the general population only about 20% will have chronic physical or emotional problems, thus a negatively based measure will provide little information about the sample as a whole. On the other hand a sample of people with serious health problems will require a highly specific tool.

4 Are the scores expressed in a way that will enable them to be linked easily with other relevant variables?

5 How have validity and reliability been tested? On what types and numbers of people? Is the population similar to your study population? Do norms exist for comparative purposes?

6 If the instrument is to be used for monitoring the effects of an intervention, will it measure aspects of health or disability that are susceptible to change within the time span of the study?

7 How appropriate is the instrument for the study population? Frail elderly people and those with poor eyesight and arthritic hands will not find self-administered questionnaires easy. Long complex questionnaires may not be suitable for ill people.

8 Have confounding variables been considered? For instance, use of other services, type of therapist, social support systems, and patient adherence to therapy.

Conclusion

In conclusion, it seems generally desirable that, when measuring health outcome, one should take a measure of functional disability and a measure of subjective health status, and assess patient expectation and satisfaction, as well as recording diagnostic criteria. However, the choice of measure is complex and merits careful consideration.

References

[1] Wilkin, D. *Theoretical and Conceptual Issues in the Measurement of Dependency*. University of Manchester: Centre for Primary Care Research, 1986.

[2] World Health Organization. *International Classification of Impairments, Disabilities and Handicaps*. Geneva: World Health Organization, 1980.

[3] Sullivan, D. F. *Conceptual Problems in Developing an Index of Health*. US Department of Health, Education and Welfare Publication No. (HRA) 74–1017, Series No. 5. Washington, DC: Department of Health, Education and Welfare, 1966.

[4] Reynolds, W. J., Rushing, W. A., Miles, D. L. The validation of a function status index. *J Health Social Behaviour* 1974; **15**: 271–89.

[5] Guttman, L. A basis for scaling quantitative data. *Am Sociol Rev* 1944; **9**: 139–50.

[6] Culyer, A. J. Need values and health status measurement. In: Culyer, A. J. and Wright, K. G. (eds.) *Economic Aspects of Health Services*. London: Martin Robertson, 1978.

[7] Williams, R. G. A., Johnston, M., Willis, L. A., Bennet, A. E. Disability: a model and measurement technique. *Br J Prev Soc Med* 1976; **30**: 71–8.

[8] Katz, S., Ford, A. B., Moskowitz, R. W., Jacobson, B. A., Jaffe, M. W. The Index of ADL: a standardised measure of biological and psychosocial function. *J Am Med Assoc* 1963; **185**: 914–19.

[9] Katz, S., Downs, T. D., Cash, H. R., Grotz, R. C. Progress in development of the index of ADL. *Gerontology* 1970; **10**: 20–30.

[10] Katz, S., Ford, A. S., Chinn, A. B., Newill, V. A. Prognosis after strokes: long term course of 159 patients. *Medicine* 1966; **45**: 236.

11 Katz, S., Vignos, P. J., Moskowitz, R. W., Thompson, H. M., Svec, K. H. Comprehensive out-patient care in rheumatoid arthritis: a controlled study. *J Am Med Assoc* 1968; **206**: 1249.

12 Katz, S., Ford, A. S., Chinn, A. B., Newill, V. A. Studies of illness in the aged: recovery after fracture of the hip. *J Gerontol* 1964; **19**: 285.

13 Katz, S., Akpom, C. A., Papsidero, J. A., Weiss, S. T. Measuring the health status of populations. In: Berg, R. L. (ed.) *Health Status Indexes*. Chicago: Hospital Research and Education Trust, 1973.

14 Fries, J. F. The assessment of disability: from first to future principles. Paper presented at the conference 'Advances in Assessing Arthritis at The London Hospital', March 1983.

15 Fries, J. F., Spitz, P., Kraines, R. G., Holman, H. R. Measurement of patient outcome in arthritis. *Arthritis and Rheumatism* 1980; **23**: 137–45.

16 Fries, J. F., Spitz, P., Young, D. Y. The dimensions of health outcomes: the health assessment questionnaire, disability and pain scales. *J Rheumatol* 1982; **9**: 789–93.

17 Meenan, R. F., Gertman, P. M., Mason, J. H. Measuring health status in arthritis: the arthritis impact measurement scales. *Arthritis and Rheumatism* 1980; **23**; 146–52.

18 Meenan, R. F., Gertman, P. M., Mason, J. H., Dunaif, R. The arthritis impact measurement scales: further investigations of a health status measure. *Arthritis and Rheumatism* 1982; **25**: 1048–53.

19 Meenan, R. F. The AIMS approach to health status measurement: conceptual background and measurement properties. *J Rheumatol* 1982; **9**: 785–88.

20 Chambers, L. W., Sackett, D. L., Goldsmith, C. H., Macpherson, A. S., Macauley, R. C. Development and application of an index of social function. *Health Service Research* 1976; **11**: 430–1.

21 Chambers, L. W., MacDonald, L. A., Tugwell, P. *et al.* The McMaster Health Index Questionnaire as a measure of quality of life for patients with rheumatoid disease. *J Rheumatol* 1982; **9**: 780–4.

22 Deyo, R. A., Inui, T. S., Leininger, J., Overman, S. Physical and psychosocial function in rheumatoid arthritis. Clinical use of a self administered instrument. *Arch Internal Med* 1982; **142**: 879–82.

23 Deyo, R. A., Inui, T. S., Leininger, J., Overman, S. Measuring functional status in chronic disease: a comparison of traditional scales and a self administered health status questionnaire in patients with rheumatoid arthritis. *Med Care* 1983; **21**: 180–92.

24 Patrick, D. Standardisation of comparative health status measures: using scales developed in America in an English speaking country. In: Sudman, S. (ed.) *Health Survey Research Methods*. Third Biannual Conference, Hyattsville, Md. National Centre for Health Services Research, PHS Publ. no 81–3268.

25 Brodman, K., Erdman, A. J., Wolff, H. G. *Cornell Medical Index Health*

Questionnaire Manual. New York: Cornell University Medical College, 1960.

26   Cairl, R. E., Pfeiffer, E., Keller, D. M., Burke, H., Samis, H. V. An evaluation of the reliability and validity of the Functional Assessment Inventory. *J Am Ger Soc* 1983; **31**: 607–12.

27   Fillenbaum, G. G., Smyer, M. A. The development, validity and reliability of the OARS multidimensional functional assessment questionnaire: disability and pain scales. *J Gerontol* 1981; **36**: 428–33.

28   Kirwan, J. R., Reeback, J. S. Using a modified Stanford Health Assessment Questionnaire to assess disability in UK patients with rheumatoid arthritis. *Ann Rheum Dis* 1983; **42**: 219–20.

29   Laing, M. H., Cullen, K., Larson, M. In search of a more perfect mousetrap (health status or quality of life instrument). *J Rheumatol* 1982; **9**: 775–9.

30   Brown, J. H., Lewis, M. D., Kazis, E. *et al.* The dimensions of health outcomes: a cross validated examination of health status measurement. *Am J Public Health* 1984; **74**: 159–61

31   Brooks, R. Health indicators in arthritis. In: Teeling Smith G. (ed.) *Measuring the Social Benefits of Medicine.* London: Office of Health Economics, 1980; 84–92.

32   Bush, J. W. General health policy model/quality of well-being (QWB) scale. In: Wenger, N. K. *et al.* (eds.) *Assessment of Quality of Life in Clinical Trials of Cardiovascular Therapies.* New York: Le Jacq, 1984.

33   Kaplan, R. M., Bush, J. W., Berry, C. C. Health status: types of validity and the index of well-being. *Health Services Research* 1976; **11**: 478–507.

34   Goldberg, D. *The Detection of Psychiatric Illness by Questionnaire.* London: Oxford University Press, 1971.

35   Bergner, M., Bobbitt, R. A., Pollard, W. E. *et al.* The Sickness Impact Profile: validation of a health status measure. *Med Care* 1976; **14**: 57–67.

36   Bergner, M., Bobbitt, R. A., Carter, W. B. *et al.* The Sickness Impact Profile: development and final revision of a health status measure. *Med Care* 1981; **19**: 787–805.

37   Hunt, S. M., McEwen, J., McKenna, S. P. *Measuring Health Status.* London: Croom Helm, 1986.

38   Chiange, C. L. *An Index of Health: Mathematical Models.* PHS Publ. no. 1000, series 2, No. 5. Washington: US Government Printing Office, 1965.

39   Chiange, C. L., Cohen, R. D. How to measure health: a Stochastic model for an index of health. *Int J Epidemiol* 1973; **2**: 7–13.

40   Hurst, J. A government economist's attitudes to the new measures. In: Teeling Smith, G. (ed.) *Measuring the Social Benefits of Medicine.* London: Office of Health Economics, 1983; 139–45.

41 Rosser, R. M., Watts, V. C. *The Sanative Output of Hospital*. Dallas: 39th Operational Research Society of America, 1971.

42 Kemp, D. A. M., Kemp, M. S., Harvey, R. O. *The Quantum of Damages*. London: Sweet and Maxwell, 1967.

43 Rosser, R. M. A history of the development of health indicators. In: Teeling Smith, G. (ed.) *Measuring the Social Benefits of Medicine*. London: Office of Health Economics, 1983; 50–62.

44 Teeling Smith, G. *Measurement of Health*. London: Office of Health Economics, 1985.

45 Rosser, R. M. Life with artificial organs – renal dialysis and transplants. In: Shepherd, E. and Watson, J. (eds.) *Personal Meanings*. Chichester: John Wiley, 1981.

7 The importance of patient selection

F. A. C. Wiegant, C. W. Kramers and R. van Wijk

Summary

Several methodological problems are encountered in the setting up of clinical trials in the field of complementary medicine. In this chapter, the problems associated with the selection of a homogeneous group of patients, which is to be included in a clinical trial, are discussed.

Three categories of clinical trials are discerned, depending on whether or not attention has been paid to the complementary therapeutic system under study when selection of patients took place. Results of some examples from these categories of trials are discussed. It will be stressed that in an optimal trial, the group of patients should not only be homogeneous from the point of view of orthodox medicine, but also from the point of view of the complementary therapist.

Finally, to achieve such a goal, several fields of research are emphasized.

Introduction

Interest in various forms of complementary medicine is growing among professional and lay people. As a result, there is increasing pressure on therapists to present evidence for the effectiveness of their therapy and/or preparations.

In order to meet the demand for more research in the field of complementary therapy, it is of course necessary to formulate research projects. In this respect, useful suggestions and an overview of the different aspects to be faced in preparing research protocols have recently been published.[1,2,3,4]

A major criticism from orthodox medicine is that most research done in the field of complementary medicine does not meet the required methodological criteria. Claims of therapeutic effectiveness will only be taken seriously when they have been subject to the same rigorous tests as those required in orthodox medicine.

The classical way to test efficacy in orthodox medicine is by clinical trials. The experiment has to follow certain methodological 'rules'. It must:

- compare the effect of treatment with the effect of no treatment (or with other treatments);
- ensure that people who receive treatment are not specifically selected into that group (randomization);
- control for the placebo effect;

- identify a clearly diagnosed illness (in this way, formation of a homogeneous group of patients can take place);
- identify a standard treatment for selected patients;
- provide for a noticeable change in the value of measured variables;
- use measures which are precise, valid and reliable.

In general, clinical trials with randomization and blinding provide the strongest evidence for a relationship between intervention and effect. The most common version of a clinical trial which satisfies these rules is the double blind trial, where neither patient nor the person using the treatment knows who is receiving the actual treatment.

One of the activities of the Research Unit for Complementary Medicine (subsidized by the Dutch Ministry of Health, Welfare and Culture) has been to assist in the formulation of research projects. Over the past few years a large number of methodological problems in the setting up of clinical studies in the field of complementary medicine were encountered.

Several articles have already been dedicated to the shortcomings of various methodological criteria when applied to complementary medicine (such as cross-over, randomization, double blind, etc.).[5,6,7,8,9,10,11,12,13,14] In our opinion, however, one of the most prominent methodological problems has not yet received sufficient attention; namely the selection of patients.

In this chapter the problems associated with the selection of a homogeneous group of patients, which is to be included in a clinical trial, are discussed. It will be stressed that a group of patients should be homogeneous not only from the point of view of orthodox medicine, but also from the point of view of the complementary therapist. Three categories of clinical trials can be discerned depending on whether or not attention has been paid to the complementary therapeutic system under study when selection of patients took place. Methodology and results of some examples from these categories of trials, in the field of homoeopathy and acupuncture, will be discussed.

Selection of patients

In order to select patients for inclusion in a clinical trial, it is of crucial importance to give as complete a description of the disease (or a description of the symptom pattern) to be treated as possible. The group of patients should be as homogeneous as possible; that is to say, all patients included in a clinical trial should show a comparable set of symptoms. Because of this homogeneity, the same (standardized) treatment can be given to all patients. When the selection criteria are not complete enough, this will result in the formation of an inhomogeneous group of patients. Applying a standard treatment to an inhomogeneous group of patients holds the risk that some patients will be treated in a non-optimal way and therefore might not react to treatment. In that case no effect of treatment will be found.

This problem of inhomogeneous groups of patients is mainly encountered in those trials in which attention has only been paid to diagnostic criteria which are used in orthodox medicine and not (or not sufficient) to the diagnostic criteria used in the complementary therapy under study (e.g. homoeopathy).

Homogeneity of groups

The problem of homogeneity is illustrated in Figure 7.1, where patients with COPD (chronic obstructive pulmonary disease) are taken as a rather similar group. Out of this group a further division can be made into three subgroups (based on a specific set of diagnostic criteria used in orthodox medicine). From the point of view of the orthodox practitioner these are homogeneous subgroups. However, from the point of view of a homoeopath or an acupuncturist, the group of patients with COPD is far from homogeneous.

The complementary practitioners are not only interested in the specific symptoms which are thought by orthodox practitioners to be of crucial importance for the diagnosis of COPD or asthma. Other factors and

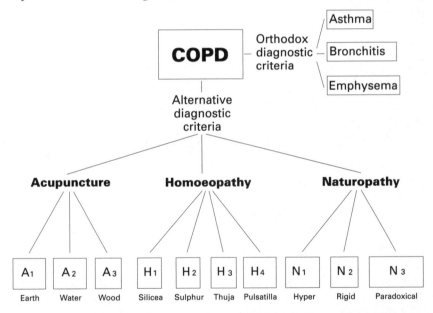

Fig. 7.1 Homogeneity of patients from the orthodox as well as the complementary medical point of view. Out of a group of patients with COPD, three more or less homogeneous subgroups can be formed, based on orthodox criteria. However, from the viewpoint of the complementary therapist (acupuncture, homoeopathy or naturopathy), these subgroups are far from homogeneous. Based on their specific diagnostic criteria, a different categorization of subgroups takes place. And seen the other way round, a subgroup that is homogeneous on complementary medical grounds is not necessarily so on orthodox grounds (see also text). An adequate selection of patients should therefore take place before patients participate in a trial to study the efficacy of a complementary therapy.

additional diagnostic criteria are also used. Based on a total individual symptom pattern, a different categorization of homogeneous groups will take place.

These symptom patterns are not only based on symptoms at the physiological level (such as alterations in the colour of the skin, tongue or iris, the number of painful spots, alterations in the pulse characteristics, etc.), but also on symptoms which are energetic, psychological (emotional, cognitive) and/or social in nature. For instance, the acupuncturist will pay attention to characteristics that can be detected by pulse and/or tongue diagnosis as well as the patient's total appearance and specific reactions to changes in the internal and external environment. These characteristics point to the functional interaction between organ systems, whether the flow of energy through the meridians is normal, etc. In this way patients can be classified according to specific syndromes, as yin- or yang-deficient, and in terms of main perverse energetic influence present (for instance, heat, damp or wind).

In homoeopathy several aspects of different levels of the human being are analysed, leading to the comparison of the symptoms of a patient with specific remedy pictures. These remedy pictures consist of symptoms which are induced in healthy persons by certain remedies. The more that symptom pattern of a patient resembles a remedy picture, the more certain the homoeopath will be regarding the prescription of the right homoeopathic remedy. In homoeopathy, a distinction can be made between several constitutional types which are more or less homogeneous (such as, for instance, phosphor, sulphur or silicea types).

In naturopathy, important aspects in diagnosis involve the examination of body fluids, the level of toxicity in tissues and the condition of the detoxifying organs (liver, intestines, kidneys, and skin), as well as the 'detoxifying' condition on the mental level (e.g. emotional expressions and type of main psychological defence mechanism used). All this is thought to determine the normal functioning and regulation of the 'basic autonomous regulatory system' (soft connective tissue including autonomic nervous system and immune system).[15] Using diagnostic methods aimed at identification of these regulatory processes, naturopaths may stress the importance of the type of reaction a patient shows to stimuli and discriminate on this basis between a normal reaction pattern, hyper-reactivity, a rigid reaction pattern or a paradoxical reaction. A treatment protocol will be determined, depending on the type of reaction pattern as well as on the degree of toxicity observed in the various organ systems of the patient.

Categories of research trials

Research trials can be categorized into three groups, depending on whether some of the above-mentioned selection criteria are used to obtain a homogeneous group of patients (from the point of view of orthodox medicine only or also from the point of view of complementary medicine).

In the first category, only selection criteria from the point of view of orthodox medicine are used. No alternative diagnosis is taken, which implies a standard treatment for all the participating patients. An individual treatment based on guidelines used within the specific therapeutic system, such as traditional acupuncture, is not allowed.

In the second category, the selection of patients is again only based on the diagnostic criteria of orthodox medicine. However, instead of giving a standard treatment to all patients, the complementary therapist is now allowed to give each patient an optimal individual treatment. Although an alternative diagnosis is completed (leading to a specific treatment protocol, such as a particular remedy or selection of acupuncture points, etc.), the whole process of diagnosis and treatment could be treated as a **black box**. This implies that no specific attention is paid to the patient's individual characteristics, which might influence the prescription of a specific complementary treatment. In many ways this is a great disadvantage: if the black box approach is used then the therapists are unable to control the details of treatment, as they would in day-to-day clinical practice.

In the third category, selection of patients is done in two steps. The first one is based on orthodox diagnostic criteria, followed by a second selection step which is dictated by the diagnostic criteria of the complementary therapy under study. Now, a group of patients is included in the trial which can be called homogeneous from both points of view; orthodox as well as complementary. Furthermore, the process of diagnosis and therapy is registered and is therefore controllable.

In this category, optimal attention is paid to the theory as well as to the specific way of working of the complementary therapy under study. Moreover, an optimal individual treatment is given according to the specific therapeutic rules, so that its effect can be studied in an optimal way.

Examples

1 Patient selection based on orthodox diagnostic criteria only

Examples of trials which belong to this category are the studies of Reilly et al.[16] and of Fung et al.[17]

Reilly et al.[16] studied the effect of a homoeopathic high potency preparation in patients with hayfever. There were 144 patients in the trial; 74 were given a homoeopathic preparation of mixed grass pollen in a 30c potency (i.e. a dilution of 10^{-60}), and 70 were given a placebo. Both groups were well matched and rigorous controls were used throughout the study. After five weeks analysis of the symptom scores showed a statistically significant improvement ($p = 0.02$) in the group of patients which were treated with a homoeopathic potency.

There is no doubt that this paper has been a landmark in homoeopathic research, since it took into account all required methodological criteria. Moreover, it showed a positive effect of a homoeopathically prepared remedy in favour of placebo.

Despite the result, the classically oriented homoeopath might object to the fact that no account has been taken of the complete symptom pattern of the individual patients since attention has only been paid to hayfever symptomatology. In their view prescription of the same homoeopathic remedy for all patients with hayfever is unlikely. A specific diagnosis from the point of view of classical homoeopathy will lead to the prescription of different remedies for each patient.

Therefore a group of patients with hayfever might be sufficiently homogeneous from the point of view of orthodox medicine but from the point of view of classical homoeopathy, this may not be the case.

The same rationale can also be used in the field of (traditional) acupuncture. The aim of Fung *et al.*[17] was to study whether real acupuncture provides a better protection against exercise-induced asthma than sham acupuncture. Twenty minutes before exercise, patients were treated on three asthma-related standard acupuncture points whereas the control group was treated on three unrelated acupuncture points in the neighbouring dermatome. They found that real acupuncture does provide a better protection against exercise-induced asthma than sham acupuncture.

Despite this result, the classically oriented acupuncturist might object that no account has been taken of the symptom pattern or specific syndrome of the individual patients. According to their view this selected group will not be homogeneous and therefore it is unlikely that the same acupuncture points should be stimulated in all patients.

Furthermore, by restricting needling sites to specific loci, limiting the number of treatment sessions and by not using traditional diagnostic practices, these kinds of clinical trials are reduced to testing the insertion of needles at particular points. In this way, acupuncture is not investigated as a treatment modality, but as a 'needling technique'.[8]

2 Patient selection based on orthodox diagnostic criteria only, followed by individual treatment within a black box

In the second category of clinical trials, the therapist is given the opportunity to apply an optimal treatment to each individual patient. However the precise way in which a diagnosis is taken and how the specific alternative therapy is applied is not registered nor studied. The whole treatment remains within a so-called 'black box'. The only relevant information in this type of study concerns the change in condition of patients before and after treatment. Examples of clinical trials which belong to this second category are the studies of Gibson *et al.*[18] and Jobst *et al.*[19]

Gibson *et al.*[18] demonstrated the superiority of individualized homoeopathy over placebo in rheumatoid arthritis. Forty six patients (receiving an orthodox first-line anti-inflammatory treatment) were divided in two matched groups. One group received a placebo, whereas the patients in the other group received a homoeopathic remedy which was prescribed according to the individual symptom patterns. Therefore most patients received different remedies, each of which had been optimally selected for that individual patient.

With respect to the result, a significant improvement was found in subjective pain, articular index, stiffness and grip strength in those patients receiving homoeopathic medicine.

The study reported by Jobst *et al.*[19] was also conducted according to the second category. Their aim was to study whether traditional acupuncture influences the perception of breathlessness in patients with chronic obstructive pulmonary disease. A treatment with either real acupuncture on individually selected acupuncture points or placebo acupuncture on non-acupuncture points was given for three weeks. After that period, they found a significant improvement in the acupuncture group with respect to the subjective perception of breathlessness.

The advantage of such studies is that instead of a standard treatment protocol, an optimal treatment is given according to the rules of the complementary therapy under study. Therefore the efficacy of a therapy is studied as a system. The disadvantage of clinical trials of this category, however, is that the diagnosis and the way in which a therapy is applied from the point of view of the complementary therapist remains unknown (i.e. hidden in the black box).

Three arguments can be formulated against the use of a black box:

1 Particularly in those trials where no effect is measured, other therapists might claim that this negative trial outcome is caused by a faulty alternative diagnosis leading to a failure to detect the characteristic symptom pattern and therefore an incorrect choice of remedies or acupuncture points to be treated. In these circumstances the quality of the therapist is at issue.

2 Fisher[20] furthermore points out the possibility that in the so-called 'one disease/any remedy' type of study, some remedies are effective whereas others may not be. One is, of course, unable to track down which remedy has been (in)effective when a black box has been used.

3 Finally, Canter[10] stresses that the task of research is not only to study the effectiveness of a certain intervention, but also to understand the strengths and weaknesses of the various approaches in complementary medicine to the promotion of human wellbeing. To develop that understanding, research should be aimed at examining the logic upon which the different complementary practices operate and studying closely the conditions under which successes and failures occur. Therefore registration of those actions which take place during the process of diagnosis and therapy is essential for the further development of research in the field of complementary medicine.

The disadvantages of the black box might be overcome in two ways:

1 By registering precisely the diagnostic outcome in terms of patient typology or syndrome, as well as all decisions leading to

the applied therapeutic protocol. In this way fellow practitioners are able to exert a control on the treatment or to check on the symptom patterns and remedies prescribed by the therapists. Then, at the end of the trial homogeneous subgroups can be formed based on alternative typology. In this way one can study whether a positive or negative effect is found in certain subgroups in comparison with control conditions.

2 A second possibility is that (before the start of the trial) selection of patients is done in two steps, the first step being based on criteria from orthodox medicine, whereas the second selection step is based on, for instance, homoeopathic criteria. Then only those patients which satisfy both sets of criteria are included in the study. The studies where this has been done belong to the third category of clinical trials.

3 Patient selection based on complementary as well as on orthodox diagnostic criteria

Examples of these trials are the fibrositis studies reported by Fisher.[21,22] Both studies were of double blind and placebo-controlled nature. In the first study,[21] only those fibrositis patients who also showed the characteristic symptomatology of one out of three homoeopathic remedies were included. In this way, 24 patients could be selected to participate in these three more or less homogeneous subgroups (as characterized by the symptomatology of Arnica, Bryonia or Rhus toxicodendron).

Moreover, an indication was given for the number of good prescribing symptoms. In other words, the 'goodness of fit' was established between the symptom pattern of a patient and the characteristic symptoms of a remedy picture. This represents, in a way, the certainty by which the correct remedy was prescribed by a homoeopath.

The three subgroups of patients with fibrositis received either a placebo or the indicated homoeopathic remedy. Several variables were measured, such as sleeping problems and pain score on 'visual analogue scales', number of painful spots and use of analgesics.

Statistical analysis was performed in two ways:

1 Comparison of control conditions versus all patients who were treated homoeopathically (irrespective of which remedy was given). In this analysis no significant difference was found with respect to sleeping and pain scores.

2 A second analysis was done including only those patients with good prescribing symptoms (meaning a good correlation between symptom pattern and corresponding remedy picture). Interestingly in this second analysis, a significant improvement was found for the homoeopathically treated group versus placebo. This result stresses the crucial importance of the proper selection of a homoeopathic remedy, since it seems that the effect of a remedy can only be detected optimally when its prescription is based on a good agreement between remedy picture and the specific symptom pattern of the patient.

In 1980 Gibson *et al.*[18] reached a similar conclusion in their study of patients with rheumatoid arthritis. They also divided their patients in two groups; those with good prescribing symptoms and those with poor prescribing symptoms. They also found that homoeopathically treated patients in the group with good prescribing symptoms showed a larger improvement (although not significant in their study) than the homoeopathically treated group with poor prescribing symptoms.

Fisher[20] proposes a distinction between a 'one disease/any remedy' type of trial and a 'one disease/one remedy' trial. However, in the latter type of trial, it is not clear whether the group of patients is homogeneous or inhomogeneous from the point of view of the complementary therapist. Theoretically both the study of Reilly *et al.*[16] as well as Fisher's second study[22] fall into this 'one disease/one remedy' type of trial.

In the field of acupuncture, we could not find a good example of a clinical trial which belongs to this third category. Some literature, however, was found in which an attempt was made to make a kind of agreement between formula acupuncture and traditional acupuncture.

Marcus *et al.*[23] studied the effect of acupuncture on migraine/headache. In all patients a standard number of four acupuncture points were treated. In addition, supplemental points were added according to the patient's symptoms. They considered the nature of the headache as well as the individual's condition in selecting a suitable number of additional points. Also, Chen[24] describes several typologies of migraine patients. She suggests the benefit of stimulation of seven points in all migraine patients. Furthermore, depending on each typology, she suggested additional specific points to be treated.

The procedure for an acupuncture study in the third category would be to select one of these typologies or syndromes out of a large group of patients with migraine. Then a standardized acupuncture treatment could be given, since all patients in the selected subgroup would be homogeneous from both points of view; orthodox and also according to traditional acupuncture. In such a trial, a standard acupuncture treatment could theoretically also be compared with placebo (although a *communis opinio* with respect to placebo treatment in acupuncture has not yet been reached[25]).

Perspective

Most clinical studies can be classified into one of the three research categories, which are characterized according to the protocol of patient selection. In summary:

Type of study	Orthodox selection criteria	Alternative selection criteria
1	yes	no
2	yes	(black box)
3	yes	yes
(4	no	yes)

The fourth category represents studies with homogeneous groups of patients only from the point of view of complementary medicine. In these studies no selection has occurred based on criteria dictated by orthodox medicine. These types of studies can only be found in journals in the field of alternative medicine and are of course only of importance for the improvement of therapeutic protocol as well as for the evolution of knowledge within the complementary therapy under study.

In the field of complementary medicine, relatively few studies have been performed according to the criteria of the third category. There are a couple of possible reasons for this:

1 Characterization of symptoms and classification in certain patient typologies or syndromes requires accurate (controllable) protocols which are not (yet) present. On the basis of these protocols, fellow therapists should be able to decide whether an adequate treatment is given.

 Computer programs may help in the process of identification of a symptom pattern and remedy selection.[26]

2 Another problem with clinical trials of the third category is that after a two-step selection, only groups of very limited size are formed. With such a small number of patients, it is impossible to use the traditional group design. The applicability of other research designs should therefore be studied, such as the single case design.[27,28] There is, however, little experience with these trials in the field of complementary medicine, but the first single case design study in the field of acupuncture has recently been published.[29]

Research priorities

Future research priorities in the field of complementary medicine should, in our opinion, include:

1 further characterization of patient typology, which is needed in order to obtain protocols for the second selection step (and which can be used for a better control by fellow practitioners on treatment strategy);

2 research on reliability and validity of diagnostic equipment used by the complementary therapist (in cases when alternative diagnostic criteria are used to select a homogeneous group of patients);

3 study of the applicability of other research designs (e.g. single case) because of the occurrence of small groups when a second selection step is implemented.

Discussion and conclusions

The need for the development of an alternative methodology has been suggested several times. In our opinion, however, the orthodox methodological criteria should be taken as a starting point which can subsequently be adapted depending on the specific situation/philosophy of the complementary therapy under study. The question of selection of patients to be included in a trial especially needs more attention and careful consideration.

The selection of patients should not only be based on orthodox diagnostic criteria but also on diagnostic criteria from complementary medicine. The proposed selection process is shown in Figure 7.2. Only after such a two-step selection procedure can a homogeneous group of patients be obtained on which the effects of a standardized therapy can be evaluated. In such an evaluation maximum attention can be paid to

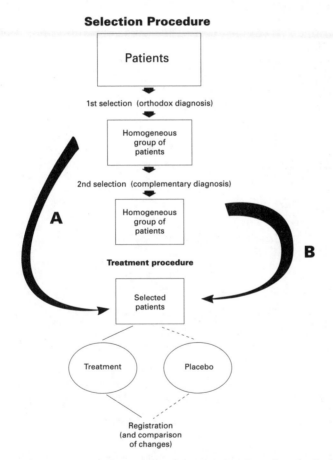

Fig. 7.2 Procedure to select patients for inclusion in clinical trials. In the first selection step, a 'homogeneous' group of patients is formed using orthodox diagnostic criteria. This group meets the criteria for a uniform orthodox treatment to be studied in a clinical trial (arrow A). However, to participate in a trial studying the effect of a complementary therapy, a second selection step should be performed. This twice-selected group now meets the criteria for a uniform complementary treatment (arrow B).

the characteristic philosophy and to the way of working, as well as to the diagnostic equipment used by the complementary practitioner.

One of the disadvantages is that a two-step selection of the research population results in small group sizes. In these circumstances one has to find alternatives for the traditional group design. One of the possibilities which remains to be explored is the single case design.

Acknowledgement

The work of the Research Unit for Complementary Medicine has been supported over the past four years by a grant (WVC86-29) from the Dutch Ministry of Health.

References

[1] Aldridge, D. A guide to preparing a research application. *Comp Med Res* 1989; **3**(3): 31–7.

[2] James, I. Tactics and practicalities. *Comp Med Res* 1989; **3**(3): 7–10.

[3] Anthony, H. M. Clinical research: questions to ask and the benefits of asking them. *Comp Med Res* 1989; **3**(3): 3–6.

[4] Crichton, N. J. The importance of statistics in research design. *Comp Med Res* 1990; **4**(2): 42–9.

[5] Heron, J. Critique of conventional research methodology. *Comp Med Res* 1986; **1**(1): 10–22.

[6] Patel, M. S. Evaluation of holistic medicine. *Soc Sci Med* 1987; **24**: 169–75.

[7] Patel, M. S. Problems in the evaluation of alternative medicine. *Soc Sci Med* 1987; **25**: 669–78.

[8] Aldridge, D., Pietroni, P. C. Clinical assessment of acupuncture in asthma therapy: discussion paper. *J Roy Soc Med* 1987; **80**: 222–4.

[9] Jingfeng, C. Toward a comprehensive evaluation of alternative medicine. *Soc Sci Med* 1987; **25**: 659–67.

[10] Canter, D. A research agenda for holistic therapy. *Comp Med Res* 1987; **2**: 104–21.

[11] Lynöe, N. Theoretical and empirical problems in the assessment of alternative medical technologies. *Scand J Soc Med* 1989; **37**: 257–63.

[12] Hornung, J. Zur Problematik der Doppelblindstudien. *Therapeutikon* 1989; **3**: 696–701.

[13] Hornung, J. Zur Problematik der Doppelblindstudien, Teil 2: Unorthodoxe Studienplan. *Therapeutikon* 1990; **4**: 355–60.

[14] Leibrich, J. Measurement of efficacy: a case for holistic research. *Comp Med Res* 1990; **4**(1): 21–5.

[15] Pischinger, A. *Das system der Grundregulation.* Heidelberg: Haug Verlag, 1975.

[16] Reilly, D. T., Taylor, M. A., McSharry, C., Aitchison, T. Is homoeopathy a placebo response? *Lancet* 1986; **2**: 881–6.

[17] Fung, K. P., Chow, O. K. W., So, S. Y. Attenuation of exercise-induced asthma by acupuncture. *Lancet* 1986; **2**: 1419–22.

[18] Gibson, R. G., Gibson, S. L. M., MacNeill, D. A., Watson-Buchanan, W. Homoeopathic therapy in rheumatoid arthritis – evaluation by double-blind clinical therapeutic trial. *Br J Clin Pharmacol* 1980; **9**: 453–9.

[19] Jobst, K., Chen, J. H., McPherson, K., Arrowsmith, J., Brown, V., Eftimiou, J., Fletcher, H. J., Maciocia, G., Mole, P., Shifrin, K. Controlled trial of acupuncture for disabling breathlessness. *Lancet* 1986; **2**: 1416–19.

[20] Fisher, P. Research into homoeopathic treatment of rheumatological disease: why and how? *Comp Med Res* 1990; **4**(3): 34–40.

[21] Fisher, P. An experimental double-blind clinical trial method in homoeopathy – use of a limited range of remedies to treat fibrositis. *Br Hom J* 1989; **75**: 142–7.

[22] Fisher, P., Greenwood, A., Huskisson, E. C., Turner, P., Belon, P. P. Effect of homoeopathic treatment on fibrositis (primary fibromyalgia). *Br Med J* 1989; **299**: 365–6.

[23] Marcus, P. Effect of treatment with acupuncture on migraine headache. *Acupunc Elec* 1979; **4**: 137–47.

[24] Chen, A. Effective acupuncture therapy for migraine: review and comparison of prescriptions with recommendations for improved results. *Am J Acup* 1989; **17**(4): 305–16.

[25] Kubiena, G. Uberlegungen zum Plazebobegriff in der Akupunktur. *Dtsch Zschr Akup* 1989; **32**(3): 52–8.

[26] Van Haselen, R., Fisher, P. Analysing homoeopathic prescribing using the Read classification and information technology. *Br Hom J* 1990; **79**: 74–81.

[27] Kazdin, A. E. *Single Case Research Designs: Methods For Clinical and Applied Settings*. New York: OUP, 1982.

[28] Aldridge, D. Single-case research designs. *Comp Med Res* 1988; **3**(1): 37–46.

[29] Vincent, C. A. The treatment of tension headache by acupuncture: a controlled single-case design with time series analysis. *J Psychosom Res* 1990; **34**: 553–61.

Section 2

8 Emerging priorities in complementary medical research

David Canter and Lorraine Nanke

Summary

The concepts underlying the questions that need to be addressed in complementary medicine are examined, with special reference to opportunities and limitations for the scientist–practitioner. The chapter shows the importance of understanding the nature of the questions asked before deciding on how to approach them. Although the clinical trial is the appropriate tool for evaluating therapy where it represents the only variable of note, most complementary therapy is multifactorial; alternative strategies are discussed. The chapter also considers the various different aspects of the 'effectiveness' of therapy.

Introduction

The aim of this chapter is to outline some basic ideas about what type of research question might fruitfully be asked in complementary medicine, and how such questions are related to research design. Examples from psychotherapy research are used where appropriate to illustrate themes of potential relevance to complementary medicine.

The scientist–practitioner model

This book is implicitly based on the ideal of the scientist–practitioner: the clinician who not only helps relieve patients' problems using the expertise of their own discipline, but also carries out research into their own practice. The model is based on the idea of a continuing dialogue between theory and practice. Clinical work provides a source of insights and hypotheses about the effects and effectiveness of particular interventions. These are then subjected to more systematic evaluation in individual cases and larger scale group studies, eventually contributing to the development of collective knowledge and improvements in practice.[1]

In relation to psychotherapy, Strupp[2] suggests that the scientist–practitioner model provides 'the opportunity for oscillation between the observation and participation, between taking part and standing back, between feeling and thinking, between (controlled) abandonment and study. It is this process of oscillation, the unique human ability to resonate, identify and therapeutically respond to themes in the patients' experience that is essential ... It should be possible to encourage research that is both rigorous and relevant to clinical and social issues' (p563).

Advantages of the model

Overcoming the clinical/research split

A major advantage of the model is that it overcomes the sterile split between clinicians and research scientists, potentially avoiding the narrowness of thought and rigidity of action which are often associated with exclusive focus on either. Scientific researchers are often criticized for producing results which seem irrelevant to clinical practice, and using measures and strategies which are beyond the scope and re- sources of clinicians. Conversely, clinicians are criticized for not using the insights acquired as a result of their experience as a basis for research, development of cumulative knowledge, or training, trusting solely on their clinical experience to evaluate their practice. The model is intended to overcome this problem by combining clinical and research functions in the same individuals where possible.

Accountability

The increasing stress on accountability in the human sciences means that particular therapeutic disciplines cannot avoid the necessity of describing and empirically validating the effects of their work. This requirement is likely to become increasingly important to patients who wish to make an informed choice between the wide diversity of treatments available. In this context, all clinical disciplines have an obligation to carry out some type of empirical research into their methods of treatment.

Lack of dependable knowledge

Perhaps the most important consideration underlying the scientist– practitioner model is the lack of dependable information currently available about the reliability and effectiveness of many diagnostic and therapeutic techniques. In 1950, Raimy[3] stated that, 'Psychotherapy is an undefined technique, applied to unspecified problems, with an unpredictable outcome. For this technique we are recommending rigor- ous training' (p. 93). It is disappointing to recognize how much this comment is still applicable to psychotherapeutic practice, and it may be useful to consider the extent to which it is also relevant to com- plementary medicine. Clinicians of all disciplines are best placed to recognize and study the important aspects of real life clinical interven- tion and change; indeed, most rely on their own experience as validation of their particular theoretical approach and techniques. Though such personal conviction may be valuable to the individual clinician and their patients, it is of little help in contributing to collective, dependable knowledge about the process of effects of different types of therapy. This requires systematic empirical investigation, producing objective results which can be evaluated by others within the discipline and the wider scientific community.

Problems of the model

A salutary lesson from clinical psychology

Unfortunately, the scientist–practitioner model remains more of an ideal than an accurate description of normal practice, even in clinical psychology which is explicitly based on this approach. Despite a thorough grounding in research methodology, very few practising clinicians actually carry out research after qualification, and many state that they would prefer less emphasis on research methodology in training.[4] Some consideration of this issue may help complementary practitioners avoid a key pitfall of the scientist–practitioner model, and help establish the research enterprise on a more productive footing.

The clinical context and experimental science

One of the major problems facing clinicians who wish to carry out research has been identified as the mismatch between the demands of clinical research and the requirements of experimental science. This was the conclusion drawn by Bergin and Strupp[5] from a survey of leading psychologists and psychiatrists. They state that 'Among researchers as well as statisticians there is a growing disaffection from traditional experimental designs and statistical procedures, which are held inappropriate to the subject matter under study. This judgement applies with particular force to the area of therapeutic change, and our emphasis on the value of experimental case studies underscores this point. We strongly agree that most of the standard experimental designs and statistical procedures have exerted, and are continuing to exert, a constricting influence on fruitful inquiry, and they serve to perpetuate an unwarranted emphasis on methodology' (p. 440). This mismatch has often been dealt with by attempting to adapt clinical questions to the Procrustean bed of experimental science. As such, it is often accepted as axiomatic in medical, psychological and biological research that the only genuinely scientific strategy is the experimental design, in which people are randomly assigned to different conditions and subjected to blind or double blind trial in order to measure the influence of a key independent variable. The independent variable in such studies is characteristically seen as the main single causal agent producing the effect, which is the observed difference between groups. The limitations of this approach have been well documented elsewhere, for example Heron,[6] but it is worth noting some of the main difficulties encountered in a clinical context here.

Conflicting priorities

A clinician's first priority is almost always the wellbeing of individual patients, and this may conflict with the requirements of strictly experimental research design. For example, treatment strategy may normally be decided on the basis of ongoing therapeutic dialogue with the patient, changing in response to the patient's reaction, and reformulations of the problem. Yet, controlled comparison between two specific techniques often requires that the treatment, or lack of treatment in the case of a control group, is determined by the requirements of the research design rather than patient need. The scientist–practitioner model is likely to be most effective when the primary clinical priority is recognized, and means found to help clinicians carry out research into what they actually do in the course of normal practice rather than tailoring practice to the experimental design.

Moral concerns

Closely related to the issue of clinicial priorities are the moral problems which can be encountered using the standard clinical trial. Firstly, there is the difficulty of obtaining patients' informed consent, as this kind of study is ideally carried out double blind, without patient or practitioner knowing which patient is receiving which treatment. Secondly, many clinicians express concern about patients in the control group being untreated, given a placebo, or receiving a treatment which may be less effective than the experimental treatment.

Single versus multiple factors

The experimental method is designed to address questions which can be answered in terms of simple cause–effect mechanisms. The clinicial trial is only able to compare simple alternative causal agents, i.e. the variable which differs between control and experimental groups, to explain observed variation in effect. This kind of question is perfectly appropriate where there are clear theoretical reasons to predict that treatment agent A will cause outcome B; for example, that a particular antibiotic will remove infection and associated symptoms, or that any difference in outcome is likely to be due to the single factor on which the control and experimental groups differ, e.g. type of treatment received. The clinical trial is particularly well suited to the traditional disease focus of orthodox medicine, in which the search for single pathogenic agents and remedies has a strong theoretical basis. However, it is less applicable to the holistic approach, which is based on a theoretical framework stressing the importance of multiple interacting factors relevant to treatment effects in each individual patient.

Clinical and statistical significance

Associated with the clinical trial methodology has been an over-reliance on statistical probability measures to compare group differences. These measures are often used inappropriately, and lead to impoverished interpretation of results, particularly in relation to small sample sizes.[7] Statistical significance is frequently confused with clinical significance, and all too often studies report only data on the probability that differential treatment outcomes are a result of chance, and assume that the treatment which produces a reliably different outcome is better. Yet, it matters little if one therapy produces effects at a statistically significant level more than other therapies, if these changes are not of sufficient magnitude to be experienced as meaningful by the patient. Even statistically significant results often account for only a small proportion of the observed variance, indicating that in such cases the single cause explanation provides an inadequate account of obtained results.[8,9]

Practical difficulties

The practical requirements of setting up clinical trials, including obtaining large numbers of matched subjects, control groups, possibly external blind raters, and large scale standardization of treatment, can place excessive and possibly unmanageable demands on practising clinicians who might otherwise be prepared to contribute to research. Further, blind administration can easily be applied to pharmacological treatments in which active and placebo substances can be made to appear identical. However, it is impossible to administer many other forms of physical or psychological treatment blind, for example massage or acupuncture; such treatments can be incorporated into standard clinical trials only if an apparently equivalent but theoretically inert form can be devised and administered to the control group.

Group versus individual differences

The practice of using group averages to compare patient groups obscures potentially important individual differences in treatment response. Kiesler[10] has described this practice as based on 'the patient uniformity myth'; that is, the assumption that the variables being studied are the only relevant differences between groups. This assumption is not warranted on empirical grounds, as there is much evidence that some patients in every study improve, some stay the same, and some get worse (for example, Garfield[11]). Barlow et al.[12] point out that the roots of the problem lie in traditional experimental research methodology, and particularly the improper use of sampling techniques. According to sampling theory, a random sample of the population of interest must be studied if adequate generalizations are to be made about the whole population. In a clinical context, this would mean drawing a sample in which all individual differences potentially relevant to treatment outcome are represented. If the treatment applied to all of these individuals produced a statistically significant effect compared to a control group, the treatment would be judged effective. However, Barlow et al. add that applied researchers have long recognized firstly the practical impossibility of obtaining a patient sample in which all potentially relevant factors are adequately represented, and secondly the theoretical problem that the sample would be so heterogeneous that few if any treatments would be likely to show statistically significant effect. An alternative strategy consistent with experimental methodology and the clinical trial has been the selection of homogeneous patient groups to minimize sources of individual variation which may confound results. This approach is also subject to the practical problem of obtaining an appropriate sample; for example, finding a group of anxiety patients who also have similar personalities, backgrounds, life circumstances and any other factors of potential relevance to treatment. Further, the results of such studies can only be generalized to patients with similar characteristics, and so are of limited value to practising clinicians. What is needed is an approach which can go beyond the comparison of group averages, to help identify which patients respond in which way to which treatment.[13]

Experimenter distortion

Experimenter distortion in research is a double-edged sword. On one hand, the most productive research is usually carried out by those with a strong interest and expertise in the subject area.[14] On the other hand, science is based on the ideal of objectivity and freedom from personal bias. Though a study may be designed on the basis of personal interests, the results should be reproducible by other independent researchers with different interests. One potent way in which the researcher can distort or influence data obtained is by conveying their expectations to patients, often inadvertently. Orne[15] suggested that subjects are usually so keen to please the researcher that they actively search for and act on clues as to how the researcher wants them to behave. These clues and hints are collectively referred to as the 'demand characteristics' of a situation. 'Demand characteristics' are clearly involved in any clinical or research enterprise involving human beings. However, tailoring treatment to fit strictly experimental research design may so alter the perceived demand characteristics for patients that results obtained may not easily generalize to the different perceived demand characteristics of the normal clinical consultation. Experimenter distortion may be one reason for the fact that one of the few reliable generalizations that can be drawn from the wealth of psychotherapy outcome research is that most studies provide some degree of support for the orientation of the researcher.

Quantitative and qualitative data

One fallacy often associated with reliance on experimental methodology is the assumption that easily quantified factors are inherently more scientific than those which are not so easily assigned to numbers. This has been likened to the fable of the drunk looking for his key under the light rather than where he lost it.[16] The important point here is that a research study should be designed to assess the factors which are likely to be relevant to the original question, rather than those which are easily measured. This applies in particular to clinical research, where qualitative changes, for example sense of wellbeing or relationships, may be of over-riding importance. Clearly, the goal of objectivity and replicability is central to any type of measurement, but different types of measurement are appropriate for different types of variable. The task is to identify ways in which relevant factors can be most reliably assessed, rather than trying to build research questions around factors which can be easily quantified.

Temporal changes

Finally, many experimental studies compare treatment outcome at one particular point in time, classifying patients in terms of extent of recovery. The usefulness of this approach may depend partly on the condition being studied; for example it makes considerable sense in relation to acute conditions such as infection, or emotional crisis reaction, but is perhaps less applicable to chronic or lifestyle-related conditions, in which longer term changes and maintenance after treatment are more significant.

A broader view of science

One major problem with the scientist–practitioner model has been identified as excessive reliance on strict experimental methodology in the clinical context. The history of science shows that this approach of transferring methodology from one field to another is rarely productive, and genuine progress is more likely when attention is first centred on the questions which need to be asked; only then can an appropriate methodology usefully be identified. In support of this suggestion, some commentators have noted that social work seems to have produced more relevant and applicable research than clinical psychology. This has been attributed to the fact that social workers, unlike clinical psychologists, do not receive a prolonged training in experimental research methodology. As a result, more emphasis is placed on asking the right questions first, and then using whatever methods seem most appropriate to finding the answer.[17]

One of the motivations underlying the tenacious hold of experimental methodology on clinical research has been the legitimate desire to carry out genuinely scientific work. The problem here is to define what 'science' really means. It has long been recognized that science does not mean building grand metaphysical systems to explain the world; that is, or at least was, philosophy. More recently, it has become apparent that science is not about collecting all the information and ending up with huge piles of data, or following a particular methodology, or using complex statistical techniques either (for example, Agnew and Pyke).[18] Rather the discipline of science consists of looking at the correspondence between the research question and the empirical data. This depends on establishing a clear question, and a methodology for obtaining data of direct relevance to the question. Data can then be used to further refine the question, leading to genuinely cumulative development in empirically based knowledge. It is the 'goodness of fit' between the question and the data that forms the basis of good scientific research.[19]

One example of how empirical observations can lead to clearer conceptual classification schemes is the discovery that some types of material leave marks on photographic plates, which led to the classification of materials in terms of whether or not they emit radiations which can be recorded. This way of thinking implies that there is some conceptual way of dividing up whatever it is you are studying, such as remedy types, acupuncture points or types of illness. The observations which are made, and the data obtained are ways of classifying the answers. Statistics is of course concerned with technical ways of classifying the data, and should ideally be used to assess the degree of correspondence between the conceptual divisions made in the research question, and the patterns which emerge from the data.[20]

Research priorities in complementary medicine

On this account of science, the most important task facing complementary medicine is to define key research questions. This involves clarification of conceptual systems used in different disciplines into a form which can be evaluated by empirical data.

Reliability of clinical judgements

When measuring stable characteristics such as personality, measurements must be stable, consistent and free from random error or chance fluctuations. For example, if a different result was obtained each time a particular individual's height was measured, something would be seriously wrong with the measuring device. The issue is more complex with regard to unstable changing characteristics such as health status which are more often the subject of clinical concern. In such cases, reliability can best be assessed in terms of inter-rater agreement in clinical judgement, or the extent to which trained clinicians will make approximately the same judgement of a particular individual characteristic. In many areas of complementary medicine fundamental questions concerning the reliability of particular clinical judgements, diagnostic tools, patient classifications or treatment effects have not been addressed by empirical research. On this basis alone, it is in many cases premature and misleading to draw too close analogies with orthodox medical research, where trials are often based on very specific research questions which have been shaped up by a wealth of accumulated data and a coherent theoretical rationale.

Such work on the reliability and validity of basic clinical tools and techniques is an essential theoretical and empirical ground-clearing exercise, which needs to be carried out on a large scale to provide a meaningful context in which to undertake and interpret more sophisticated studies such as clinical trials. Unless we know that clinicians are talking about the same thing when they refer to, for example, particular homoeopathic types or cranial rhythms, studies based on such classifications will be very difficult to interpret. Similarly, it is essential to determine how much each of these classifications corresponds to clinically important differences between patients, which make a real difference when taken into account in treatment planning. Such data is best obtained by trained clinicians carrying out studies to check the types of clinical judgement made in their own area of expertise.

Basic clinical questions

Kazdin[21] has identified a range of questions which have provided a useful basis for psychotherapy outcome research, and which may also be of relevance to complementary medicine.

Does treatment work?
The question here is whether patients change for the better as a result of treatment; would it make any difference if the patient was simply left alone? This simple question is often lost in a range of complex statistical manipulations yet it is the most fundamental issue in clinical research.

Patel[22] has proposed that multidimensional cost-benefit analysis is the most useful approach to treatment evaluation. This should include the cost of treatment required to produce particular therapeutic effects, in terms of time, money, other resources, and possible negative consequences for the patient. Clearly, all other things being equal, the least costly treatment alternative is to be preferred. Similarly, many different aspects of outcome should be taken into account in treatment evaluation. Patel suggests that holistic practitioners may see a higher proportion of positive treatment effects that are gradual and relatively intangible in nature, such as emotional and physical wellbeing, healthy lifestyle, and more satisfying relationships. Though such factors may be more difficult to assess than specific symptom reduction, they must be included in any comprehensive evaluation of treatment outcome and effectiveness. There are several important questions related to the key issue of treatment effectiveness.

Patient deterioration

Do some patients get worse as a result of treatment? This possibility is often obscured by the use of group averages which do not differentiate between those patients who do particularly well and those who do particularly badly as a result of a particular intervention. There may also be a reluctance on the part of therapists of all persuasions to examine treatment failures. Though this tendency is understandable it may well be based on a fundamental misunderstanding.

Any effective intervention is likely to have the potential for causing negative as well as positive consequences depending on context use. In the case of complementary medicine and psychotherapy, as with much of orthodox medicine, the question is to identify those applications which maximize positive and minimize negative consequences, rather than abandoning the treatment. The identification of deterioration in individual patients in response to treatment is an essential part of mapping out the optimal range of applications for particular treatments and specifying contraindications.

Durability

The temporal aspects of treatment and recovery are often overlooked in comparisons of outcome in patient groups at a particular point in time. This approach is most useful in relation to acute conditions which can be described as 'cured' or otherwise following a limited period of treatment. For patients who do not fall into this category, closer examination of the nature of changes occurring over periods of time may help to clarify the processes involved in recovery. For example, some treatment approaches, such as homoeopathic medicine and psychoanalytic psychotherapy, predict temporary exacerbation of problems in some cases as part of the process of genuine recovery. These exacerbations are therefore not contraindications for treatment, but signs that it may be having a longer-term therapeutic effect.

Conversely, there is the important question of durability of treatment effects. There are real clinical and practical difficulties involved in producing and evaluating long-term effects, but they are an important aspect of comprehensive treatment evaluation. For example, research into the addictive disorders has shown relatively good short-term effects following treatment, followed by consistently high relapse rates within three months following treatment. It would be of interest to determine whether positive lifestyle changes are adopted as a result of complementary medical treatment, and if so whether they are equally ephemeral or more enduring.

Comparative effectiveness

The question here is which of a range of treatments is most effective for a particular condition; there are two related issues involved here. Firstly, there is a need for direct assessment of the nature and extent of effects produced by different treatments. Secondly, there is a need for conceptual clarification. Complementary medicine includes a wide diversity of disciplines which share some basic common features such as concern with treating the whole person, as well as unique conceptualizations of human disease and distress, and associated interventions. Complementary disciplines are derived from diverse cultures and historical periods, often related to more primitive ideas and practices. An important part of comparative research must be the appraisal of the conceptualizations and procedures of each discipline, both in their own terms and in relation to each other, in order to provide a meaningful context within which comparative outcome studies can be designed and interpreted.

Causal mechanisms

What aspects of treatment are necessary, sufficient or facilitative of therapeutic change? This is a more focused question about the effects of particular components of the therapeutic package. It has attracted increasing attention in view of meta analyses of psychotherapy outcome studies, which tend to show fairly similar results despite differences in therapist, theoretical approach, and type of intervention.[23] These findings strongly suggest that treatment may not always work for the theoretical reasons that therapists believe. Comparison of differential outcomes following treatment does not by itself answer the question of what were the 'active ingredients' of treatment.

This question is usually addressed by identifying the main components of treatment, and assessing outcome in patient groups receiving systematically different combinations of these components. For example, in homoeopathy it would be possible to compare three groups of patients receiving only constitutional, only pathological, or both types of remedy. Similar studies could be carried out including, for example, different lengths of consultation, advice on health maintenance, and physical examination, in combination with other treatment techniques. Often such research showing that particular aspects of treatment are associated with particular effects is accepted as adequate justification of clinical practice, though there may be considerable debate about the precise causal mechanisms involved.

Which therapist factors are important?

Within complementary medicine there has been much debate about the relative contribution of personal and professional qualifications to the therapeutic process. For example, homoeopathic medicine is practised by both medically qualified and lay clinicians, though the clinical importance of this difference remains unclear.

Psychotherapy research has shown that a wide range of practitioner qualities can affect the process and outcome of therapy, including personality, interpersonal style, beliefs, values, gender, power, attractiveness, socio-economic status, and length and type of professional experience.[24] Of particular relevance is the fact that studies carried out in this area have shown little evidence that theoretical orientation of psychotherapists influences treatment outcome.[25]

On the basis of these findings, it could be hypothesized that the diversity of theoretical orientations and techniques associated with complementary medicine obscures a greater similarity in types of personal qualities and approach relevant to the treatment process. The questions here are: what influence do the personal qualities of therapists have on treatment outcome, and do they bear any systematic relation to professional discipline or training?

Patient factors
As with therapists, a wide range of patient characteristics have been shown to affect treatment outcome. One particularly interesting finding in psychotherapy research is that patients' perception of therapist qualities, specifically warmth, empathy and genuineness, are predictive of treatment success or failure in a variety of therapeutic contexts.[26] By contrast, direct measures of therapist verbal and non-verbal behaviour thought to be expressive of these qualities have not shown consistent links with outcome.[27]

On the basis of such findings, Kendall and Norton-Ford have proposed the hypothesis that patients' perceptions of therapy may have a more important influence on treatment outcome than specific therapist actions or interventions.[28] Put another way, the patients' perception of therapy may be an important mechanism accounting for treatment effects.

Partly as a result of its search for objective and easily quantifiable effects, and partly due to the influence of 'passive patient/active therapist' expectations, psychological research has only recently begun to take account of the patients' perspective. However, as Joynson[29] has pointed out, one of the unique and most important characteristics of human beings is their capacity for self-understanding and control. Any approach which tries to understand or predict human response without taking this important source of data into account is bound to meet with limited success.

Alternative strategies

Any research activity has two components, which jointly contribute to defining the meaning of the research question. The *strategy* or *design* refers to the overall plan of campaign, according to which the study will be carried out and data collected. The *tactics* refer to more detailed methodology employed to achieve the wider objectives, including how the researcher will interact with patients in order to study them, the precise data to be obtained, and the type of analysis to be carried out. Tactical issues are well documented in most research methodology texts, and will not be dealt with further here.

The clinical trial described above is only one of a range of potential research strategies, each of which has a different optimal range of application and different associated advantages and disadvantages. The following list is intended to give an idea of some alternatives to the clinical trial which have proved useful in psychotherapy research and may be of value to complementary medicine.

Single case design

It is often useful to ask what is happening to this patient? What am I doing to them? What experiences are they going through? How do they understand what is happening to them? Are any events in their lives relevant to my intervention? The detailed analysis of individual cases can be used to illustrate certain principles, provide accounts of descriptive procedures, provide a focus for debate about the way in which particular problems can be managed, and generate hypotheses about significant factors in treatment response which could form the basis for subsequent studies using larger samples.[30] This type of clinical vignette is commonly used for teaching purposes, though its potential in written form has been less well exploited.

This type of research may be particularly useful for holistic practitioners, who are concerned that the important role played by individual differences in treatment is obscured by use of standardized measuring techniques or average scores. It allows more detailed inclusion of the experience of both therapist and patient during treatment. A range of tactics can be used in the single case study, ranging from a narrative biographical format, to a controlled study in which the individual is used as their own control, and response compared at different stages of treatment, and to different types of intervention.[31]

The main limitation of this approach is that it may be unrepresentative and reflect the idiosyncracies of a particular therapeutic intervention in a way which cannot be generalized to other contexts. This does not invalidate single case studies provided they are not used to address general questions such as the efficacy of particular treatments.

Questionnaires

Given the importance of subjective and experiential factors to the treatment process, the development of questionnaires to assess such material can potentially make an important contribution to research. However, they also introduce a range of new problems. It is a very common occurrence for people to mistake substantive questions about what they are intending to study for practical problems about the phrasing of questionnaire items. Partly for this reason, it is often preferable to find other ways of obtaining this data where possible, such as direct observations or measurements. William James, one of the founders of modern psychology, recognized this point as long ago as the 1890s in his statement,[32] 'Because of its ease of use, the questionnaire is the bane of modern society'.

The questionnaire is a complex and subtle instrument and nothing is more cost-effective when you get it right, but getting it right is often a tedious process which involves precise definition of the focus of research interest, eliminating sources of potential ambiguity and bias, and a design which is clear, simple, easy to use and interesting to complete.

Field study

This involves careful analysis of an ongoing situation into which some kind of change is introduced; for example, changes in referral rates from other practitioners following provision of different types of information. The stress here is on examining naturally occurring changes and developments, rather than introducing changes for the purpose of research. The main advantage of this strategy is its focus on authentic real life events in the clinical situation. Conversely, the main disadvantage is the researchers' lack of direct control over the events being studied, so that it may be difficult to identify the nature and direction of causal relationships.

Laboratory model

This involves setting up experiments in carefully controlled situations, such as the clinical trial. The main question which this strategy is designed to address is the extent to which a particular causal agent is responsible for a particular effect. The limitations have been described above.

Consultancy activities

In this situation the question is, 'How can I facilitate or improve a particular intervention process? What can I do to make it more effective?' As with field studies, the main advantage of this approach is its close contact with real life situations where the researchers' main aim is to improve a particular situation.

Conclusions

The main point made in this chapter is that priority should be given to defining research questions which can be answered by empirical data. Methodology should be selected to meet the requirements for the substantive clinical question, rather than to conform to the perceived requirements of experimental science. In this respect, experimental methodology and the clinical trial have a legitimate and important role to play, but exclusive reliance on these strategies can have a constricting influence on the research enterprise in complementary medicine. Some examples of research questions and strategies which have proved useful in psychotherapy research, and may have some application in complementary medicine, were briefly outlined.

References

1   Barlow, D. H., Hayes, S. C., Nelson, R. O. *The Scientist–Practitioner.* Oxford: Pergamon, 1984; 3–33.

2   Strupp, H. H. Clinical research, practice, and the crisis of confidence. *Consult Clin Psychol* 1981; **49**: 216–20.

3   Raimy, V. C. *Training in Clinical Psychology* (Boulder Conference). New York: Prentice-Hall, 1950.

4   Garfield, S. L., Kurtz, R. M. Clinical psychology in the 1970s. *Am Psychol* 1976; **31**: 1–9.

5   Bergin, A., Strupp, H. *Changing Frontiers in the Science of Psychotherapy.* Chicago: Aldine, 1972.

6   Heron, J. Critique of conventional research methodology. *Comp Med Res* 1986; **1**: 12–22.

7   Carver, R. P. The case against statistical significance testing. *Harvard Educ Rev* 1978; **48**: 378–99.

8   Cowger, C. D. Statistical significance tests: scientific ritualism or scientific method? *Soc Serv Rev* 1984; 359–72.

9   Meehl, P. E. *Clinical Versus Statistical Prediction.* Minnesota: University of Minnesota Press, 1954.

10   Kiesler, D. J. Some myths of psychotherapy research and the search for a paradigm. *Psychol Bull* 1965; **65**: 110–36.

11   Garfield, S. L. Evaluating the psychotherapies. *Behav Therap* 1981; **12**: 295–308.

12   In 1, p. 31.

13   Paul, G. Strategy of outcome research in psychotherapy. *J Cons Psychol* 1967; **31**: 109–19.

14   Campbell, J. P., Daft, R. L., Hulin, C. L. *What to Study: Generating and Developing Research Questions.* Beverly Hills, Calif.: Sage, 1982; Chapter 5.

15   Orne, M. On the social psychology of the psychology experiment: with particular reference to Demand Characteristics and their implications. *Am Psychol* 1962; **17**: 776–83.

16   Ornstein, R. *The Psychology of Consciousness.* Harmondsworth: Penguin, 1986.

17   In 1, p. 21.

18   Agnew, N. M., Pyke, S. W. *The Science Game: An Introduction to Research in the Behavioral Sciences.* Englewood Cliffs, NJ: Prentice-Hall, 1969.

19   Canter, D. C. (ed.) *Facet Theory: Approaches to Social Research.* Berlin: Springer Verlag, 1985.

20   Canter, D. C. A research agenda for holistic therapy. *Comp Med Res* 1987; **2**(1): 104–16.

21 Kazdin, A. E. *Research Design in Clinical Psychology.* New York: Harper and Row, 1980.

22 Patel, M. S. Evaluation of holistic medicine. *Soc Sci Med* 1987; **24**(2): 169–75.

23 Shapiro, D. A., Shapiro, D. Meta analysis of comparative therapy outcome research: replication and refinement. *Psychol Bull* 1982; **92**: 581–604.

24 Parloff, M. B, Waskow, I. E., Wolf, B. E. Research on therapist variables in relation to process and outcome. In: Garfield, S. L., Bergen, A. E. (eds.) *Handbook of Psychotherapy and Behavior Change.* 2nd edition. New York: Wiley, 1978.

25 Kendall, P. C., Norton-Ford, J. D. Therapy outcome research methods. In: Kendall, P. C., Butcher, J. N. (eds.) *Handbook of Research Methods in Clinical Psychology.* New York: Wiley, 1982.

26 Gurman, A. The patient's perception of the therapeutic relationship. In: Gurman, A., Razin, A. (eds.) *Effective Psychotherapy: a Handbook of Research.* New York: Pergamon, 1977.

28 Kendall, P. C., Butcher, J. N. (eds.) *Handbook of Research Methods in Clinical Psychology.* New York: Wiley, 1982.

29 Joynson, R. B. *Psychology and Common Sense.* London: Routledge & Kegan Paul, 1977. Chapter 1.

30 Kazdin, A. E. Single case experimental designs. In: Kendall, P. C., Butcher, J. N. (eds.) *Handbook of Clinical Psychology.* New York: Wiley, 1982; 461–91.

31 Mitchell, M., Jolley, J. *Research Design Explained.* New York: Holt, Rinehart & Winston, 1988; 235–42.

32 James, W. *Principles of Psychology.* New York: Holt, 1890.

9 Some methodological problems in the assessment of complementary therapy

Honor M. Anthony

Summary

The increased interest of the public and the medical profession in complementary forms of therapy introduces an urgent need for proper assessment of efficacy. This growth in popularity suggests that complementary therapies are effective in some circumstances, but without objective assessment neither the public nor the medical profession can be sure. Rigorous scientific assessment is required, but the nature of complementary therapy is such that double blind randomized controlled trials, as usually conducted, are rarely applicable, and alternative approaches are needed. At its best, complementary therapy is designed individually for each patient, and few treatments can readily be applied 'blind'. These are the main problems in trial design but complementary therapists are also aware of the importance of body–mind interactions: they see the 'placebo effect' as an integral part of treatment which needs investigation, and they question the validity of clinical trials in which the patient's will is not fully engaged through lack of information, and of those not asking the patients if they feel better. The problems are examined and alternative approaches suggested. The chapter raises the question of whether they are only problems for complementary medicine.

Introduction

There is an urgent need for proper assessment of the efficacy of complementary therapies: more patients are consulting such practitioners and two studies have shown that a substantial proportion of general practitioners think that complementary therapies help some of their patients,[1,2] although the report published in 1986 by the British Medical Association[3] showed not only official scepticism but also a degree of ignorance. Most complementary therapists do not have the advantages of a tradition of research, close links with institutions where research is done, or access to research-funding bodies. The Research Council for Complementary Medicine (RCCM) was set up jointly by the orthodox profession and the main groups of complementary therapists in the United Kingdom to fill these gaps, but soon found that research methodology presented as great a problem. The journal *Complementary Medical Research*, set up to publish good research into the efficacy of complementary therapies, has included the proceedings of two conferences on research methodology in its early issues.[4,5]

The problem

Complementary therapists find a number of problems in designing and executing clinical trials using standard methodology.[4]

1 The central problem hinges on the conviction of complementary therapists that treatment strategies must take account as much of the individual as of the disease, condition or symptoms. They usually plan therapy individually for each patient, and to them the testing of a standard therapy for a standard 'disease' would fall so far short of optimal therapy that the results would be irrelevant.

2 Treatment often consists of a number of therapeutic components; decisions about the use of some may not be made at the outset, but later as a result of continued observation of the patient and the response to earlier components.

3 'Blind' designs are rarely possible with respect either to the therapist or to the patient. Most complementary therapies involve some physical treatment, instruction or training which cannot be disguised, and although placebo 'treatments' have been devised for some of these (for example, the use of false acupuncture points), their validity has been questioned.

4 Complementary therapists recognize the effects of the *therapist* as an integral part of treatment and, although they appreciate the need for evaluation of the safety and efficacy of individual components of therapy, they would expect that the overall effectiveness of management be judged from assessment of the whole therapeutic encounter.

5 In general, complementary therapists are aware of the interactions of mind and body, and of their influence on illness and recovery; this position receives support from recent evidence concerning the interaction of the brain and the immune system.[6,7] Some therapists would go so far as to doubt the validity of any trial in which the patient's potential for self-healing is not fully harnessed,[8] as it cannot be if patients are unaware of the specific treatment they are receiving, or if some patients suspect that they are 'only the control'. This is an extreme view, but I know of no evidence to indicate that it is safe to discount it: it derives support from studies of the placebo response.[9]

6 Finally, there are problems with endpoints. Complementary practitioners rarely treat patients with life-threatening disease, and survival is an unlikely endpoint in their studies. The aims of treatment range from eradication of the cause of the symptoms to no more than bringing about a reduction in the discomfort experienced from unchanged pathology, and/or of the disruption of their lives caused by the 'disease'. Objective measures of improvement will sometimes be available, but often they will not, and in any case the therapist would rarely be satisfied with an objective criterion alone without finding out how the patient rated the improvement. Both subjective data and multiple endpoints are generally viewed with disfavour in clinical trials.

The problems outlined above mean that the double blind randomized controlled trial, in its standard form, is often not applicable to trials in complementary medicine. However, many of the problems so evident to complementary practitioners are *also* problems at times for orthodox medicine,[10] and there are doubts also about the applicability of standard trials methodology to some treatment situations within orthodox medicine. These centre on the appropriateness of the type of question usually asked, and of the disease model implied. For the model where a potent treatment 'cures' the condition the simple question 'Is treatment A or treatment B more effective in the treatment of patients with this complaint?' is appropriate, provided that it is accompanied by questions about the side effects of treatment. A randomized, controlled trial is the method of choice in answering this question, as long as the subgroups resulting from randomization are comparable with respect to important prognostic variables. With this simple model comparability can be checked by examining the distribution of markers of the severity of the disease and of standard demographic factors. There are some treatment situations which conform to this simple model, but there are many others which do not; situations in which recovery is influenced as strongly by the *patient* as by the *treatment*. This is the most common model for treatment in complementary medical practice and is being increasingly recognized in orthodox practice.[11] Here the problems of ensuring and demonstrating the comparability of the treatment and control groups (or two treatment groups) are much more difficult; the larger the number of variables that are recognized as influencing outcome, the greater the chance that some of them will be maldistributed, even in studies involving large numbers of patients. This is a threat to the validity of the results (a *hidden* threat unless the distribution of all these factors is examined), especially if there is a chance of interaction between the therapy and some of the characteristics. This is precisely the implication of the contention of complementary[5] and some orthodox[11] practitioners that for optimal results therapy must be designed for each individual. Clinical hunches of this kind probably lie behind the difficulty many orthodox doctors find in complying with the protocols of clinical trials.

The evidence

Individuals vary in their genetic make-up and in experience, habits, housing, personal relationships, food, stress, exercise, attitude and so on. We are bound to take seriously the experience of complementary therapists that assessments of the characteristics of the individual are an essential preliminary to planning optimal therapy.[5] Some complementary disciplines have specific ways of making these assessments; traditional Chinese acupuncturists and herbal therapists assess patients on the 'Eight Conditions' or the 'Five Elements',[12] and homoeopaths on various modalities,[13] in each case building up a picture of the patient from observation, smell and touch, and from enquiries concerning details which would seem bizarre to those with a Western background. Other disciplines assess in terms of stance, movement, psychological factors or reserve.[5] They use these assessments because they find them useful, a clinical judgement, in some cases with impressive historical support, but with little objective evidence. Before the advent of the modern range of potent treatments, orthodox doctors too were well aware of the importance of the individual in the response to treatment, since much of their practice consisted of no more than helping the patient to get better. Much of this traditional wisdom was lost when doctors came to rely on potent treatments, because it appeared that *treatment* did the healing. It has gradually become apparent that this is only a half-truth. In the 1960s Feinstein showed that, even for cancer patients, factors related to the resistance of the patient added substantially to the accuracy of prognoses based on the extent and type of tumour,[14] and Meyer and Haggerty[15] found that acute and chronic stress were both associated with the occurrence of pharyngitis in a longitudinal study, but that the numbers and type of streptococci in the throat were not. Much more evidence that psychosocial factors influence the onset and course of disease, and recovery, has been reported since,[16–19] and the multifactorial nature of illness and recovery is recognized increasingly.[20]

In addition to studies of psychosomatic diseases, in which personal factors are seen as a *cause* of illness,[16–18] there are reports that individual characteristics influence the course of other illnesses and the responses of patients to therapy in other conditions, and are associated with non-specific differences in susceptibility, prognosis or response to therapy. The prognostic implications of the associations with *susceptibility* are not always clear, but in chronic diseases susceptibility tends to mark the presence of adverse factors, of poor resistance leading to more rapid progression, or of idiosyncratic enzyme patterns. Much of the information is derived from studies set up with quite different aims; this means that the data is difficult to find, may be incomplete, and may only be a fraction of what might be uncovered if studies were set up to look for it. The data is reviewed in more detail elsewhere.[21]

Until the advent of antibiotics, infant boys had a higher death rate from infections than infant girls, enough to affect the sex ratio of the population, and females still show greater longevity. Females, whether rabbit or human, are better antibody producers,[22] and this may partly explain the difference; females are also more prone to autoimmune diseases.[23] The HLA antigens are the transplantation antigens detected on leucocytes; some are associated with differences in the pattern of immune reactivity,[24,25] with susceptibility to various autoimmune diseases,[23] and infectious diseases,[26] or with poor resistance;[27] some appear to mark a greater risk of side effects of anti-rheumatic therapy.[28] Blood group associations with disease, involving the ABO and rhesus and some of the minor systems, have been reviewed extensively:[29] the most striking associations seem to be expressed through differences in the immune system,[24,29] and in clotting.[29] Blood group O was associated with a poorer response to immunomodulation in two studies in patients with malignant disease.[30,31] Left-handedness was associated with certain autoimmune diseases and with severe migraine.[32] Increasing numbers of minor enzyme anomalies are being reported: most affect single conditions only but some have wider implications, for instance through effects on the activation or excretion of drugs, or poor utilization of food, or through impairment or distortion of immune function resulting in poor resistance or unwanted reactions (including reactions to drugs) not all of which are strictly 'immunological'.[33] The tendency to atopy, which is inherited, contributes to drug reactions, and to other hyper-responsiveness, which in turn contributes to the occurrence and progression of lesions resulting from exposure to inhaled organic pollutants (for example, grains, fibres and cigarette smoke) and related 'idiopathic' conditions, many of which show more rapid progression in individuals with evidence of a more cellular, or of an atopic, response.[34–36] The quality of the 'stress' response is another important variable, perhaps of greater significance than the degree of stress itself.[37–39] Since improved stress management resulted in clinical improvement in hypertension,[19] one must assume that the way the patient copes with stress affects outcome in other illnesses with a stress component.

Medical investigations therefore confirm the practitioners' contention that individuals differ in ways that may affect their response to therapy in a wide range of conditions. Some of the associations may reflect direct influences on effector mechanisms, but others seem to be merely marker associations: from the point of view of understanding mechanisms the distinction may be important but for utilitarian purposes it is the consistency of the association that matters.

Significance for methodology

Accepting the premise that individual factors influence the outcome of therapy and may determine the most appropriate treatment strategy has implications for the planning of therapy trials. According to the principles of statistics, all such factors should either be recorded and examined in the analysis, or be balanced out. In keeping with this, Feinstein published a series of papers in 1968 in which he called for the recording and analysis of all relevant information about patients,[40] pointing out that with the advent of computers this had become feasible. Now, more than 20 years later, with computers much more accessible and easier to use, the data recorded in clinical trials is still restricted usually to accepted prognostic factors as assessed in clinical medicine with an emphasis on information about the *disease*. Little data about the individual patient (except standard demographic data and inclusion and exclusion criteria) is usually recorded, even where 'host' characteristics are of proven prognostic importance.[14] Data on the significance of both individual characteristics and host responses has tended to be overlooked: for example, information on immunocompetence is not considered obligatory in cancer trials, or about stress management in cardiac trials, in spite of the evidence that they affect prognosis. There has been little effort to explore the range of individual factors that can be adequately assessed, or of the methodological problems involved. Recording and evaluating characteristics of the individual which may mark different responses to illness and to therapy could be employed within the context of the randomized clinical trial, where this strategy is applicable, and this should be done. Trials on this pattern could start to ask, 'How can we tell which patients, if any, will be helped by this treatment?' (subject, of course, to the accrual of adequate numbers of patients). It is, after all, individual patients that the clinician has to treat, and guidance about the treatment of individual patients that is sought from clinical trials.

The *nature* of the variables also has implications for the planning of therapy trials. Some may be passive markers of differences in natural history; for these the standard approach of balancing out confounding variables is adequate, but it seems that others mark subgroups with different *needs* for therapy, or different responses to it: for these it is essential to record the variable and examine its effects, since 'balancing out' would give different overall results dependent on the patient mix. When one of the characteristics (such as coping behaviour) influences treatment strategy, and is a subsidiary target for therapy, as well as an endpoint criterion, any assessment error is liable to be magnified, and objective and/or independent and/or reduplicated assessment is essential. There is even a possibility that some characteristics mark groups of patients in which treatment has contrary effects, helping some and harming others: then different trials could show results ranging from 'advantage' through 'no effect' to 'harm' according to the proportion of patients with that characteristic. Failure to record that variable, or to analyse its effects, would give conflicting and misleading results, capable of obscuring the whole issue. I have had experience of this effect in two immunomodulating trials that were conducted in lung cancer: in each, patients with weak immunocompetence, who had a poorer prognosis anyway,[41] tended to do even worse when treated.[30,42] I was working in the north of England, in areas with poor dietary habits, and in particular low vitamin C intake; many lung cancer patients showed markedly low vitamin C levels, verging on the scorbutic, associated with low values on immunocompetence parameters.[43] The findings suggest that the poor results in our study, compared to parallel studies in areas with better eating habits,[44] may have been due to their inability to respond to immunomodulation, since vitamin C is used up in resistance reactions. Similar factors probably lie behind other contradictory findings, but if the relevant factors are not recorded, the possibility cannot be examined.

Examining multiple variables

There has been an unwillingness to look at large numbers of variables in clinical trials, and in particular to look for interactions, on the grounds that if you look at enough factors some will appear significant. This is certainly a real risk for a single study (particularly serious if multiple separate analyses are performed), but if overall patterns are looked for, the likelihood of identical patterns occurring by chance alone is surely *inversely* related to the number of variables forming the pattern, and to the number of parallel groups examined. Also the number of patients needed for significant results should *decrease* as the variance attributed to chance is reduced by attributing it to other variables which can be included in the analysis. Biologists are used to attributing much of the confounding variation to 'chance', but how much is really chance? Some chance events may interfere with trials (accidental injury or death for example), but most other variation comes from differences between people or in the way they are treated. Before computers made the examination of complex interactions feasible, relying on randomization to balance out these differences was the best that could be managed. Now that it is possible to record and analyse multiple factors, trials recording minimal details about the patients and relying on the inclusion of large numbers of patients to 'balance out' other variables should be limited to those instances where interactions between the response to therapy and any other characteristics (including individual characteristics) have been actively excluded, to reduce the risk of misleading and contradictory results. In other instances we should record and analyse a comprehensive range of factors describing both the condition and the patient, including markers for *all* factors which have been shown to influence outcome or response to therapy, or are identified on theoretical grounds (for example, looking at gender in any condition in which immune mechanisms are concerned, because of the differences in the immune system between the sexes). In addition to recording disease status, and immunological and/or stress status where relevant, the range of variables should include general data about the individual (such as that collected by the set of questionnaires developed at Surrey[45]), and, for complementary medicine, the traditional assessments used by the various disciplines, in defined, categorized and codified form. The analysis should include examination for interactions; looking for consistency patterns in parallel studies, or in randomly assigned subgroups of single studies, would avoid attributing unwarranted weight to chance associations.

This approach can only be challenged on theoretical grounds by those who dismiss the evidence that there are patterns behind the differences in response of different patients, but on practical grounds there may be doubts about methods of data collection and analysis (considered later), and about how much of the variability of response between individuals could be represented using a manageable number of readily assessable variables. This needs investigation in detailed studies. Until such results are available it will remain a matter for conjecture, but, based on the surprisingly consistent patterns which emerged from this type of approach in lung cancer patients,[41] I suspect that an unexpectedly high proportion of the variability might be explained in this way.

Excluding observer bias

Where 'blinding' techniques are not applicable, other ways of reducing observer bias must be employed. The most important of these is that an independent assessor who is unaware of the treatment status of the patient should undertake both initial and final assessments. The inclusion of overlapping assessments,[46] patients' diary records of pain, analgesic use, activities and so on, and the views of the patients' relatives or close friends (as well as those of the patients) concerning changes in condition, should be considered, in addition to whatever objective assessments are available. *All* these endpoints must then be included in the analysis, not just the most favourable. These precautions may actually be *more* effective than a blind strategy, since there are often signs which disclose the treatment to the therapist, if not to the patient; this can result in a 'paper' blindness, even with the most rigorous trial management.

Other approaches

All these strategies can be applied within the randomized controlled trial, and at present this must be the plan of choice wherever the requirements of the randomized trial do not violate the concepts of the therapy tested: for example, in studies comparing the efficacy of management by one complementary discipline with that of another or of orthodox medicine allowing open-ended treatment protocols (using more than one therapist of each kind, preferably with contrasting styles, to give partial control of the therapist effect); or in studies of the *safety* of individual components of therapy (provided that inclusion and exclusion criteria were carefully drawn); or in studies where one treatment modality predominates and the others can be standardized. However, assessment of the efficacy of individual therapeutic techniques which are seen as only part of a multi-pronged strategy requiring different mixes for patients with different characteristics presents problems for the randomized controlled trial, unless it is possible to limit the study to homogeneous subgroups. One approach might be to randomize patients to two groups, both treated by open-ended protocols, with the test treatment banned from one of the groups – full recording of characteristics, indications for each part of the treatment, the exact treatments given, and of outcome would be needed.

What other approaches could be employed? Some simple strategies might be relevant in certain circumstances. For example, testing the efficacy of a treatment according to how well it was initially deemed appropriate (as long as the conditions for appropriateness were without implication for outcome), or treating each of two affected limbs with different topical preparations,[47] or random blind allocation for each patient of the order of giving the therapies to be compared,[48] applicable only to therapies with short-term, reversible effects. In other cases evidence of effectiveness may come from investigations showing relevant biological or biochemical effects.

There are other situations where none of these strategies is appropriate and where a randomized controlled trial is ruled out because it cannot be applied without violating the central tenets of the therapy tested. For example, where studies are aiming at assessing and improving complex treatment strategies involving a number of interacting components used either in different ways, or to a different extent in different patients; where the effect of giving information, advice or training is to be tested; and wherever it proves impossible to devise a logical test strategy which adequately reflects the clinical treatment situation. In the former case logistics may preclude the limitation of the study to a subgroup in which similar treatment would be appropriate, even if such a subgroup can be identified. There are difficulties in the design of studies of the effects of giving information or advice partly because randomization at one centre carries a high probability that information will 'leak' to the control group (randomizing *centres* may avoid this but only at the expense of the comparability of the groups), but also because of the impossibility of conforming to even the minimal ethical standard of telling the patients of their inclusion and the aim of the study, since telling control patients that information was being withheld would be both unethical and counterproductive: this problem is particularly acute for those who consider it unethical not to ensure that patients' potential for self-healing is fully engaged.

We are left with the question as to whether it is possible to design a rigorous study without using the randomized controlled format. I think it may be, at least in theory. In studies in which multiple variables are included, the most interesting, and probably the most informative, results are likely to come from detailed analyses within the groups rather than from comparison of 'test' and 'control' groups. Comparison with a concurrent control group actually introduces the need for randomization to exclude allocation bias. If there is sufficient background knowledge of the effects of all the other factors which influence outcome, single-group therapy studies become a valid way of examining effectiveness partly because the accumulated data describes the range of variation within the population allowing a valid comparison taking *all* factors influencing outcome into account, and partly because such a format might be expected to generate its own controls. There is a sense in which this strategy can be considered as utilizing a natural control group from within the population whenever subgroup differences in response occur. For example, in patients with the same condition, if those with a certain characteristic (A) respond consistently to one treatment (X) and not to another (Y), and those with characteristic B respond to Y and not to X, then they control each other. Provided that controls for observer bias have been incorporated, the validity of the observation depends not on comparison with an artificially engendered control group, but on whether the finding applies consistently when different groups of patients are observed. Exhaustively analysed single-group trials might command as much rigour as trials based on comparisons, but their validity would depend on identification, and inclusion, of most of the factors which influence outcome. Different criteria for demonstrating efficacy would be required since these would depend on the internal consistency of the relationship of the treatment response with each of the other factors in groups of patients treated in the same way, and/or in detecting consistent differences in the relationship of these factors to the endpoint variables in the treated population compared to the reference populations.

At first sight this strategy appears to lose out through not using a simultaneous control group from which to derive a firm estimate of comparative efficacy. However, this is less of a detriment than it appears. In most trials efficacy is expressed in terms of the *proportion* of patients benefiting and/or the *extent* of benefit and the frequency or severity of side effects. The approach outlined would aim not just to estimate the proportion benefiting, but also to describe the subgroup of patients who benefit. Strictly speaking it would only be able to compare the *amount* of improvement in responding individuals if *all* the factors which influence outcome had been identified and accurately assessed in each of the studies concerned, but then the quantitative comparison of effect in a controlled trial, relying on chance to distribute unrecorded factors with an influence on outcome between the groups, can also only give a tentative estimate, which may be quite misleading. In each case confidence in the result requires that repeated studies give consistent results. If repeated studies of different therapies give rise to different, but in each case consistent patterns, the resulting quantitative estimate might well be as reliable as that from a controlled trial.

The results of randomized controlled trials could be considered as pointing towards this strategy. If some patients benefit and others do not (or not sufficiently to satisfy the criteria) and some suffer side effects and others do not, there must be a reason, either in the way the treatment was given, or in the state or the constitution of the patients. If, for example, only seven out of ten patients benefited in a study whose results were deemed significantly positive, extrapolation to the population at large implies that there would be large numbers of potential patients who could expect no advantage from this treatment. This situation can only be remedied by finding out the characteristics that distinguish those individuals who respond (or do not respond), or who suffer side effects. Most previous attempts to do this have tended to concentrate on differences in the *condition*: the evidence suggests that further attempts should focus on the characteristics of the *individual*.

Practical considerations

Whether such studies form part of a randomized trial or not, three difficulties are immediately apparent: getting large quantities of good quality data; deciding which variables should be recorded, and of analysis. Good quality data requires good planning and discipline,[40] dedicated personnel, and the recording of each factor in the simplest terms available, concentrating on questionnaires, observations and on routine tests.[21] These should be evaluated in terms of reliability and marker potential rather than physiological role. Canter and his associates have developed methods for the recognition and validation of multiple variables based on Facet Theory;[49] they have investigated the application of these methods to clinical trials.[45,46] These methods have advantages over the combination of partial correlation analysis based on non-parametric matrices[50] and log-rank survival analysis,[51] which I have used in the past in studies of lung cancer patients.[41] Other methods may also be applicable, but on the whole distribution-free methods are preferred because of the nature of many of the variables. Establishing standard accepted strategies for handling large numbers of variables in clinical trials would encourage researchers to adopt this approach. Standard methods for handling multiple outcome variables are also needed to accommodate the insistence of complementary therapists, and others, that the patient's opinion of the extent of benefit must form an integral part of the assessment of the outcome of therapy, even if objective criteria are available.

Conclusions

Experience, both in complementary and in orthodox clinical practice, and investigations indicate that individuals vary in their response to illness and to therapy. These variations need to be taken into consideration in clinical trials to a greater extent than they are at present. The number and severity of side effects from drugs that have been tested in clinical trials before release[33] is a cogent argument for reconsidering our methods.

As a result of criticisms, mainly from the behavioural sciences, Kramer and Shapiro published a review[10] of the scientific challenges in the application of clinical trials, which considered some of the problems which worry complementary therapists; in particular they recognized psychological factors as possible confounding factors. However, the central difficulty was not mentioned; they did not face up to the fundamental possibility that all treatments do not suit all patients equally well, just because they have the same 'disease'. This is the central problem that I think we all have to face.

References

[1] Wharton, R., Lewith, G. Complementary medicine and the general practitioner. *Br Med J* 1986; **292**: 1499–1500.

[2] Anderson, E., Anderson, P. General practitioners and alternative medicine. *J Roy Coll Gen Pract* 1987; **37**: 52–5.

[3] Payne, J. (ed.) *Report of the Board of Science Working Party.* London: British Medical Association, 1986.

[4] Evans, B. (ed.) Proceedings of the 1st Conference on Research Methodology for Complementary Medicine. *Comp Med Res* 1986; **1**: 1–87.

[5] Anthony, H. M. (ed.) The patient as individual and statistic; Proceedings of the 2nd Conference on Research Methodology for Complementary Medicine. *Comp Med Res* 1987; **2**: 48–121.

[6] Solomon, G. F. The emerging field of psychoneuroimmunology. *Advances* 1985; **2**: 6–19.

[7] Stein, M., Keller, S. E., Scheifer, S. E. Stress and immunomodulation: the role of depression and neuroendocrine function. *J Immunol* 1985; **135**: 827–33.

[8] Heron, J. Critique of conventional research methodology. *Comp Med Res* 1986; **1**: 12–22.

[9] Lewith, G. T. Every doctor a walking placebo. *Comp Med Res* 1987; **2**: 10–18.

[10] Kramer, M. S., Shapiro, S. H. Scientific challenges in the application of randomised trials. *J Am Med Assoc* 1987; **252**: 2739–63.

[11] Southgate, L. Individual characteristics assessed and used in practice: 3. Orthodox medicine (General Practice). *Comp Med Res* 1987; **2**: 59–63.

12 Mole, P. Individual characteristics assessed and used in practice; 2. Traditional Chinese Acupuncture. *Comp Med Res* 1987; **2**: 56–9.

13 Davey, R. Individual characteristics assessed and used in practice: 5. Homoeopathy. *Comp Med Res* 1987; **2**: 66–70.

14 Feinstein, A. R. Symptoms as an index of biological behaviour and prognosis in human cancer. *Nature* 1966; **209**: 241–5.

15 Meyer, R. J., Haggerty, R. J. Streptococcal infections in families. Factors altering individual susceptibility. *Pediatrics* 1962; **29**: 539–49.

16 Henry, J. P. The relation of social to biological processes in disease. *Soc Sci Med* 1982; **16**: 369–80.

17 Martin, R. D. A critical review of the concept of stress in psychosomatic medicine. *Perspect Biol Med* 1984; **27**: 443–64.

18 Marmot, M. G. Psychosocial factors and blood pressure. *Prev Med* 1985; **14**: 451–65.

19 Patel, C., Marmot, M., Terry, D. J., Carruthers, M., Hunt, B., Patel, M. Trial of relaxation in reducing coronary risk; four year follow-up. *Br Med J* 1985; **290**: 1103–6.

20 Roe, W. Science in the practice of medicine: its limitations and dangers. *Perspect Biol Med* 1984; **27**: 386–400.

21 Anthony, H. M. Measuring differences between individuals: medical measurements. *Comp Med Res* 1987; **2**: 82–93.

22 Fudenberg, H. H., Pink, J. R. L., Strites, D. P., Wang, A. C. *Basic Immunogenetics*. New York: Oxford University Press, 1972.

23 Bodmer, W. (ed.) HLA and autoimmune disease. *Br Med Bull* 1978; **34**: 213–316.

24 Petranyi, G., Ivanyi, P., Hollan, S. R. Relations of HLA and Rh systems to immune reactivity. *Vox Sanguinis* 1974; **26**: 470–82.

25 Van Rood, J. J. HLA as regulator. *Ann Rheum Dis* 1984; **43**: 665–72.

26 Van Eden, W., de Vries, R. R. P., van Rood, J. J. HLA and infectious diseases. *Prog Clin Bio Res* 1982; **103**: B37–54.

27 Matthey, F., James, D. G. The patient with poor resistance. *Br J Clin Pract* 1985; **39**: 171–6.

28 Bardin, T., Dyll, A., Debeyre, N., Ryckewaert, A., Legrand, L., Marcelli, A., Dausset, J. HLA system and side effects of gold salts and D-penicillinase treatment of rheumatoid arthritis. *Ann Rheum Dis* 1982; **41**: 599–601.

29 Mourant, A. E., Kopec, A. C., Domaniewska-Sobczak, K. *Blood Groups and Diseases*. Oxford: Oxford University Press, 1978.

30 Anthony, H. M. Blood groups and the response to immunotherapy. *Cancer Immunol Immunopathol* 1981; **11**: 287–9.

31 Harris, R., Zuhrie, S. R., Freeman, C. B., Read, A. P., MacIver, J. E.,

Geary, C. C., Delamore, I. W., Tooth, J. A. A successful randomized trial of immunotherapy versus no maintenance in acute myelogenous leukaemia. In: Terry, W. D., Rosenberg, S. A. (eds.) *Immunotherapy of Cancer*. North Holland: Elsevier, 1982; 11–16.

32 Geschwind, N., Behan, P. Lefthandedness: association with immune disease, migraine, and developmental learning disorders. *Proc Nat Acad Sci* 1982; **79**: 5097–100.

33 Dukor, P. (ed.) *Pseudo-allergic Reactions*. Vols 1 (1980), 2 (1980), 3 (1982). Basle: Karger.

34 Crystal, R. G., Bitterman, P. B., Rennard, S. I., Hance, A. J., Keogh, B. A. Interstitial lung disease of unknown cause. 2. Disorders characterised by chronic inflammation of the lower respiratory tract. *New Eng J Med* 1984; **310**: 235–44.

35 Chan-Yeung, M., DeBuncio, A. Leukocyte count, smoking and lung function. *Am J Med* 1984; **75**: 31–7.

36 Anthony, H. M. Reactive changes in the blood of smokers and the development of arterial disease and COPD, a review. *Rev Environmental Health* 1989; **3**: 25–86.

37 Laudenslager, M. L., Ryan, S. M., Drugan, R. C., Hyson, R. L., Maier, S. F. Coping and immunosuppression: inescapable but not escapable shock suppresses lymphocyte proliferation. *Science* 1983; **221**: 568–70.

38 Blizard, D. A., Freedman, L. S., Liang, B. Genetic variation, chronic stress and the central and peripheral noradrenergic systems. *Am J Physiol* 1981; **245**: R600–605.

39 Besedovsky, H., del Rey, A., Sorkin, E., Da Prada, M., Burri, R., Honegger, C. The immune response evokes changes in the brain noradrenergic neurons. *Science* 1983; **221**: 564–6.

40 Feinstein, A. R. The epidemiology of cancer therapy 2. The clinical course: data decisions and demarcations. *Ann Int Med* 1969; **123**: 323–44.

41 Anthony, H. M., Madsen, K. E., Mason, M. K., Templeman, G. H. Lung cancer, immune status, histopathology and smoking. *Br J Dis Chest* 1981; **75**: 40–54.

42 Anthony, H. M. Yorkshire trial of adjuvant therapy with Levamisole in surgically-treated lung cancer. In: Terry, W. D., Rosenberg, S. A. (eds.) *Immunotherapy of Cancer*. North Holland: Elsevier, 1982; 135–40.

43 Anthony, H. M., Schorah, C. J. Severe hypovitaminosis C in lung cancer patients: the utilisation of Vitamin C in surgical repair and lymphocyte-related host resistance. *Br J Cancer* 1982; **46**: 354–67.

44 Amery, W. K. Double-blind Levamisole trial in resectable lung cancer. *Ann New York Acad Sci* 1976; **277**: 260–8.

45 Booker, K., Canter, D. Measuring differences between individuals; psychological measurements: the Surrey Experience of Treatment Battery (SET). *Comp Med Res* 1987; **2**: 94–103.

46 Canter, D. A research agenda for holistic therapy studies. *Comp Med Res* 1987; **2**: 104–16.

47 Alexander, K. Traditional medicine. *Missionary Herald* 1985; April: 68–9.

48 Guyatt, G., Sackett, D., Taylor, D. W., Chong, J., Roberts, R., Pugsley, S. Determining optimal therapy – randomised trials in individual patients. *New Eng J Med* 1986; **314**: 889–92.

49 Canter, D. (ed.) *Facet Theory*. New York: Springer-Verlag, 1984.

50 Nie, N. H., Jenkins, J. G., Steinbrunner, K., Bent, D. H. *Statistical Package for the Social Sciences*. 2nd ed. New York: McGraw Hill, 1975; 288, 302.

51 Peto, R., Pike, M. C., Armitage, P., Breslow, N. E., Cox, D. R., Howard, S. V., Mantel, N., McPherson, K., Peto, J., Smith, P. J. Design and analysis of randomised trials requiring prolonged observation of each patient. *Br J Cancer* 1977; **34**: 585–612, and **35**: 1–39.

10 Tactics and practicalities

Ian James

Summary

In planning a study and writing the protocol, getting the question right at the outset is the key to success. This will of course determine the exact design. The various types of study design are outlined in this chapter ranging from the simple fact-finding exercise to the complicated double blind trial. The importance of randomization and techniques to avoid bias are emphasized. Errors due to poor patient selection and inappropriate measurements have all too often marred trials in the past. The advantages and disadvantages of using visual analogue scales or graded scales is dealt with. Accuracy in recording the data is essential. Thought should be given at an early stage to the design of the data sheet on which the results are to be recorded. Some ways of getting out of trouble once the trial has started are also outlined.

Introduction

The first thing to be decided is who exactly is going to do the research. Are you going to do it by yourself? Who else is going to be involved with you? Presumably the general field of your interest will have been defined, but it is as well to ask yourself if all the aspects of your study are covered by the necessary experience. If your research experience, or experience of some essential technique, is limited, then it may be a good idea to collaborate with someone who has that relevant experience. Doing research by oneself is not easy. Things do not always go well and it is very easy for one person working alone to lose heart. This is much less likely to occur with a team of researchers. If you combine with others it is very important that they be involved from the very earliest stages of planning.

Asking the right question

If you ask experienced research workers what single factor more than any other is likely to be associated with success, they will tell you that it is the formulation of the question. Getting the question exactly right may take weeks of intensive work, but it is always worth it. Not only should the question you are trying to answer be carefully constructed, but it should also be written down. Ideally this should be accomplished in one sentence. Inexperienced investigators always try and answer too many questions or questions which are poorly defined. Make sure your question is answerable with the facilities at your disposal.

A design of the study

The question posed will of course determine the design of the study. If inexperienced investigators have heeded the advice given above then the design should be fairly simple. The simplest format is the simple fact-finding exercise. Such a task is an essential prerequisite to a more complicated investigation anyway. It should go without saying that a good simple study is far more valuable than a poorly designed and badly carried out complicated one.

Simple fact-finding exercise

This entails assessing cases in greater detail than is usual in clinical practice. It also means recording your findings in a way that you can subsequently handle. One has to develop ways of assessing patients and of making appropriate measurements. The variability of the disease and of the various measurements is assessed. The natural history of the disease should become clearer. In these initial fact-finding studies the number of patients to be studied is usually determined in an arbitrary fashion. However, such data does enable one to calculate the numbers required for comparative trials. Trials which can never hope to recruit adequate numbers should not be started. Preliminary studies of this type are therefore an essential.

Simple comparative open trial

The problem with all studies of treatment is that we each have biases of some sort or another. Either we think our treatment is fantastic or that some other therapy is dangerous. Often these judgements are subjective, based on very little evidence, and in fact may lead to really dangerous misconceptions. The clinical trial is a device to get over bias.

Formally defined, a clinical trial is a comparison of treatments in groups of patients by controlling or equalizing all variables except the administration itself. In the simplest case there is some form of comparison of one treatment with another. Even under these circumstances patients should be allotted randomly to each of the groups.

Randomization is one of the most important factors in the elimination of bias. One of the simplest ways of carrying out randomization is by the sealed envelope technique. If 50 patients are to be studied and half are to be given one form of treatment and the other half are to be given another form of treatment, then the first thing to do is to obtain 50 envelopes. Into the first 25 one places a card on which is written the word 'Treatment 1' and into the second 25, a card on which is written 'Treatment 2'. The envelopes are sealed and then shuffled. The outsides of the envelopes are then numbered consecutively. The envelopes are opened in this order when needed and the appropriate treatment given.

Simple single blind comparative trial

Bias can be decreased further by using a simple single blind format. The investigator knows what treatment the patient has been given but the patient does not. This type of trial randomization is as important as the double blind trial and the use of an independent assessor (i.e. not the therapist) decreases errors due to bias to an even greater extent.

Double blind trial

This is a system favoured for many drug trials. Neither the patient nor the investigator is aware of what treatment the patient is taking. For many types of complementary medicine this type of design is unfortunately difficult to use. The reason for this is that it is often impossible to disguise the fact that some form of treatment has been administered. It is not always possible to give a convincing sham treatment alternative.

Cross-over versus non-cross-over design

In the non-cross-over trial one group of patients is given the treatment to be tested and the other some form of dummy treatment or placebo. Alternatively, the new treatment may be compared with older treatments already established as being effective.

In the cross-over trial one group of patients is initially given the experimental treatment and the other dummy or standard treatment. Once the effect of these has been established the group given dummy treatment is changed to active treatment and vice versa.

The advantages of the non-cross-over trial are that there are no carry-over effects from one treatment period to another, and the timing of treatment can be precisely regulated to the natural history of the disease process. It has the disadvantage that between-patient variability is increased. The advantages of the cross-over trial are that fewer patients are required and that variability between patients is lessened. The disadvantage of a cross-over trial is that sometimes it is impossible. Carry-over effects from one treatment to another can complicate the interpretation.

The pseudo-cross-over trial

For want of a better term there is another design which might be called the pseudo-cross-over trial. In this format the main comparison is between parallel groups, one given treatment, the other not. The statistical analysis is that of a non-cross-over trial. After the treatment period, however, the patients are crossed over so that those who were denied treatment initially are now given it. One also has an opportunity of following those given treatment initially to see if the beneficial effects are maintained. This trial gets round a number of ethical and practical problems and may be particularly suitable for complementary studies.

Investigators should perhaps be reminded that it is unethical not to tell the patient that for a part of the time he or she will not be on treatment. Most patients are sympathetic to the idea that one is trying to evaluate therapy so long as they do not suffer particularly in any way.

Patients to be studied

Other than for the simplest fact-finding investigation, the type of patient you are going to study needs to be defined. The use of patients who are too sick or not sick enough may result in a very misleading answer.

Inclusion and exclusion criteria need to be agreed by all the investigators and written down.

How drop outs or withdrawals are to be handled statistically should be decided before the trial begins.

Techniques to be used

The exact techniques to be used must be agreed by all the investigators; how they are to be administered, by whom and how often, for how long.

Measurements

What measurements are needed to answer the question? Again, one has to decide how often these should be made and exactly how they are going to be performed.

It is frequently said that objective measurements such as pulse and blood pressure are better than subjective assessments but this is not necessarily so. Certainly measurements or assessments must be appropriate to the question being asked.

The use of visual analogue scales

Visual analogue scales can be used by an observer or by the patient. They are useful to assess things such as pain or wellbeing. On the left hand side of a 10 cm line is marked 'No pain' and on the right side is marked 'Pain as bad as I have ever experienced'. The subject marks the line to indicate the severity of his symptoms. Such a technique can be used to compare the responses of groups of patients to different treatments or to follow the response of an individual patient sequentially.

The use of graded scales

These scales again can be used by an observer or by the patient. A simple tick box format can be employed. Grade 0 may be 'No pain' and grade 5 may be 'Pain as bad as ever experienced'. Personally I find this type of scale easier to administer and easier to handle statistically. There are some who argue that the analogue gives greater accuracy, but I remain unconvinced. There is some evidence that nervous subjects tend always to mark the centre of visual analogue scales.

For both scales, if the measurements are subject to bias then the assessment should be made by someone other than the principal investigator or therapist. Assessments need to be frequent enough to give adequate data but not so frequent that they cause the patient unnecessary hardship. If the patient is so put off that they never come back no one benefits from the exercise. Recruitment for most trials is difficult enough anyway.

In order to calculate the required numbers for a trial, it is necessary to make an estimate of the order of improvement in the most important measurements or calculate the percentage of patients likely to derive benefit from the new therapy over the old.

The protocol

Before commencing to do a study, a full protocol has to be written which needs to address itself to all the above factors. The list below gives a basic outline.

Protocol content checklist

1   *Title*
    Title, date, draft number or final version, index/contents.

2   *Personnel identification*
    Principal organizing and responsible personnel involved, their position, function, address and telephone numbers.

3   *Objectives*
    Primary question or questions being asked.

4   *Rationale*
    How did the idea originate? Relevant previous findings, ethical issues and their resolution, expected application of results or advance in knowledge.

5   *Design*
    Uncontrolled/controlled; cross-over/matched pair/parallel group; fixed number/sequential; open or single/double blind; use of randomization; number of patients; number of observers; duration of treatment and study. Ethics: is the study compatible with the Declaration of Helsinki?

6   *Patient selection*
    Criteria for admission; exclusion; confirmation of informed consent.

7   *Definition of treatment*
    Method should be defined. Is a placebo treatment possible? How often is treatment given and by whom? How long does treatment continue for? How does one handle other therapy? Should it be stopped? Is it ethical to do this?

8   *Patient management*
    a) Order of events: patient enrolment; follow-up visits; investigations to be undertaken; record completion.
    b) Investigations: what measurements are to be made? What apparatus is necessary?
    c) Records: what records are to be kept? Description of presentation; content; responsibilities and methods of completion.
    d) Adverse events: how should they be recorded?
    e) Method of obtaining informed consent.

9   *Responsibilities*
    Who is responsible for what? Who is to obtain ethical approval?

Who is to do the statistical analysis? Who is going to write the report? Is patient insurance adequate?

10   *Statistical considerations*
   a) Study size.
   b) Sample population.
   c) Randomization.
   d) Analysis.

11   *References and bibliography*

Recording data

Certain details need always to be considered when designing the record form. It is wise to consider initially what facts have to be recorded and then to decide how exactly this should be done, and in what order. It is as well to allow space on the form for things which are measured on the same occasion to be grouped together. The last thing one wants when busy is to spend time thumbing through a bulky protocol trying to find where exactly one should record the facts. If one is going to photostat the forms it is sometimes a good idea to use different coloured paper for different visits. Patient identification and personal details should be on the first page, ideally with a telephone number.

The design of the form is extremely important. One should keep the questions clear so that the responses are obvious to the person filling it in. How to record baseline measurements, measurements on subsequent evaluation, treatment particulars, and treatment response all need to be decided. A simple yes/no tick box approach is usually best.

Always leave enough space on the form so that it does not appear cramped. This is very important, especially if a visual analogue scale is being employed. Always try out a pilot form first and be prepared to modify it in the light of experience.

Troubleshooting

Common problems include the following:

a) We've got a splendid idea but we've no money
If the idea is truly splendid then finding the money should be no problem. The policy of the RCCM is to give assistance in appropriate situations to inexperienced investigators. If it is possible to find someone with research experience to put in a joint application, so much the better.

b) We had plenty of patients before we started the trial but now they have all disappeared
There are three possible answers to such a problem:

   1 It sometimes helps to set aside a special time and place to carry out the study. Certainly one must not be in a hurry when asking a patient if he or she would participate. If this is rushed in any way you are very likely to get a refusal.

2 Can you increase your recruitment either by searching out other collaborators or by letting others know of your research interests? Can you increase the numbers by offering to pay busfares of older patients, etc.?

3 Finally, you may have to relax your entry criteria. This is not an ideal solution but at least it is better than the trial collapsing. Making exclusion criteria too rigorous for no very good reason is an extremely common error. If too many patients start the study, but drop out for one reason or another, are you expecting too much from them? Are all the visits necessary? Do you have to make as many measurements each time?

c) We are worried about patient insurance
This can be a very nasty question indeed to answer. Perhaps the simplest way around the problem is to persuade someone in the conventional field who has to be covered anyway to join your research.

Further reading

Pocock, S. J. *Clinical Trials: A Practical Approach*. Chichester: Wiley, 1983.

Grahame-Smith, D. G., Aronson, J. K. *The Oxford Textbook of Clinical Pharmacology and Drug Therapy*. Oxford: OUP, 1984; 204–22.

James, I. M. The appropriate use of conventional research methodology. *Comp Med Res* 1986; **2**(1): 7–11.

Glenny, H., Nelmes, P. *Handbook of Clinical Drug Research*. Oxford: Blackwell Scientific, 1986.

11 Clinical research: questions to ask and the benefits of asking them

Honor M. Anthony

Summary

There is an urgent need for more (and for more appropriate) research into holistic forms of therapy, including complementary therapies, but clinical research involves substantial investment of time, effort, and money, which may be wasted if inappropriately complex studies are embarked on by those with little experience of research of this kind. This chapter discusses the value of simple studies, for their own sake, as a preparation for controlled studies, and as a way of starting in research.

Introduction

This chapter aims to give information and advice about the planning of studies, to help people with little experience to get started. There is no need to stress the importance of doing research, or the benefits overall that it can bring. Instead we need to look closely at the types of study with which to start and the sort of information you might expect to obtain. The eventual aim of most clinical research is to demonstrate the effectiveness of therapy in a rigorous trial (either in overall terms, or in relation to a certain treatment in a certain condition), and to go on from there to work towards improving the quality of the care provided, its effectiveness, its acceptability, and the goodness of 'fit' between the treatment and the patient. Most of this will probably be best tackled using controlled trials, either double blind or using some other technique to eliminate bias. But a controlled trial is of no value, and may be actually misleading, unless it is based on firm foundations: it is mainly the foundations we are concerned with here.

The results of research are only as good as the data that is collected – rubbish in, rubbish out – no matter how carefully controlled the study is. And 'rubbish' in the results of clinical trials is not only a waste of time, energy and money, it is also dangerous. So this chapter will concentrate on the art and discipline of making good clinical observations and on recording them in such a form that they can be meaningful when analysed, and will encourage you to set about the task of planning studies of this sort. But researchers go on learning about how to do research (and about how not to do it) for most of their working lives, so you should view your first study as a step in the process, not as reaching the end.

1 Starting in clinical research

The main characteristic of the studies we suggest you should start with is that they observe what happens in the course of therapy, rather than interfere with it. This may be in preparation for a controlled trial, but may not, because observation also has roles to play in its own right – estimating satisfaction with therapy, or collecting information needed for judging manpower needs, or space requirements for therapy centres, and for judging the need for (and the success of) dissemination of information either to individuals or for political purposes. These may be good initial projects.

How do you decide where to start? There are a number of starting points. You may have made an unexpected observation, which has demanded to be studied, or you may have questions or doubts about the applicability of a certain treatment to some patients, about the reliability of certain clinical findings, or about the effectiveness or acceptability of a treatment you use, or your main concern may be to prove to the deaf world that your therapy is more effective in certain difficult conditions than other therapies. So what kind of study should you start with?

2   Questionnaire studies

One possibility is that of collecting other peoples' views – a questionnaire study. This might ask patients about what it is like to be ill, about their experiences of therapy, or about how effective it has been. Replies might point out deficiencies in the organization of care, or in the explanations given, or suggest minor modifications of treatment schedules which might make considerable differences to the patients. A strong case can be made for always including a questionnaire about outcome and about any side effects of therapy in any study of the effectiveness of therapy: this should preferably be filled up independently by the patient and a close relative or friend. Even if objective measures demonstrate improvement after treatment, all trials should find out whether the patients feel better and whether it has enabled them to live a more normal life.

Questionnaire studies directed at the general public or at other health professionals might show up misconceptions about your type of therapy, or about the sort of patients you treat, and might discover what information should be made available, or what data is most likely to convince others of the value of what you do. Such studies can have important political implications.

3   Recording cases

Or you may wish to collect data about the types of case treated by your kind of therapist, and about satisfaction with the treatment. This would be a hybrid study, in which the therapist keeps records of the cases, their treatment, and the outcome as he sees it, and the patient is asked for his view too. Any study aiming to assess the numbers of patients treated (or the numbers of different types of patient treated) needs to base the count on a clear baseline (either all patients seen, or all seen one day a week, or some other unit, whatever is feasible in the time you have available). You need to differentiate clearly between new patients and those returning for more treatment; this sounds easy, but actually needs quite a lot of thought. If a patient you are treating comes back with pain at a different site, is that part of the 'old' condition or does he become a 'new' patient? The answer probably depends on an analysis of the causes, but you may need to make yourself some rules which are relevant to your type of practice. In addition, it is important to remember that the time of the year, the day of the week, and the time of the day can all influence the sort of patients who attend, and therefore influence the count. School age children will tend to ask advice about chronic complaints in the school holidays; a count of attendance by hayfever patients in December will bear no relation to one in June (an obvious example, but many other conditions also vary from time to time).

4 Reliability of observation

An important group of studies that are often overlooked are those concerned with the reliability of clinical observation and investigation. There are a number of examples in the literature, pointing to the fact that observations are rarely as reliable as we expect, unless special steps are taken to standardize. Three questions need to be faced about most of the observations we make. Is the observation consistent (that is, would the same observer get the same answer on different occasions with the same condition)? This is easy to test with 'traits' (such as height) that remain constant from day to day, but more difficult with 'state' characteristics (such as pulse rate or mood) which vary. Is there a reliable way of recording the observation? (Perhaps just Yes/No or Yes/Unsure/No is sufficient, or can you grade it and, if so, is it consistent, and are you sure of the order? Or can it be measured, and if so is the measurement reliable?) And thirdly, do others find the same and can you agree on your gradings? With practice, even simple descriptive gradings can often be applied consistently by several people. It is better to use a simple assessment that can be applied consistently than a very accurate-sounding measurement that is unreliable. Checking whether you are safe to rely on the assessment of some of your key observations is a good way to start in research.

5 Reliability of diagnosis and prognosis

Other studies that are often overlooked are those elucidating the factors that determine the decisions about whether the patient has the condition in question, how severe it is, and what its prognosis is likely to be. These are central to all trials, and it is essential to assess and record the main factors of each kind. A clinical trial usually compares a new treatment with an established treatment or with no treatment, and relies heavily on the comparability of two groups of patients. If the patients do not actually have the same condition, or if differences in severity are overlooked, the trial may be a nonsense. This sounds simple, but unless you can identify the condition and assess its severity reliably, it is a real risk. Moreover, patients do not come in nicely labelled, comparable packages: they are all different, but their differences tend to make patterns, and some of the patterns may be related to their suitability for some treatments, or to the way in which they respond to treatment, or to their inherent capacity for recovery. Unrecognized differences on some of these factors give rise to contradictory and confusing results of clinical trials. Randomization and blind designs eliminate the human biases – the biases introduced by the researchers or the patients, either intentionally or more usually unintentionally. But randomization does not ensure that the two groups are truly comparable unless large numbers of patients are involved. If you record all the major factors that influence outcome it is possible to check that different responses in the two groups are not caused by inequality of the groups on these factors, and so strengthen the case that they result from the different treatment. It also allows you to start to ask more questions; questions about whether each treatment is equally effective for the different sorts of people included in the study, or whether one of the characteristics defines a group of people who respond better to one of the treatments. We say then that the characteristic interacts with the treatment.

Holistic practitioners of all kinds claim to take all sorts of facts about the individual patient into consideration in making decisions about therapy, implying that they believe these factors to interact with some of their therapies. It is essential that these factors are assessed and recorded if trials are to be designed that test these therapies rigorously on their own terms. Working out how to assess and record these characteristics of the individual is a high priority; if they influence the choice of treatment it is presumably because they are believed to determine response to therapy and this needs to be confirmed or refuted. This is a task that groups of therapists might consider tackling, particularly perhaps the practitioners of traditional Chinese medicine and of homoeopathy, each with their very distinctive assessment system. But the task is not limited to them, and should be considered by all holistic practitioners. It can be thought of as the challenge of incorporating observations based on the art of therapy into a rigorous scientific study.

6   Defining treatments

A related type of study, which all practitioners might undertake, would look at what treatments you actually use and what determines your treatment decisions in practice. One of the main reasons why clinicians tend to be sceptical about the results of clinical trials is because the formalized treatment schedules tested often overlook the details which influence the decisions of clinicians from day to day. The fact, for instance, that you do not like to give one treatment to anyone under 12 years old, or that you avoid another treatment in redheads, or in people who are tall and thin, is essential information for planning a good trial. It is surprising how few practitioners of any sort are actually aware of the full range of factors involved in decisions like this until faced with actual cases. So keeping records of cases, treatments, and the reasons for choosing that treatment can be a rewarding exercise that can produce some surprises if you question yourself closely enough.

7 Adverse effects of therapy

Another group of studies concerns the ill effects of treatment. Complementary therapists have been heard to claim that their treatments never have ill effects, and some of the orthodox community to counter this by saying 'No, only effective treatments have side effects'. Both are biased overstatements. Some effective therapies may be genuinely free of ill effects, but most treatments that have effects may have ill effects if applied inappropriately, or unskilfully, or without tact and understanding, and sometimes for no apparent reason. So every therapy needs to look for ill effects; to *look* for them because most are not found without a lot of effort. The patient who does not come back may have been cured, or they may have been made worse and not want any more – we all need to find out which. This can best be done by including outcome in studies; schemes such as the Yellow Card scheme for recording the side effects of drugs are less effective; no attempt is made to follow up all the patients and only a proportion of doctors remember to notify even the acute side effects, let alone the longer-term or delayed effects that are much more difficult to associate with the therapy.

8 Preparation for a controlled trial

If you wish to prepare for a controlled trial, what should you do? Firstly decide which condition you wish to study, preferably in collaboration with some colleagues. The condition chosen will probably either be one you treat very effectively, or one that you suspect of inhomogeneity, because some patients do well and others do badly. Work out how you define the condition, what observations you need to establish it, and how you would assess its severity. Decide how you can record each of these factors. And then list all of the factors you have been taught (or have since recognized through experience) to take into account in deciding therapy, and those you think influence prognosis. Discuss these with other people, and consult the literature. Are there established ways of assessing/measuring these factors? Are the methods suitable for your patients? Do you need to develop ways of assessing or recording? Do you need to test the reliability of your measurements? How do you know if the patients are better? If you are not sure on any of these points, set up a simple study to find out.

Then consider the therapies you would give. Are there some patients you would not give any of the therapies to? If so, those patients must be excluded. You may need to record your treatment decision over a period of time to find out.

When you have worked out what you think you should do, design forms on which to do it; perhaps forms that can go in the patients' notes and become part of your clinical record. Make sure that there are clear categories whenever they are suitable (as these are the only items you can analyse satisfactorily), with open recording when necessary. Such forms may improve your clinical recording, and may even make it quicker. Try the forms out. Make a list of the patients you record in this way; after five or ten examine what you have done and see whether you need to add other factors or change the categories, etc. The improved data set may actually show the importance of some of the factors you have recorded (even if you were doubtful about including them), or show the reason for differences in outcome.

You may decide to do this in combination with a colleague in your own discipline, in a different complementary discipline, or in orthodox medicine. In some cases you may need to arrange for both disciplines to assess all the patients at the beginning, with independent assessment at the end, so that you can compare results. Are there some types of patient who respond better, or worse, to your sort of treatment? This sort of study can provide valuable insight into the treatment process, but unless you have data about patients who are untreated, or treated in a standard way, you cannot *prove* that it is your treatment that is making them better, although you may get very close to it, particularly when the complaints treated are chronic and are monitored long-term both before and after the therapy.

9   The basis of good clinical studies

Carrying out a good clinical trial of any kind depends on accuracy of observation, clarity of recording, good understanding of the condition to be studied and of the factors that influence its natural history, and understanding how treatment decisions are reached, as well as accurate information about the numbers and the characteristics of patients with the condition available for inclusion. It is a waste of time, money and energy to try and do a controlled trial without information and experience in these areas.

Conclusion

The importance of good clinical research in complementary medicine at the present time can hardly be overemphasized; complementary practitioners believe their therapies to be effective but there is little objective evidence to support that belief. The fact that such studies must stand up to rigorous scrutiny may give the impression that only randomized controlled trials are of any value, and the urgency of the need for evidence may encourage inexperienced researchers to embark on trials of this kind. Complementary therapists actually need to undertake *more* preparation than those involved in standard drug trials before setting out on a controlled trial, in order to make sure that it addresses the *real* therapy situation. Such preparatory studies offer a good introduction to research, and in more developed form may uncover important factors about therapy that controlled trials which follow the standard pattern cannot address, because of their structure.

Further reading

Anthony, H. M. Some methodological problems in the assessment of complementary therapy. *Stat Med* 1987; **6**: 761–71.

Davies, T. M. E. *A Guide to Biomedical Research*. Oxford: Blackwell Scientific, 1984.

Guyatt, G., Sackett, D. *et al.* Determining the optimal therapy – randomised clinical trials in individual patients. *New Eng J Med* 1986; **314**: 889–92.

Kazdin, A. E. *Single-case Research Designs: Methods for Clinical and Applied Settings*. New York: OUP, 1982.

Powell-Tuck, J., McRae, K. D. *et al.* A defence of the small clinical trial: evaluation of three gastroenterological studies. *Br Med J* 1986; **292**(6520): 599–602.

Proceedings of the 2nd RCCM Methodology Conference: The Patient as Individual and Statistic. *Comp Med Res* 1987; **2**(1).

Proceedings of the 3rd RCCM Methodology Conference: How Do We Know It Works? Measures of Outcome. *Comp Med Res* 1988; **2**(3).

12 Single case research designs

David Aldridge

Summary

Single case research designs are a part of a whole spectrum of research methods. Such designs have the advantage of being adaptable to the clinical needs of the patient and the therapeutic approach of the practitioner. There are various possibilities for experimental rigour which include both randomization and blind assessment. The designs are appropriate for the development of research hypotheses, testing those hypotheses in daily clinical practice and refining clinical techniques. Single case designs, if systematically replicated, could provide an ideal developmental collaborative research tool for uniting clinicians from differing backgrounds.

Introduction

This chapter attempts to describe a methodological approach suitable for some research initiatives in complementary medical practice. Currently, much of the methodological debate is about the use of randomized controlled clinical trials as group designs, as if no other clinical research strategies are available. We have a spectrum of clinical research methods which are applicable for studying complementary medical practices. Each method has its own range of applicability, and each generates differing sets of data. Each method has a different range of validity and ethical constraints. In this chapter, one group of the available research methods is introduced, that of single case study designs.[1-8]

The folklore of single case study methods suggests that these designs emerged from the practice of experimental psychology and psychoanalysis. Such a myth ignores the simple fact that human ideas have been conveyed in story form for centuries. 'Once upon a time . . .' until 'They lived happily ever after' reflects this basic form. When clinicians of whatever therapeutic persuasion gather together for their clinical discussions, they focus on cases, whether these be diverse, difficult or dangerous. Even research scientists at conferences adopt a style, usually when away from the podium, which reflects the human story as epitomized by the single case. Single cases bring an important facet to clinical research – that of personal application.

Case reports have always been used as guides to the study of rare clinical situations, for the reporting of new information about side effects of treatment or for introducing views which challenge the existing theories of disease. The clinical account of single cases was once the primary form of medical knowledge.[9] Although now often unfairly dismissed as 'unscientific', the single case report is important in that it can suggest new hypotheses for investigation or relate a particular case to a given body of knowledge. It is this hypothesis-generating function and comparative analysis which converts a clinical anecdote into a valuable single case study.[10,11] The difficulty of accepting clinical descriptions lies at the heart of controversies surrounding scientific medicine when it is practised in the clinic. There is often a split between clinicians and researchers; the researcher emphasizing correlation, generalization and statistical significance, the clinician emphasizing application, specificity and significance for the patient. This dichotomy reflects the historical shift in medicine to a pathophysiological explanation of disease and treatment.[9] However, medical knowledge is unavoidably clinical and patient-dependent; it is not a matter of scientific principles alone.[10]

Single case study designs are an attempt to formalize clinical stories. These designs take as their basis the clinical process where the illness is assessed and diagnosed, a treatment is prescribed, the patient is monitored during the application of that treatment, and the success of the treatment is then evaluated. However, the validity of this therapeutic 'success' is open to question. There may be a subjective bias influenced by the expectations of the clinician and the patient. Similarly, the patient may appear to improve through willingness to please the physician. In some cases, the disease may have run its course and improvement would have occurred without a therapeutic intervention.

Finally, the initial assessment of the patient may have represented temporary extreme values which are lessened at a subsequent assessment, i.e. a 'regression towards the mean'. The experimental approach attempts to accommodate these difficulties by 'systematically varying the management of the patient's illness during a series of treatment periods'[12] using randomization of treatment periods and blind assessment.

Single case research designs are not a unified approach. There are differing levels of formality and experimentation. The three approaches introduced in this chapter are:

- Randomized single case study designs, often called N = I studies[12–14]

- Single case experimental designs[15]

- Diary or calendar methods.[16]

General approach

A common feature of these designs is that they adhere to the practice of the clinician. An advantage is that there are no difficulties of recruiting large groups of patients, or having to collect and analyse large data sets.

A criticism of group designs is that they mask individual change.[17,18] Improvement or deterioration is not evident for particular patients. Furthermore, the results of large-scale trials are not always easy to translate into clinical terms for the practitioner. Single case designs highlight individual change in daily clinical practice. Furthermore, the dilemma of clinical priorities or research priorities is minimized. This type of research is applied as part of the clinical treatment and is relevant to both clinician and patient. In some cases patient and clinician are the researchers.[12]

The principal feature of single case study designs is that they are feasible. The problems of recruitment are minimized, the study is cheap and the results are generally evident. Much research flounders because of the difficulties of finding large groups of patients with similar symptoms, a lack of resources (time, personnel and money) or an absence of clear statistical analysis which is often compounded by initial confusions in the methodological approach.

In this approach each person serves as his or her own control. Effective treatments are linked with specific patient characteristics which are immediately relevant to the clinician and the patient. Any decisions about the design of the trial, and the choice of outcome measures, can be made with the patient.[14] It is this practical cooperation which makes these designs favourable for complementary practitioners. The primary focus of the research is upon the treatment benefit for the individual, whereas conventional studies are more concerned with changes in groups of patients. A weakness of single case designs is that, while individual change is specific, it is difficult to argue for a general validity of the treatment.

Randomized single case designs

The first step in this approach is to identify the target behaviour. This can be a symptom or physical sign, a result of a test, or an indicator suggested by the patient. This is negotiated with the patient and is understood by both clinician and patient as being appropriate and relevant to the patient's wellbeing or clinical improvement. A critical feature of this target behaviour is that it will be susceptible to rapid improvement when therapy begins.

This target behaviour then becomes the *baseline* measure in an initial period of observation, which is sometimes called the 'A' phase. The intention of this phase is to enable a stable pattern or trend to emerge. This is based on the natural frequency of the symptoms. Any treatment effects can then be seen clearly in contrast to this baseline. Barlow and Hersen[15] recommend a minimum of three observation points in a given period of time.

It is important that the method of measuring the observed behaviour is specified accurately. There can of course be more than one form of assessment; the clinician may want to rely upon physiological, immuno-logical or biochemical markers while the patient may devise a self-report index. Apart from its clinical value, the choice of measure has a secondary research value. If the case study is to be part of a systematic research approach, the measure will need to be replicable. Similarly, if the research is also intended to speak to other practitioners it is important to develop a measure which they can validate.

The development of a specific evaluative index,[5,19−21] or battery of tests, is an important task which challenges the clinician to relate theory to clinical practice. The main requirement of such an index is that it will be sensitive to change over time and will include all the clinically important effects. It is important to be able to link those clinical changes to the treatment.

The next step is to introduce the agreed treatment variable. There can be multiple treatment courses during this period, and these can include placebo. In the randomized case design these treatment courses are randomly assigned. This design is strengthened by the possibility for the patient and the clinician to be blind to the treatment variable if a medicament is used. Where the patient and clinician cannot be blind to the treatment intervention, an external assessor can be blind to the treatment period. Such an external assessor can also act as a monitor of the trial and halt it if it is in the best interests of the patient.

An important feature of these methods is that they are flexible without losing rigour. A multi-cross-over model has been developed[22] which is only partly randomized but there are regular interchanges between treatment periods with active drug and placebo. Such a trial is evaluated on the number of times the active drug is associated with fewer symptoms than the placebo period(s).

Single case experimental designs

Where the treatment variables cannot be randomized, single case experimental designs are used. The intention is to stay as close to experimental method as possible with an assessor blind to the treatment phase.

The initial baseline 'A' period is followed by a treatment period, 'B'. This is an improvement on the case history in that it offers comparative data in two clear phases. This design can be extended by an additional assessment 'A' phase. There are problems here in that a decision about when to stop treatment has to be made, and the treatment may not be continued to conclusion. This is compounded by the difficulty of ending on a 'no treatment' phase.

If a further treatment period is introduced, then an 'A-B-A-B' design occurs. The intention in these designs is to keep the length of the treatment phases identical.[22]

These designs can become quite complex. An example of an 'A-C-A-B-C-B-C-B' design is demonstrated by Rose.[23] The 'A' phase refers to the baseline phase of the behaviour of a girl on a particular diet which contained no artificial flavours or colours, and no natural salicylates. The 'B' phase was another type of baseline and involved the introduction of an oatmeal biscuit which contained no additives. The 'C' phase included the introduction of an oatmeal biscuit which contained an artificial yellow dye. This biscuit appeared to be the same as the other biscuit. The girl's behaviour was then observed by her parents and others who were blind to the introduction of the biscuit containing artificial colouring. In the 'C' phases of the experiment the girl became hyperactive, leading to the author concluding that artificial colouring led to her hyperactivity.

A further elaboration of this method is to introduce composite treatments. Parts of the treatment can then be omitted or included systematically. For example, after the baseline data is gathered, 'A', then a composite treatment is administered, 'BC'. This could be a treatment which included manipulation of the body and a medicament. In the following phase the medicament could be withdrawn, the 'B' phase. The next phase returns to the composite treatment. This then becomes an 'A-BC-B-BC' design.

These composite designs are particularly useful when the practitioner–patient relationship is assumed to be a significant part of the treatment.

Multiple baseline designs have been used to test some psychological behaviour approaches.[15,24-26] The treatment variable stays the same, but there are multiple baseline target behaviours of differing duration. Ideally these target behaviours are specific and independent.

The application of the treatment variable is staggered. First, after assessment, the treatment is applied to one particular target behaviour. If the target behaviours are independent then the chosen target behaviour will change and the others remain stable. The behaviours are constantly monitored. Then the treatment variable is also applied to a second target behaviour which should demonstrate a change at the onset of therapy. This treatment may be administered by another therapist. The other target variables continue to be monitored and treated in turn.

Clinical applications

As might be expected of research methods that were developed from the field of psychology, the majority of the clinical literature has its origin in psychological or psychotherapeutic applications[4,8,27-30] (see Table 12.1).

Single case studies have been used to assess the impact of behaviour therapy for the treatment of mental handicap,[31] epileptic seizures,[32] infantile autism,[33,34] obsessive ruminations and compulsive behaviour,[35,36] delusional experiences,[37] neurotic patients,[38] pain,[39] depression,[4] agoraphobia and panic disorders,[40] anxiety-based disorders,[41] and multiple personality disorder.[42] They lend themselves well to individual problems where diagnostic categories are broad yet symptoms are idiosyncratic, and where it is necessary to combine both behavioural and existential considerations.[43]

These techniques are also seen as useful for encouraging structured learning. Milne[44] used single case designs to introduce behaviour therapy techniques and skills to nurses. With their emphasis on methodological awareness[39] and formal experimental decisions while retaining the patient as the primary focus of research, these methods are particularly useful for teaching and developing research methods.[45]

Table 12.1 Single case investigations of psychological problems

Psychological and psychotherapeutic applications	Arnold, 1989; Goth, 1985; Kazdin, 1983; Tracey, 1985; Wilson, 1984; Wilson, 1987
Mental handicap	Hoefkens, 1990
Epilepsy	Brown, 1989
Infantile autism	Bernard-Opitz, 1989; Gillberg, 1984
Compulsive behaviour	Salkovskis, 1983; Salkovskis, 1989
Delusional experience	Brett-Jones, 1987
Neurosis	Kockott, 1983
Depression	Goth, 1985
Panic disorders	Cottraux, 1984
Anxiety	Hayes, 1983
Multiple personality	Coons, 1986
Structured learning	Milne, 1984

In more recent years, the field of neurology has also developed these single case approaches (see Table 12.2). In assessing the cognitive competence of patients following brain injury, and the effects of therapeutic interventions intended to remedy the effects of injury, it has been important to develop specific, often idiosyncratic, indices and treatment plans. These methods have been applied to the study of amnesia,[46] echolalia,[47] aphasia,[48] apraxia and alexia,[30] problems after stroke,[49] attentional difficulties[50] after brain injury and memory problems.[51]

The study of individual brain-damaged persons has also led to inferences about normal cognitive functions,[52,53] although the validity of these assumptions has been challenged.[54] The reasoning behind this challenge reflects both the strength and the weakness of this approach;

Table 12.2 Single case investigations of neurological problems

Echolalia	Diesfeldt, 1986
Aphasia	Karanth, 1988
Apraxia and alexia	Wilson, 1987
Problems after stroke	Edmans, 1989
Attentional difficulties	Gray, 1989
Brain injury and memory problems	McLean, 1987
Normal cognitive functions	Caramazza, 1986; McCloskey, 1986; Marshall, 1984

namely, while arguing for the specific validity as applied to individual patients, it is not acceptable to argue for a generalized validity as applied to the group. However, twelve patients were studied using single case designs to see how they coped with the stress of being diagnosed as having breast cancer.[55] This design used standardized diaries during the first 90 days after diagnosis and surgery to obtain a multivariate description of individual mood states and coping responses. By using such a time-based approach which evaluates different modes of coping, it is possible to propose specific intervention strategies for individuals, albeit with a common problem. The secret lies in understanding what is common to the methodological approach and what is specific to the treatment intervention, what is common to the overall problem and what is specific to the individual patient in the way in which they respond to such problems. Unfortunately, many arguments revolve around either the group or the individual without realizing that there are intermediate levels; i.e. not all individuals behave idiosyncratically, or all the same, and there may be clusters of common responses.

Diary and calendar recording

Although a research approach in itself, the patient diary can also be part of the evaluative index mentioned in the previous approaches. The patient diary is rather a catch-all term in that some researchers will collect daily data according to specific rating scales. These could be more appropriately termed calendar methods. An extension of daily rating and subjective commentary would be appropriately called a diary. The detailed daily recording of patient commentaries involving introspective accounts may be likened to a journal and is the least formal, in experimental terms, of the three approaches mentioned here.

In diary studies the principal collector of data is the patient. One of the tasks of research scientists working in the field of clinical practice is to learn what happens in the context of the patient's daily life and to make some attempt to dicover how his or her problem impinges upon his or her daily routine. Similarly, it is important to discover who in the family of that person is involved at the time of onset of the symptoms and in the management of those symptoms. The use of subjects making their own assessments of symptomatology is not new,[16] and offers a non-intrusive means of gathering data. Perhaps as significantly, the diary also offers the patient a neutral stance whereby the symptoms are assessed methodically and in accordance with a particular framework designed to be ultimately beneficial.

Health care diaries have been used to discern the content of clinical practice with all its diversity of complaints and problems.[56–59] Most symptom episodes are transient and limited in extent.[60,61] Retrospective interviews cannot provide sufficient or precise data about the events which precede the onset of symptoms or the details of the management of such episodes.

The use of diaries has several advantages. First, there is the opportunity to provide a daily scoring which eliminates recall error and in general produces consistent reporting. Second, there is a comprehensive view of the person's health and the relational context of that health status *vis à vis* other family members.[62] Third, symptoms are treated as episodes rather than static events.[63,64] Fourth, diffuse conditions are included which may not be disabling or necessitate intervention but which contribute to the profile of the patient's symptomatology.

A benefit of using calendar and diary methods is also one of the drawbacks. The data is rich and varied but this can cause problems for analysis, i.e. there can be too much data. Furthermore, patients can become sensitized to their own problems and hence concentrate more and more on those problems. This is a confounding factor for single case research designs in general where the research process itself becomes a treatment variable. However, for discovering what a patient considers to be important about the treatment process, diary methods are very useful.

Diary applications

Diary methods have been applied in several broad approaches (see Table 12.3). First, they are not always single case specific and can be used in clinical controlled trials.[65–73] The benefit they bring to clinical trials is that they can be used to study a subpopulation of a large group for assessing validity and reliability,[74] and for assessing quality of life.[75,76]

Table 12.3 Diary applications

Use in clinical controlled trials	Burkhardt, 1983; Gandolfo, 1987; Grammer, 1987; Guyatt, 1988; Horan, 1990; Johnston, 1988; Prida, 1987; Richter, 1987; Sinaki, 1989
Assessing validity	Toporoff, 1990
Assessing quality of life	Aaronson, 1989; Oleske, 1990
Alcohol problems	Blose, 1987; Brenner, 1987; Cole-Hamilton, 1986; Corti, 1990; de Castro, 1990; de Castro, 1990; Epperlein, 1987; Fauske, 1990; Griffin, 1986; Griffin, 1987; Gruchow, 1983; Heller, 1988; Hilton, 1989; Hilton, 1989; Matthews, 1987; Muller, 1989; Sellers, 1988; Skog, 1986; Starrin, 1990
Allergy	Chu, 1989; Creticos, 1989; Ferguson, 1988; Gong, 1988; Grammer, 1987; Horan, 1990; Joad, 1986; Kjellman, 1986; Meltzer, 1988; Osur, 1989; Pierson, 1988; Schatz, 1988; Shirakawa, 1988; Spector, 1986; Tinkelman, 1990
Asthma	Aldridge, 1987; Ferguson, 1988; Gong, 1988; Gregg, 1985; Gustafsson, 1986; Janson, 1990; Joad, 1986; Katz, 1986; Lebowitz, 1987; Meltzer, 1988; Rachelefsky, 1986; Schatz, 1988; Schwartz, 1990; Shirakawa, 1988; Spector, 1986; Stafford, 1988; Tinkelman, 1990

Table 12.3 – *cont.*

Cancer	Aldridge, 1988; Feinstein, 1966; Forbes, 1987; Lavigne, 1986; Love, 1989; Oleske, 1990; Robinson, 1989; Rose, 1987; Toporoff, 1990; Wittig, 1989
Diet and nutrition	Allison, 1986; Bandini, 1990; Boyd, 1988; Brewer, 1988; Cole-Hamilton, 1986; Cotugna, 1990; Cugini, 1987; Cuppari, 1989; Dietrich, 1988; Dunbar, 1986; Frenkiel, 1986; Haymes, 1989; Heaney, 1990; Heller, 1988; Huss-Ashmore, 1989; Jackson, 1986; Jones, 1986; Kindstedt-Arfwidson, 1988; King, 1988; Krall, 1987; Laidlaw, 1988; Levine, 1989; Lindsay, 1986; Lissner, 1988; Marable, 1988; Parker, 1988; Rose, 1987; Rubenstein, 1989; Rush, 1988; Salomon, 1990; Saudek, 1989; Shutler, 1989; Stevens, 1989; Toporoff, 1990; Wing, 1986; Witschi, 1987; de Castro, 1990; Grimm, 1990; Ho, 1988; Kamat, 1987; Kaplan, 1989; Schweiger, 1988
Heart disease	Barry, 1988; Crake, 1987; Hougham, 1989; Hougham, 1989; Mahapatra, 1987; O'Keefe, 1987; Prida, 1987; Quyyumi, 1987; Sharma, 1988; Simon, 1989; Sklar, 1989; Stone, 1988; Uusitalo, 1986; Vetrovec, 1986; Anastasiades, 1990; Brenner, 1987; Dalton, 1986; Forbes, 1987; Freeman, 1987; Gruchow, 1983; Halberg, 1989; Heller, 1988; Helman, 1987; Isolauri, 1986; Kalkwarf, 1989; Lambert, 1989; LeBlanc, 1986; Lindemans, 1986; Lynch, 1977; Margraf, 1987; Reynolds, 1989; Schulz, 1989; Walker, 1979; Walker, 1982
Stress	Barry, 1988; Bentzen, 1989; Bolger, 1989; Chapar, 1988; Cooney, 1986; Cooper, 1987; Dimsdale, 1988; Dooley, 1989; Freeman, 1987; Fukui, 1987; Griffin, 1986; Griffin, 1987; Hicks, 1987; Kiernan, 1989; Kirsch, 1987; Laessle, 1987; Love, 1989; Magos, 1986; Milton, 1987; Neugebauer, 1989; Nulty, 1987; Prior, 1987; Realini, 1990; Sampson, 1989; Schweiger, 1988; Scott, 1990; Verbrugge, 1989; Ward, 1983; Wilson, 1990; Wittig, 1989; Zastowny, 1986
Sleep disturbance	Alward, 1990; Barry, 1988; Davies, 1986; Fry, 1986; Hicks, 1987; Hoelscher, 1988; Janson, 1990; Kirsch, 1987; Meuleman, 1987; Milton, 1987; Minors, 1989; Moller, 1989; Morin, 1989;

Table 12.3 – *cont.*

	Otsuka, 1990; Renfrew, 1987; Reynolds, 1989; Robinson, 1989; Scott, 1990; Stanton, 1989; Weissman, 1989; Winer, 1990
Menopause	Buckley, 1989; Sinaki, 1989; Griffin, 1986; Lissner, 1988; Smith, 1987

Second, they are applicable for particular complex clinical problems which may also have psychological and social implications; alcohol abuse,[77–95] allergy,[67,69,96–108] asthma,[98–100,102,105–7] cancer,[39,55,74,76,118–123] diet and nutrition,[74,79,82,88,123–160] heart disease,[71,78,87,88,120,161–189] stress,[6,55,85,86,121,160,161,176,190–212] sleep disturbance[112,122,161,186,198,200,202,208,213–225] and menopause.[73,85,145,226–228] These methods, with their emphasis on contextual details, have also been widely applied to the study of children.[33,34,39,98,101,103,111,115,124,139,149,156,159,192,194,197,212,229–243]

Third, the patient diary in clinical practice has been found to be adaptable for patient reports and specific measures. Morin[220] investigated the clinical efficacy of a behavioural management programme for treating insomnia secondary to chronic pain. Treatment consisted of a combination of stimulus control and sleep restriction procedures. Daily sleep diaries and all-night polysomnographic measures were used to document changes in sleep/wake patterns.

Writing pain journals, for example, serves several purposes for both the patient and the practitioner.[244] Diaries reveal feelings and experiences on a subjective level, and information about medications, pain duration and other factual information on an objective level. The benefits can be immediate and therapeutic, or retrospectively useful to the patients.

There have been criticisms of diaries; for instance, that not all subjects are totally objective in their reporting of medication use,[107] and that it is sometimes difficult to relate diary material (including symptoms) to objective measures.[245] In an attempt to counteract such discrepancies, computerized methods have been used with some effect to improve and simplify diary methods,[99,107,137,182,246] but these are generally restricted to clearly defined measurable data sets of physiological variables. As in all research methods, it is necessary to discern the appropriate form of data collection methods for the study in hand.

Finally, diaries provide an opportunity to see the way in which problems develop over time and the way in which treatment initiatives can influence such developments. When studying complex chronic problems, the chronological information also illustrates how psychological or social factors enhance or complicate the clinical picture.[81,82,112,128,135,211,247,248,249,250]

Statistical analysis

In single case designs there are possibilities for a statistical analysis of each single study.[1,14,251] However, the main appeal of working in this way is that daily measures are plotted on a chart and can be seen by eye.[252,253] Clinical improvement can also be assessed by reports from the patient and various persons connected with the patient (spouses, relatives, experts) who can also suggest that the change is of applied significance. Statistical analysis can be used where subtle significant changes occur in the data which are not immediately visually apparent, or where many variables are collected from an individual and need to be correlated one with another.

The most familiar tests are the *t* and F test depending on the number of different conditions or phases. The main difficulty in applying these tests is an artefact of the research design itself. The collection of data over time may mean that the data is serially dependent. Serial dependence occurs when successive observations in a time series are correlated, and this dependence seriously violates the premise of analysis of variance. It is necessary in these studies to test data for auto-correlation.

If the data is serially dependent then it is possible to perform a *time series analysis* of the data. This provides a *t* test and important information about the different characteristics of behaviour change across phases. Such time series analysis requires large samples of data points to select the processes within the series itself.

A difficulty which can arise in single case studies is when they are used following a period of standard treatment which has not worked. Some general improvement may occur which is nothing to do with the treatment being used but is a 'regression towards the mean', i.e. the tendency of an extreme value to be closer to the mean on remeasurement. This can be overcome by including a wash-out period between the treatments. Such a period would serve to establish the patient's eligibility for the trial. Following this there would be a set of measurements which would be considered as the baseline data.

The consistent recording of longitudinal multiple data in these studies requires great perseverance on behalf of the collector and the patient. This is mitigated by the sample size of one. Any systematic replication needs to bear in mind this necessity for perseverance and patient compliance before a multicentre study is carried out. There may be a temptation by some researchers to lump together single case designs and treat them as a group. To do so contains all the pitfalls of *post hoc* hypothesizing, loses the primary advantage of individual consideration and means handling vast amounts of often disparate data. It is vitally important that the research design is clearly thought out before the research begins.

The application of time series analysis

Time series analysis is a developing field. In particular, methods have been developed which allow for missing data, and also do not require that data be collected at precisely equal intervals. A problem of clinical data collection is that it is not always feasible to take measures at the same time each day, and when it is possible, this data may not reflect the chronobiological status of the subject in terms of circadian rhythmicity. However, recent methods do expect that data has a deterministic cycle within a known period.[221,254,255,256,257,258]

The monitoring of single patients using time series analysis has been emphasized in clinical cardiology. A marked circadian rhythm in the frequency of myocardial infarction and sudden death has been observed,[221] as has close coupling between variation in heart rate and ambulatory ischaemia in patients with severe coronary artery disease,[181] and recurrent ischaemic attack subject to seasonal pattern.[259]

It is this ability to search for patterns over varying time periods[182] which is the strength of time series analysis; i.e. time itself is treated as an important variable. For patients with chronic problems, it is these

Table 12.4 Statistical analysis of rhythmical fluctuation

Cyclical variation	Berman, 1981; Lentz, 1990; Minors, 1988; Otsuka, 1990; Taylor, 1990; Teicher, 1990
Myocardial infarction and sudden death	Otsuka, 1990
Coronary artery disease	Lambert, 1989
Recurrent ischaemic attack	Fersini, 1987
Foetal heart rate	Dalton, 1986
Patterns of muscle activity	Gianutsos, 1986; Graupe, 1985; Moss, 1983; Sigge, 1988
Stress profiles	Cooney, 1986
Cognitive stressors	Ward, 1983
Short and long-term blood pressure monitoring	Cugini, 1987; Halberg, 1989
Energy consumption and the menstrual cycle	Lissner, 1988
Growth hormone release	Togo, 1988; Asplin, 1989; Hartman, 1990; Hindmarsh, 1988; Ho, 1988; Winer, 1990
Insulin secretion	Moran, 1987; O'Rahilly, 1988
Thyrotrophin and cortisol release	Wheatley, 1989 Vance, 1989
Correlation with plasma lipids	Desoye, 1987

patterns of changes involving multiple variables over time which are the key to understanding therapeutic change, or the lack of it. Time series analysis of stress profiles,[193] for example, permits statistical conclusions to be made on the stress profile of a single individual, thereby providing an objective basis for treatment decisions.

The analysis of time series data has led to an understanding of changes in individual physiology (see Table 12.4). Such studies include the monitoring of foetal heart rate rhythms,[175] patterns of muscle activity,[24,260–262] short[129] and long-term blood pressure monitoring,[177] and epinephrine and norepinephrine responses to cognitive stressors.[210]

In addition, many hormones are secreted as periodic impulses or oscillations and the discernment of the attributes of these oscillations is of clinical importance. A variety of studies has developed ways of assessing this rhythmic fluctuation in terms of energy consumption and the menstrual cycle,[145] adolescent growth spurt[263] and growth hormone release in general,[157,225,235,264,265] insulin secretion,[266,267] thyrotrophin[268] and cortisol[269] release, and correlations of hormones with plasma lipids.[270] With the ability to monitor and analyse multiple variables collected over time from the same patient, we have the possibility to strengthen the evidence for therapeutic interventions which claim to influence these regulatory mechanisms, and to correlate changes in subsystems one with another; and, using single case experimental designs, relate those changes to particular treatment interventions.

Conclusion

The disadvantages of these single case approaches are as follows:

In the main, these approaches are inappropriate for the *comparison* of 'global' treatments. An example of a 'global' treatment is psychotherapy, or a natural medicine approach which includes a plant extract, an organ extract, a change in diet and medication. However, single case approaches are important tools for discerning what are the active ingredients in a 'global' treatment, and for discerning individual treatment strategies.[8,43]

There can be carry-over effects from one therapeutic phase to another. The therapeutic effect of the first treatment may persist during the administration of the second treatment. This can be mitigated by including a delay between treatment periods. However, some preparations may stay in the body for a long time. In such cases it may be necessary to consider multiple baseline studies in several patients. This moves away from the true single case design and a group design may be more appropriate.

Other treatments may produce an irreversible effect. For example, there may be a change in patient attitude, a change in circumstance or a clinical insight on the part of the patient. These changes are problematical in any research. Patients cannot be inhibited from reflecting upon their own lives. The use of single case research designs, by concentrating on symptomatic relief and the possibility of immediate observable improvement, may itself promote clinical insights.[271]

Perhaps the major criteria for using a single case design are that the treatment should exert its effect in a moderately short time, and the effect will be temporary and reversible once treatment is discontinued. If not, then a group design must be considered. These single case methods are generally reliant upon a stable baseline period in the 'A' phase. This means that they are not particularly relevant to acute or labile problems. They are appropriate for chronic problems, or patterns of recurring behaviour which have become stable over time.

The advantages of these single case research designs are their flexibility of approach, the opportunity to include differing levels of rigour and the emphasis on providing the best clinical care for the individual patient. Such designs are appropriate for practitioners wishing to introduce research into their own practice, and particularly for developing hypotheses which may be submitted for other methods of clinical validation at a later date.[253,272] As a teaching tool they bridge the gap between general principles and clinical practice. The clinician is encouraged to fit particular knowledge into a broader context of scientific principles. Occasionally these principles are challenged by particular clinical instances. To detract from such singular empirical observation is folly as it makes claims for scientific knowledge which science as a discipline of knowing itself finds inadmissible. Ideally scientific knowledge is always provisional and open to refutation.

Furthermore, with the development of statistical methods suitable for the monitoring of subjective, rhythmic or episodic data, which is not dependent upon the collection of equally spaced recording and which provides a method which can not only detect change but also discriminate between those changes[221,252,255,258] even when they occur in the 'normal' range, clinicians have an opportunity to further validate their clinical finding. What we must keep in mind is that the pattern of reactivity in the individual is something like a weather pattern; it constantly changes, never achieving a steady state.[273] This analysis is pertinent to the individual in that they are always compared to their own individual physiology.

If the clinician does need to relate this individualized data to other forms of research then it is possible to make a prognosis from the baseline data and clinical history comparative with group statistics; e.g. survival data utilizing cancer site and staging. This prognosis can be made blind to the patient and practitioner using an expert external assessor and the progress of the individual patient then compared with a group trend. It is possible then to assess individual patients according to precise survival statistics where available, and to have an external individual assessor who can also make a clinical prognosis from expert knowledge. A group of single case studies of individual patients who are individually treated with a particular common approach and assessed according to standardized outcome measures can then be compared with their individualized expert prognoses and group survival statistics. Individualized treatment is thereby retained but incorporated within a larger framework of knowledge. If these individuals can then be matched with other patients who are treated at another clinic, fulfilling the same entrance criteria of site, staging and spread, then a further level of rigour is added.

Coda

The development of a bureau which could provide research advice and coordinate research activities seems to be a necessary next step in developing a coherent national research strategy. This can then be extended throughout Europe such that other international partners can cooperate in coherent research endeavours. This will foster a climate of research cooperation while raising the standard of clinical research itself.

A necessary factor in the development of these single case research methods, and in the whole development of clinical research methodology, will be the development of clinical trials design software and the appropriate statistical computing methods. This means the development of information technology in cooperation with the development of research methodology. Both information technology and clinical trials methodology are encompassed within the context of a cooperative scientific community which will need financial resources. Such resources are dependent upon long-term strategies within a European context, the development of which will depend upon individual national lobbies.

It is imperative that we develop:

1 a central research agency for the consultation, coordination and analysis of single case designs, preferably with connections in other European countries. This would include cooperating professionals from varying institutions. Such an agency would then coordinate research initiatives in smaller institutions, give advice and support on research methods, and help with the analysis of data;

2 methods of data acquisition, statistical research, statistical analysis and data presentation suitable for clinicians to use in their daily practice;

3 criteria for the establishment of standardized baselines according to clinical parameters;

4 data suitable for the establishment of prognostic variables; and a panel of external expert assessors;

5 life quality scales and health status instruments sensitive to change according to various chronic clinical problems.

References

[1] Barlow, D. H., Hersen, M. *Single Case Experimental Designs: Strategies for Studying Behaviour Change.* New York: Pergamon Press, 1984.

2   Kazdin, A. *Research Design in Clinical Psychology*. New York: Harper and Row, 1980.

3   Kazdin, A. *Single Case Research Designs: Methods for Clinical and Applied Settings*. New York: OUP, 1982.

4   Goth, N. Single case studies in clinical psychology and medicine. *Z Arztl Fortbild Jena* 1985; **79**(22): 973–6.

5   Crane, D. Single-case experimental designs in family therapy research: limitations and considerations. *Fam Process* 1985; **24**(1): 69–77.

6   Laessle, R. Course-oriented single-case studies in clinical practice – methodology and examples for use. *Psychiatr Neurol Med Psychol Leipz* 1987; **39**(7): 385–98.

7   Schroeder, H., Wildman, B. Single case designs in clinical settings. *Hosp J* 1988; **4**(4): 3–24.

8   Wilson, G., Bornstein, P. Paradoxical procedures and single-case methodology: review and recommendations. *J Behav Ther Exp Psychiatry* 1984; **15**(3): 195–203.

9   Hunter, K. Anecdotes in medicine. *Perspect Biol Med* 1986; **29**(4): 619–30.

10 Hunter, K. A Science of individuals: medicine and casuistry. *J Med Philosophy* 1989; **14**: 193–212.

11 Simpson, R., Griggs, T. Case reports and medical progress. *Perspect Biol Med* 1985; **28**(3): 403–5.

12 Guyatt, G., Satchett, D., Taylor, D., Chong, J., Roberts, R., Pugsley, S. Determining optimal therapy randomized trials in individual patients. *New Eng J Med* 1986; **314**: 889–92.

13 Louis, T., Lavori, P., Bailar, J., Polansky, M. Cross-over and self-controlled trials in clinical research. *New Eng J Med* 1984; **310**: 24–31.

14 McLeod, R., Taylor, D., Cohen, Z., Cullen, J. Single patient randomised clinical trials. *Lancet* 1986; **29**: 726–8.

15 Barlow, D., Hersen, M., Jackson, M. Single-case experimental designs. *Arch Gen Psychiat* 1973; **23**: 319–25.

16 Murray, J. The use of health care diaries in the field of psychiatric illness in general practice. *Psychol Med* 1985; **11**: 551–60.

17 Aldridge, D., Pietroni, P. Research trials in general practice: towards a focus on clinical practice. *Fam Prac* 1987; **4**: 311–15.

18 Wulff, H. Single case studies. An introduction. *Scand J Gastroenterol Suppl* 1988; **147**: 7–10.

19 Anthony, H., Parsons, F. Why measure outcomes? *Comp Med Res* 1988; **2**(3): 1–12.

20 Anthony, H. Measuring differences between individuals – medical measurements. *Comp Med Res* 1987; **2**(1): 82–93.

21   Kirshner, B., Guyatt, G. A methodological framework for assessing health indices. *J Chron Dis* 1985; **38**: 27–36.

22   Johannessen, T., Fosstvedt, D., Petersen, H. Experience with a multi-crossover model in dyspepsia. *Scand J Gastroenterol Suppl* 1988; **147**: 33–7.

23   Rose, T. The functional relationship between artificial food colors and hyperactivity. *J Appl Behav Anal* 1978; **11**: 439–46.

24   Gianutsos, J., Eberstein, A., Krasilovsky, G., Ragnarsson, K., Goodgold, J. Visually displayed EMG feedback: single case studies of hemiplegic upper extremity rehabilitation. *Cent Nerv Syst Trauma* 1986; **3**(1): 63–76.

25   Murphy, R., Doughty, N., Nunes, D. Multi-element designs: an alternative to reversal and multi-element evaluative strategies. *Ment Retard* 1979; **17**: 23–27.

26   Robertson, I., Gray, J., McKenzie, S. Microcomputer-based cognitive rehabilitation of visual neglect: three multiple-baseline single-case studies. *Brain Inj* 1988; **2**(2): 151–63.

27   Arnold, E., Grawe, K. Descriptive single case analyses – a strategy for studying effectiveness correlations in psychotherapy. *Z Klin Psychol Psychopathol Psychother* 1989; **37**(3): 262–76.

28   Kazdin, A. Single-case research designs in clinical child psychiatry. *J Am Acad Child Psychiat* 1983; **22**(5): 423–32.

29   Tracey, T. The N of 1 Markov chain design as a means of studying the stages of psychotherapy. *Psychiatry* 1985; **48**(2): 196–204.

30   Wilson, B. Single-case experimental designs in neuropsychological rehabilitation. *J Clin Exp Neuropsychol* 1987; **9**(5): 527–44.

31   Hoefkens, A., Allen, D. Evaluation of a special behaviour unit for people with mental handicaps and challenging behaviour. *J Ment Defic Res* 1990; **34**(3): 213–28 (discussion 229–35).

32   Brown, S., Fenwick, P. Evoked and psychogenic epileptic seizures: II. Inhibition. *Acta Neurol Scand* 1989; **80**(6): 541–7.

33   Bernard-Opitz, V., Roos, K., Blesch, G. Using computers with autistic handicapped children. *Z Kinder Jugenpsychiatr* 1989; **17**(3): 125–30.

34   Gillberg, C., Winnergard, I., Wahlstrom, J. The sex chromosomes – one key to autism? An XYY case of infantile autism. *Appl Res Ment Retard* 1984; **5**(3): 353–60.

35   Salkovskis, P. Treatment of an obsessional patient using habituation to audiotaped ruminations. *Br J Clin Psychol* 1983; **22**(Pt 4): 311–3.

36   Salkovskis, P., Westbrook, D. Behaviour therapy and obsessional ruminations: can failure be turned into success? *Behav Res Ther* 1989; **27**(2): 149–60.

37   Brett-Jones, J., Garety, P., Hemsley, D. Measuring delusional

experiences: a method and its application. *Br J Clin Psychol* 1987; **26**(Pt 4): 257–65.

38 Kockott, G. Behavior therapy in sex deviations – an orienting overview. *Psychiatr Prax* 1983; **10**(3): 78–82.

39 Lavigne, J., Schulein, M., Hahn, Y. Psychological aspects of painful medical conditions in children. II. Personality factors, family characteristics and treatment. *Pain* 1986; **27**(2): 147–69.

40 Cottraux, J. Agoraphobia and panic attacks. Biological and behavioral approaches. *Encephale* 1984; **10**(1): 13–19.

41 Haves, S., Hussian, R., Turner, A., Anderson, N., Grubb, T. The effect of coping with statements on progress through a desensitization hierarchy. *J Behav Ther Exp Psychiat* 1983; **14**(2): 117–29.

42 Coons, P. Treatment progress in 20 patients with multiple personality disorder. *J Nerv Ment Dis* 1986; **174**(12): 715–21.

43 Butcher, P. Existential-behaviour therapy: a possible paradigm? *Br J Med Psychol* 1984; **57**(Pt 3): 265–74.

44 Milne, D. The development and evaluation of a structured learning format introduction to behaviour therapy for psychiatric nurses. *Br J Clin Psychol* 1984; **23**(Pt 3): 175–85.

45 Aldridge, D. Research strategies in a hospital setting. *Comp Med Res* 1989; **3**(2): 20–24.

46 Warrington, E., McCarthy, R. The fractionation of retrograde amnesia. *Brain Cogn* 1988; **7**(2): 184–200.

47 Diesfeldt, H. A psycholinguistic study in a patient with echolalia. *Tijdschr Gerontol Geriatr* 1986; **17**(5): 191–200.

48 Karanth, P., Rangamani, G. Crossed aphasia in multilinguals. *Brain Lang* 1988; **34**(1): 169–80.

49 Edmans, J., Lincoln, N. Treatment of visual perceptual deficits after stroke: four single case studies. *Int Disabil Stud* 1989; **11**(1): 25–33.

50 Gray, J., Robertson, I. Remediation of attentional difficulties following brain injury: three experimental single case studies. *Brain Inj* 1989; **3**(2): 163–70.

51 McLean, A. J., Stanton, K., Cardenas, D., Bergerud, D. Memory training combined with the use of oral physostigmine. *Brain Inj* 1987; **1**(2): 145–59.

52 Caramazza. A. On drawing inferences about the structure of normal cognitive systems from the analysis of patterns of impaired performance: the case for single-patient studies. *Brain Cogn* 1986; **5**(1): 41–66.

53 McCloskey, M., Sokol, S., Goodman, R. Cognitive processes in verbal-number production: inferences from the performance of brain-damaged subjects. *J Exp Psychol Gen* 1986; **115**(4): 307–30.

[54] Marshall, J., Newcombe, F. Putative problems and pure progress in neuropsychological single-case studies. *J Clin Neuropsychol* 1984; **6**(1): 65–70.

[55] Wittig, R. Adjustment, stress and coping with stress in breast cancer. Results of single case studies. *Z Klin Psychol Psychopathol Psychother* 1989; **37**(3): 303–16.

[56] Beresford, S., Walker, J., Banks, M., Wale, C. Why do women consult doctors? Social factors and the use of the general practitioner. *Br J Soc Prev Med* 1977; **31**: 220–26.

[57] Scambler, A., Scambler, G., Craig, D. Kinship and friendship networks and women's demand for primary care. *J Roy Coll Gen Pract* 1981; **31**: 746–50

[58] Freer, C. Self care: a health diary study. *Med Care* 1980; **18**: 853–61.

[59] Robinson, D. *The Process of Becoming Ill.* London: Routledge and Kegan Paul, 1971.

[60] Dunnell, K., Cartwright, A. *Medicine-takers, Prescribers and Hoarders.* London: Routledge and Kegan Paul, 1972.

[61] Horder, J., Horder, E. Illness in general practice. *Practitioner* 1954; **173**: 177–85.

[62] Monck, E., Dobbs, R. Measuring life events in an adolescent population: methodological issues and related findings. *Psychol Med* 1985; **15**: 841–50.

[63] Aldridge, D., Rossiter, J. Difficult patients, intractable symptoms and spontaneous recovery in suicidal behaviour. *J Syst Strat Ther* 1985; **4**: 66–76.

[64] Aldridge, D., Rossiter, J. A strategic assessment of deliberate self harm. *J Fam Ther* 1984; **6**: 119–32.

[65] Burkhardt, R., Kienle, G. Basic problems in controlled trials. *J Med Ethics* 1983; **9**: 80–84.

[66] Gandolfo, J., Farthing, M., Powers, G., Eagen, K., Goldberg, M., Berman, P., Kaplan, M. 4-Aminosalicylic acid retention enemas in treatment of distal colitis. *Dig Dis Sci* 1987; **32**(7): 700–4.

[67] Grammer, L., Shaughnessy, M., Bernhard, M., Finkle, S., Pyle, H., Silvestri, L., Patterson, R. The safety and activity of polymerized ragweed: a double-blind, placebo-controlled trial in 81 patients with ragweed rhinitis. *J Allergy Clin Immunol* 1987; **80**(2): 177–83.

[68] Guyatt, G., Sackett, D., Adachi, J., Roberts, R., Chong, J., Rosenbloom, D., Keller, J. A clinician's guide for conducting randomized trials in individual patients. *Can Med Assoc J* 1988; **139**(6): 497–503.

[69] Horan, R., Sheffer, A., Austen, K. Cromolyn sodium in the management of systemic mastocytosis. *J Allergy Clin Immunol* 1990; **85**(5): 852–5.

70 Johnston, D., Troyer, I., Whitsett, S. Clomipramine treatment of agoraphobic women. An eight-week controlled trial. *Arch Gen Psychiat* 1988; **45**(5): 453–9.

71 Prida, X., Gelman, J., Feldman, R., Hill, J., Pepine, C., Scott, E. Comparison of diltiazem and nifedipine alone and in combination in patients with coronary artery spasm. *J Am Coll Cardiol* 1987; **9**(2): 412–9.

72 Richter, J., Dalton, C., Bradley, L., Castell, D. Oral nifedipine in the treatment of noncardiac chest pain in patients with the nutcracker esophagus. *Gastroenterology* 1987; **93**(1): 21–8.

73 Sinaki, M., Wahner, H., Offord, K., Hodgson, S. Efficacy of nonloading exercises in prevention of vertebral bone loss in postmenopausal women: a controlled trial. *Mayo Clin Proc* 1989; **64**(7): 762–9.

74 Toporoff, E., Hebert, J. A proxy approach to the determination of total caloric intake for use in cancer epidemiology. *Nutr Cancer* 1990; **13**(1–2): 35–49.

75 Aaronson, N. Quality of life assessment in clinical trials: methodologic issues. *Controlled Clin Trials* 1989; **10**(4 Suppl): 195S–208S.

76 Oleske, D., Heinze, S., Otte, D. The diary as a means of understanding the quality of life of persons with cancer receiving home nursing care. *Cancer Nurs* 1990; **13**(3): 158–66.

77 Blose, J., Holder, H. Liquor-by-the-drink and alcohol-related traffic crashes: a natural experiment using time-series analysis. *J Stud Alcohol* 1987; **48**(1): 52–60.

78 Brenner, M. Economic change, alcohol consumption and heart disease mortality in nine industrialized countries. *Soc Sci Med* 1987; **25**(2): 119–32.

79 Cole-Hamilton, I., Gunner, K., Leverkus, C., Starr, J. A study among dietitians and adult members of their households of the practicalities and implications of following proposed dietary guidelines for the UK. British Dietetic Association Community Nutrition Group Nutrition Guidelines Project. *Hum Nutr Appl Nutr* 1986; **40**(5): 365–89.

80 Corti, B., Binns, C., Howat, P., Blaze Temple, D., Kai-Lo, S. Comparison of 7-day retrospective and prospective alcohol consumption diaries in a female population in Perth, Western Australia – methodological issues. *Br J Addict* 1990; **85**(3): 379–88.

81 de Castro, J., Orozco, S. Moderate alcohol intake and spontaneous eating patterns of humans: evidence of unregulated supplementation. *Am J Clin Nutr* 1990; **52**(2): 246–53.

82 de Castro, J. Social, circadian, nutritional, and subjective correlates of the spontaneous pattern of moderate alcohol intake of normal humans. *Pharmacol Biochem Behav* 1990; **35**(4): 923–31.

[83] Epperlein, T. Initial deterrent effects of the crackdown on drinking drivers in the state of Arizona. *Accid Anal Prev* 1987; **19**(4): 285–303.

[84] Fauske, S., Haug, K., Bovim, G. The process of change – a therapeutic model in alcohol abuse. *Tidsskr Nor Laegeforen* 1990; **110**(14): 1841–4.

[85] Griffin, M., Mendelson, J., Mello, N., Lex, B. Marihuana use across the menstrual cycle. *Drug Alcohol Depend* 1986; **18**(2): 213–24.

[86] Griffin, M., Mello, N., Mendelson, J., Lex, B. Alcohol use across the menstrual cycle among marihuana users. *Alcohol* 1987; **4**(6): 457–62.

[87] Gruchow, H., Rimm, A., Hoffmann, R. Alcohol consumption and ischemic heart disease mortality: are time-series correlations meaningful? *Am J Epidemiol* 1983; **118**(5): 641–50.

[88] Heller, R., O'Connell, D., Roberts, D., Allen, J., Knapp, J., Steele, P., Silove, D. Lifestyle factors in monozygotic and dizygotic twins. *Genet Epidemiol* 1988; **5**(5): 311–21.

[89] Hilton, M. A comparison of a prospective diary and two summary recall techniques for recording alcohol consumption. *Br J Addict* 1989; **84**(9): 1085–92.

[90] Hilton, M. Trends in drinking problems and attitudes in the United States: 1979–1984. *Br J Addict* 1988; **83**(12): 1421–7.

[91] Matthews, R., Scully, C., Levers, B., Hislop, W. Clinical evaluation of benzydamine, chlorhexidine, and placebo mouthwashes in the management of recurrent aphthous stomatitis. *Oral Surg Oral Med Oral Pathol* 1987; **63**(2): 189–91.

[92] Muller, A. Business recession, alcohol consumption, drinking and driving laws: impact on Oklahoma motor vehicle fatalities and fatal crashes. *Am J Public Health* 1989; **79**(10): 1366–70.

[93] Sellers, E., Kadlec, K., Kaplan, H., Naranjo, C. Limitations in the measurement of urine ethanol in clinical trials to monitor ethanol consumption. *J Stud Alcohol* 1988; **49**(6): 567–70.

[94] Skog, O. An analysis of divergent trends in alcohol consumption and economic development. *J Stud Alcohol* 1986; **47**(1): 19–25.

[95] Starrin, B., Larsson, G., Brenner, S., Levi, L., Petterson, I. Structural changes, ill health, and mortality in Sweden, 1963–1983: a macroaggregated study. *Int J Health Serv* 1990; **20**(1): 27–42.

[96] Chu, T., Yamate, M., Biedermann, A., Wolfe, J., Goldsobel, A. Once versus twice daily dosing of terfenadine in the treatment of seasonal allergic rhinitis: US and European studies. *Ann Allergy* 1989; **63**(6, Pt 2): 612–15.

[97] Creticos, P., Marsh, D., Proud, D., Kagey-Sobotka, A., Adkinson, N. J., Friedhoff, L., Naclerio, R., Lichtenstein, L., Norman, P. Responses to ragweed-pollen nasal challenge before and after immunotherapy. *J Allergy Clin Immunol* 1989; **84**(2): 197–205.

[98] Ferguson, A. Persisting airway obstruction in asymptomatic children with asthma with normal peak expiratory flow rates. *J Allergy Clin Immunol* 1988; **82**(1): 19–22.

[99] Gong, H. J., Simmons, M., Clark, V., Tashkin, D. Metered-dose inhaler usage in subjects with asthma: comparison of Nebulizer Chronolog and daily diary recordings. *J Allergy Clin Immunol* 1988; **82**(1): 5–10.

[100] Joad, J., Ahrens, R., Lindgren, S., Weinberger, M. Extrapulmonary effects of maintenance therapy with theophylline and inhaled albuterol in patients with chronic asthma. *J Allergy Clin Immunol* 1986; **78**(6): 1147–53.

[101] Kjellman, N., Gustafsson, I. Topical sodium cromoglycate in atopic dermatitis. A disappointing but informative trial. *Allergy* 1986; **41**(6): 423–8.

[102] Meltzer, E., Storms, W., Pierson, W., Cummins, L., Orgel, H., Perhach, J., Hemsworth, G. Efficacy of azelastine in perennial allergic rhinitis: clinical and rhinomanometric evaluation. *J Allergy Clin Immunol* 1988; **82**(3, Pt 1): 447–55.

[103] Osur, S., Volovitz, B., Dickson, S., Enck, D., Bernstein, J. Eustachian tube dysfunction in children with ragweed hayfever during natural pollen exposure. *Allergy Proc* 1989; **10**(2): 133–9.

[104] Pierson, W. Objective measurements of nasal airway testing. *J Allergy Clin Immunol* 1988; **81**(5, Pt 2): 949–52.

[105] Schatz, M., Harden, K., Forsythe, A., Chilingar, L., Hoffman, C., Sperling, W., Zeiger, R. The course of asthma during pregnancy, post partum, and with successive pregnancies: a prospective analysis. *J Allergy Clin Immunol* 1988; **81**(3): 509–17.

[106] Shirakawa, T., Kusaka, Y., Fujimura, N., Goto, S., Morimoto, K. The existence of specific antibodies to cobalt in hard metal asthma. *Clin Allergy* 1988; **18**(5): 451–60.

[107] Spector, S., Kinsman, R., Mawhinney, H., Siegel, S., Rachelefsky, G., Katz, R., Rohr, A. Compliance of patients with asthma with an experimental aerosolized medication: implications for controlled clinical trials. *J Allergy Clin Immunol* 1986; **77**(1, Pt 1): 65–70.

[108] Tinkelman, D., DeJong, R., Lutz, C., Spangler, D. Evaluation of tremor and efficacy of oral procaterol in adult patients with asthma. *J Allergy Clin Immunol* 1990; **85**(4): 719–28.

[109] Aldridge, D., Pietroni, P. The clinical assessment of acupuncture for asthma therapy. *J Roy Soc Med* 1987; **80**: 222–4.

[110] Gregg, I. The quality of asthma in general practice – a challenge for the future. *Fam Pract* 1985; **2**: 94–100.

[111] Gustafsson, P., Kjellman, N., Cederblad, M. Family therapy in the treatment of severe childhood asthma. *J Psychosom Res* 1986; **30**(3): 369–74.

112 Janson, C., Gislason, T., Boman, G., Hetta, J., Roos, B. Sleep disturbances in patients with asthma. *Respir Med* 1990; **84**(1): 37–42.

113 Katz, R., Rachelefsky, G., Siegel, S., Spector, S., Rohr, A. Twice-daily beclomethasone dipropionate in the treatment of childhood asthma. *J Asthma* 1986; **23**(1): 1–7.

114 Lebowitz, M., Collins, L., Holberg, C. Time series analyses of respiratory responses to indoor and outdoor environmental phenomena. *Environ Res* 1987; **43**(2): 332–41.

115 Rachelefsky, G., Rohr, A., Katz, R., Wo, J., Gracey, V., Spector, S., Siegel, S., Mickey, M. Sustained-release theophylline preparations in asthmatic children. A short-term comparison of two products and the relationship of serum theophylline levels and pulmonary function changes. *Am J Dis Child* 1986; **140**(4): 336–40.

116 Schwartz, J., Zeger, S. Passive smoking, air pollution, and acute respiratory symptoms in a diary study of student nurses. *Am Rev Respir Dis* 1990; **141**(1): 62–7.

117 Stafford, C. New concepts in chronic asthma. What is the impact on therapy? *Postgrad Med* 1988; **84**(4): 85–6, 91–6, 98.

118 Aldridge, D. Families, cancer and dying. *J Instit Religion & Med* 1988; **3**: 312–22.

119 Feinstein, A. Symptoms as an index of biological behavior in human cancer. *Nature* 1966; **209**: 241–5.

120 Forbes, J., McGregor, A. Male unemployment and cause-specific mortality in postwar Scotland. *Int J Health Serv* 1987; **17**(2): 233–40.

121 Love, R., Leventhal, H., Easterling, D., Nerenz, D. Side effects and emotional distress during cancer chemotherapy. *Cancer* 1989; **63**(3): 604–12.

122 Robinson, R., Blake, G., Preston, D., McEwan, A., Spicer, J., Martin, N., Wegst, A., Ackery, D. Strontium-89: treatment results and kinetics in patients with painful metastatic prostate and breast cancer in bone. *Radiographics* 1989; **9**(2): 271–81.

123 Rose, D., Boyar, A., Cohen, C., Strong, L. Effect of a low-fat diet on hormone levels in women with cystic breast disease. I. Serum steroids and gonadotropins. *J Natl Cancer Inst* 1987; **78**(4): 623–6.

124 Allison, M., Walker, V. The sodium and potassium intake of 3 to 5 year olds. *Arch Dis Child* 1986; **61**(2): 159–63.

125 Bandini, L., Schoeller, D., Cyr, H., Dietz, W. Validity of reported energy intake in obese and nonobese adolescents. *Am J Clin Nutr* 1990; **52**(3): 421–5.

126 Boyd, N., McGuire, V., Shannon, P., Cousins, M., Kriukov, V., Mahoney, L., Fish, E., Lickley, L., Lockwood, G., Tritchler, D. Effect of a low-fat high-carbohydrate diet on symptoms of cyclical mastopathy. *Lancet* 1988; **2**(8603): 128–32.

[127] Brewer, J., Williams, C., Patton, A. The influence of high carbohydrate diets on endurance running performance. *Eur J Appl Physiol* 1988; **57**(6): 698–706.

[128] Cotugna, N., Vickery, C. Diabetic diet compliance: student dietitians reverse roles. *Diabetes Educ* 1990; **16**(2): 123–6.

[129] Cugini, P., Kawasaki, T., Leone, G., Di Palma, L., Letizia, C., Scavo, D. Discrimination and spectral resolution of ultradian and circadian periodicities for 24-hour blood pressure patterns on sodium manipulation in normotensive humans. *Jpn Circ J* 1987; **51**(11): 1296–304.

[130] Cuppari, L., Draibe, S., Ancao, M., Sigulem, D., Sustovich, D., Ajzen, H., Ramos, O. Nutritional assessment of chronic renal patients in hemodialysis programs. A multicenter study. *AMB Rev Assoc Med Bras* 1989; **35**(1): 9–14.

[131] Dietrich, A., Nelson, E., Kirk, J., Zubkoff, M., O'Connor, G. Do primary physicians actually manage their patients' fee-for-service care? *JAMA* 1988; **259**(21): 3145–9.

[132] Dunbar, J. Practical aspects of dietary management of hypertension: compliance. *Can J Physiol Pharmacol* 1986; **64**(6): 831–5.

[133] Frenkiel, P., Lee, D., Cohen, H., Gilmore, C., Resser, K., Bonorris, G., Marks, J., Schoenfield, L. The effect of diet on bile acid kinetics and biliary lipid secretion in gallstone patients treated with ursodeoxycholic acid. *Am J Clin Nutr* 1986; **43**(2): 239–50.

[134] Haymes, E., Spillman, D. Iron status of women distance runners, sprinters, and control women. *Int J Sports Med* 1989; **10**(6): 430–3.

[135] Heaney, R., Davies, K., Recker, R., Packard, P. Long-term consistency of nutrient intakes in humans. *J Nutr* 1990; **120**(8): 869–75.

[136] Huss-Ashmore, R., Goodman, J., Sibiya, T., Stein, T. Energy expenditure of young Swazi women as measured by the doubly-labelled water method. *Eur J Clin Nutr* 1989; **43**(11): 737–48.

[137] Jackson, B., Dujovne, C., DeCoursey, S., Beyer, P., Brown, E., Hassanein, K. Methods to assess relative reliability of diet records: minimum records for monitoring lipid and caloric intake. *J Am Diet Assoc* 1986; **86**(11): 1531–5.

[138] Jones, S., Owens, H., Bennett, G. Does behaviour therapy work for dietitians? An experimental evaluation of the effects of three procedures in a weight reduction clinic. *Hum Nutr Appl Nutr* 1986; **40**(4): 272–81.

[139] Kindstedt-Arfwidson, K., Strandvik, B. Food intake in patients with cystic fibrosis on an ordinary diet. *Scand J Gastroenterol Suppl* 1988; **143**: 160–2.

[140] King, W., Fadal, R., Ward, W., Trevino, R., Pierce, W., Stewart, J., Boyles, J. J. Provocation-neutralization: a two-part study. Part II.

Subcutaneous neutralization therapy: a multi-center study. *Otolaryngol Head Neck Surg* 1988; **99**(3): 272–7.

141 Krall, E., Dwyer, J. Validity of a food frequency questionnaire and a food diary in a short-term recall situation. *J Am Diet Assoc* 1987; **87**(10): 1374–7.

142 Laidlaw, S., Shultz, T., Cecchino, J., Kopple, J. Plasma and urine taurine levels in vegans. *Am J Clin Nutr* 1988; **47**(4): 660–3.

143 Levine, S., D'Elia, J., Bistrian, B., Smith-Ossman, S., Gleason, R., Mitch, W., Miller, D. Protein-restricted diets in diabetic nephropathy. *Nephron* 1989; **52**(1): 55–61.

144 Lindsay, D. Estimation of the dietary intake of chemicals in food. *Food Addit Contam* 1986; **3**(1): 71–88.

145 Lissner, L., Stevens, J., Levitsky, D., Rasmussen, K., Strupp. B. Variation in energy intake during the menstrual cycle: implications for food-intake research. *Am J Clin Nutr* 1988; **48**(4): 956–62.

146 Marable, N., Kehrberg, N., Judd, J., Prather, E., Bodwell, C. Caloric and selected nutrient intakes and estimated energy expenditures for adult women: identification of non-sedentary women with lower energy intakes. *J Am Diet Assoc* 1988; **88**(6): 687–93.

147 Parker, S., Sussman, G., Krondl, M. Dietary aspects of adverse reactions to foods in adults. *Can Med Assoc J* 1988; **139**(8): 711–18.

148 Rubenstein, L., Calkins, D., Young, R., Cleary, P., Fink, A., Kosecoff, J., Jette, A., Davies, A., Delbanco, T., Brook, R. Improving patient function: a randomized trial of functional disability screening. *Ann Intern Med* 1989; **111**(10): 836–42.

149 Rush, D., Horvitz, D., Seaver, W., Leighton, J., Sloan, N., Johnson, S., Kulka, R., Devore, J., Holt, M., Lynch, J. The National WIC Evaluation: evaluation of the Special Supplemental Food Program for Women, Infants, and Children. IV. Study methodology and sample characteristics in the longitudinal study of pregnant women, the study of children, and the food expenditures study. *Am J Clin Nutr* 1988; **48**(2 Suppl): 429–38.

150 Salomon, P., Kornbluth, A., Janowitz, H. Treatment of ulcerative colitis with fish oil n-3-omega-fatty acid: an open trial. *J Clin Gastroenterol* 1990; **12**(2): 157–61.

151 Saudek, C. Data source automation: new technology for the management of patient-generated test results. *Diabetic Med* 1989; **6**(5): 394–9.

152 Shutler, S., Bircher, G., Tredger, J., Morgan, L., Walker, A., Low, A. The effect of daily baked bean (Phaseolus vulgaris) consumption on the plasma lipid levels of young, normo-cholesterolaemic men. *Br J Nutr* 1989; **61**(2): 257–65.

153 Stevens, V., Rossner, J., Greenlick, M., Stevens, N., Frankel, H., Craddick, S. Freedom from fat: a contemporary multi-component

weight loss program for the general population of obese adults. *J Am Diet Assoc* 1989; **89**(9): 1254–8.

154 Wing, R., Nowalk, M., Epstein, L., Koeske, R. Calorie-counting compared to exchange system diets in the treatment of overweight patients with type II diabetes. *Addict Behav* 1986; **11**(2): 163–8.

155 Witschi, J., Capper, A., Hosmer, D. J., Ellison, R. Sources of sodium, potassium, and energy in the diets of adolescents. *J Am Diet Assoc* 1987; **87**(12): 1651–5.

156 Grimm, H. Nutrition and food on youths' hikes in the first 3rd of the 20th century. *Arztl Jugendkd* 1990; **81**(2): 128–38.

157 Ho, K., Veldhuis, J., Johnson, M., Furlanetto, R., Evans, W., Alberti, K., Thorner, M. Fasting enhances growth hormone secretion and amplifies the complex rhythms of growth hormone secretion in man. *J Clin Invest* 1988; **81**(4): 968–75.

158 Kamat, S., Doshi, V. Sequential health effect study in relation to air pollution in Bombay, India. *Eur J Epidemiol* 1987; **3**(3): 265–77.

159 Kaplan, B., McNicol, J., Conte, R., Moghadam, H. Overall nutrient intake of preschool hyperactive and normal boys. *J Abnorm Child Psychol* 1989; **17**(2): 127–32.

160 Schweiger, U., Laessle, R., Schweiger, M., Herrmann, F., Riedel, W., Pirke, K. Caloric intake, stress, and menstrual function in athletes. *Fertil Steril* 1988; **49**(3): 447–50.

161 Barry, J., Selwyn, A., Nabel, E., Rocco, M., Mead, K., Campbell, S., Rebecca, G. Frequency of ST-segment depression produced by mental stress in stable angina pectoris from coronary artery disease. *Am J Cardiol* 1988; **61**(13): 989–93.

162 Crake, T., Quyyumi, A., Wright, C., Mockus, L., Fox, K. Treatment of angina pectoris with nifedipine: a double blind comparison of nifedipine and slow-release nifedipine alone and in combination with atenolol. *Br Heart J* 1987; **58**(6): 617–20.

163 Hougham, A., Hawkinson, R., Crowley, J., Wilson, R., Glode, J., Hilty, R., Hughes, S., Koeppl, C., Kovaric, T., Wyskoarko, N. Improved skin adherence and patient acceptance in a new transdermal nitroglycerin delivery system. *Clin Ther* 1989; **11**(1): 23–31.

164 Hougham, A., Hawkinson, R., Crowley, J., Wilson, R., Brown, S., Dougherty, P., Fogel, M., Hash, V. J., Rietbrock, M. Improved comfort and patient acceptance in a novel transdermal nitroglycerin delivery system. *Clin Ther* 1989; **11**(1): 15–22.

165 Mahapatra, R., Mahapatra, D., Yaden, S. Clinical experience with a transdermal nitroglycerin system. *Angiology* 1987; **38**(4): 277–86.

166 O'Keefe, J., Creamer, J., Banim, S. Efficacy of nisoldipine combined with beta-adrenergic-blocking drugs in the treatment of chronic stable angina. *Clin Cardiol* 1987; **10**(6): 345–50.

167   Quyyumi, A., Crake, T., Wright, C., Mockus, L., Fox, K. Medical
       treatment of patients with severe exertional and rest angina: double
       blind comparison of beta blocker, calcium antagonist, and nitrate. *Br
       Heart J* 1987; **57**(6): 505–11.

168   Sharma, M., Voyles, W., Prasad, R., Teague, S., Thadani, U. Long-
       term bepridil monotherapy for angina pectoris. *Am J Cardiol* 1988;
       61(15): 1210–13.

169   Simon, J., Gibbs, R., Crean, P., Mockus, L., Wright, C., Sutton, G.,
       Fox, K. The variable effects of angiotensin converting enzyme
       inhibition on myocardial ischaemia in chronic stable angina. *Br Heart
       J* 1989; **62**(2): 112–17.

170   Sklar, J., Dennish, G., Glode, J., Wyskoarko, N., Giles, T., Freedman,
       D., Buhite, S., Koretz, S., Roe, R. Usefulness of nicardipine as
       monotherapy for chronic, stable angina. *Am J Cardiol* 1989; **63**(17):
       1203–7.

171   Stone, P., Ware, J., DeWood, M., Gore, J., Eich, R., Pietro, D., Parisi,
       A., Nesto, R., Boden, W., Sharma, S. The efficacy of the addition of
       nifedipine in patients with mixed angina compared to patients with
       classical exertional angina: a multicenter, randomized, double-blind,
       placebo-controlled clinical trial. *Am Heart J* 1988; **116**(4): 961–71.

172   Uusitalo, A., Arstila, M., Bae, E., Harkonen, R., Keyrilainen, O.,
       Rytkonen, U., Schjelderup Mathiesen, P., Wendelin, H. Metoprolol,
       nifedipine, and the combination in stable effort angina pectoris. *Am J
       Cardiol* 1986; **57**(10): 733–7.

173   Vetrovec, G., Parker, V. Alternative medical treatment for patients
       with angina pectoris and adverse reactions to beta blockers.
       Usefulness of nifedipine. *Am J Med* 1986; **81**(4A): 20–7.

174   Anastasiades, P., Johnston, D. A simple activity measure for use
       with ambulatory subjects. *Psychophysiology* 1990; **27**(1): 87–93.

175   Dalton, K., Denman, D., Dawson, A., Hoffman, H. Ultradian
       rhythms in human fetal heart rate: a computerised time series
       analysis. *Int J Biomed Comput* 1986; **18**(1): 45–60.

176   Freeman, L., Nixon, P., Sallabank, P., Reaveley, D. Psychological
       stress and silent myocardial ischemia. *Am Heart J* 1987; **114**(3):
       477–82.

177   Halberg, E., Jardetzky, N., Halberg, F., Soong, L., Halberg, F., Wu, J.,
       Zhou, S., Jardetzky, O. Magnetic resonance spectroscopy and
       ambulatory cardiovascular monitoring noninvasively gauge timing
       of phosphate metabolism and circulation. *Chronobiologia* 1989; **16**(1):
       1–8.

178   Helman, C. Heart disease and the cultural construction of time: The
       type A behaviour pattern as a western culture-bound syndrome. *Soc
       Sci Med* 1987; **25**: 969–79.

179   Isolauri, J., Harju, E., Markkula, H. Gastrointestinal symptoms after
       colon interposition. *Am J Gastroenterol* 1986; **81**(11): 1055–8.

180 Kalkwarf, H., Haas, J., Belko, A., Roach, R., Roe, D. Accuracy of heart-rate monitoring and activity diaries for estimating energy expenditure. *Am J Clin Nutr* 1989; **49**(1): 37–43.

181 Lambert, C., Coy, K., Imperi, G., Pepine, C. Influence of beta-adrenergic blockade defined by time series analysis on circadian variation of heart rate and ambulatory myocardial ischemia. *Am J Cardiol* 1989; **64**(14): 835–9.

182 LeBlanc, A. Quantitative analysis of cardiac arrhythmias. *Crit Rev Biomed Eng* 1986; **14**(1): 1–43.

183 Lindemans, F., Rankin, I., Murtaugh, R., Chevalier, P. Clinical experience with an activity sensing pacemaker. *PACE* 1986; **9**(6, Pt 2): 978–86.

184 Lynch, J. *The Broken Heart: the Medical Consequence of Loneliness.* New York: Basic Books, 1977.

185 Margraf, J., Taylor, B., Ehlers, A., Roth, W., Agras, W. Panic attacks in the natural environment. *J Nerv Ment Dis* 1987; **175**(9): 558–65.

186 Reynolds, V., Marriott, F., Shawkat, F., Eggerman, M., Nikolaou, V. Heart-rate variation, age, and behaviour in elderly women. *Ann Hum Biol* 1989; **16**(3): 265–73.

187 Schulz, S., Westerterp, K., Bruck, K. Comparison of energy expenditure by the doubly labeled water technique with energy intake, heart rate, and activity recording in man. *Am J Clin Nutr* 1989; **49**(6): 1146–54.

188 Walker, B., Sandman, C. Human visual evoked responses are related to heart rate. *J Compar Physiol Psychol* 1979; **93**: 717–29.

189 Walker, B., Sandman, C. Visual evoked potentials change as heart rate and carotid pressure change. *Psychophysiology* 1982; **19**: 520–7.

190 Bentzen, N., Christiansen, T., Pedersen, K. Self-care within a model for demand for medical care. *Soc Sci Med* 1989; **29**(2): 185–93.

191 Bolger, N., DeLongis, A., Kessler, R., Schilling, E. Effects of daily stress on negative mood. *J Pers Soc Psychol* 1989; **57**(5): 808–18.

192 Chapar, G., Friedman, S., Horwitz, J. Relationship between psychosocial variables and school absenteeism in kindergarten children. *J Dev Behav Pediatr* 1988; **9**(6): 352–8.

193 Cooney, J., Clarke, J., Morris, G. Analysis of the physiological stress profile: the interrupted time-series design. *Biofeedback Self Regul* 1986; **11**(3): 231–45.

194 Cooper, P., Bawden, H., Camfield, P., Camfield, C. Anxiety and life events in childhood migraine. *Pediatrics* 1987; **79**(6): 999–1004.

195 Dimsdale, J., Stern, M. E. The stress interview as a tool for examining psychologic reactivity. *Psychosom Med* 1988; **50**: 64–71.

196 Dooley, D., Catalano, R., Rook, K., Serxner, S. Economic stress and suicide: multilevel analyses. Part 1: Aggregate time-series analyses

of economic stress and suicide. *Suicide Life Threat Behav* 1989; **19**(4): 321–36.

197   Fukui, T. Health diary study of Japanese residents in Greater Boston: variables related to high incidence of health problems. *Cult Med Psychiatry* 1987; **11**(4): 509–20.

198   Hicks, R., Garcia, E. Level of stress and sleep duration. *Percept Mot Skills* 1987; **64**(1): 44–6.

199   Kiernan, M., Toro, P., Rappaport, J., Seidman, E. Economic predictors of mental health service utilization: a time-series analysis. *Am J Community Psychol* 1989; **17**(6): 801–20.

200   Kirsch, C., Blanchard, E., Parnes, S. A multiple-baseline evaluation of the treatment of subjective tinnitus with relaxation training and biofeedback. *Biofeedback Self Regul* 1987; **12**(4): 295–312.

201   Magos, A., Brincat, M., Studd, J. Trend analysis of the symptoms of 150 women with a history of the premenstrual syndrome. *Am J Obstet Gynecol* 1986; **155**(2): 277–82.

202   Milton, J., Gotman, J., Remillard, G., Andermann, F. Timing of seizure recurrence in adult epileptic patients: a statistical analysis. *Epilepsia* 1987; **28**(5): 471–8.

203   Neugebauer, R. Reliability of seizure diaries in adult epileptic patients. *Neuroepidemiology* 1989; **8**(5): 228–33.

204   Nulty, D., Wilkins, A., Williams, J. Mood, pattern sensitivity and headache: a longitudinal study. *Psychol Med* 1987; **17**(3): 705–13.

205   Prior, J., Vigna, Y., Sciarretta, D., Alojado, N., Schulzer, M. Conditioning exercise decreases premenstrual symptoms: a prospective, controlled 6-month trial. *Fertil Steril* 1987; **47**(3): 402–8.

206   Realini, J., Walters, M. Vaginal diaphragm rings in the treatment of stress urinary incontinence. *J Am Board Fam Pract* 1990; **3**(2): 99–103.

207   Sampson, G. Premenstrual syndrome. *Baillieres Clin Obstet Gynaecol* 1989; **3**(4): 687–704.

208   Scott, G., Richards, M. Night waking in infants: effects of providing advice and support for parents. *J Child Psychol Psychiat* 1990; **31**(4): 551–67.

209   Verbrugge, L. The twain meet: empirical explanations of sex differences in health and mortality. *J Health Soc Behav* 1989; **30**(3): 282–304.

210   Ward, M., Mefford, I., Parker, S., Chesney, M., Taylor, C., Keegan, D., Barchas, J. Epinephrine and norepinephrine responses in continuously collected human plasma to a series of stressors. *Psychosom Med* 1983; **45**(6): 471–86.

211   Wilson, P., Borland, M. Vaginal cones for the treatment of genuine stress incontinence. *Aust NZ J Obstet Gynaecol* 1990; **30**: 157–60.

212   Zastowny, T., Kirschenbaum, D., Meng, A. Coping skills training for

children: effects on distress before, during, and after hospitalization for surgery. *Health Psychol* 1986; **5**(3): 231–47.

213 Alward, R., Monk, T. A comparison of rotating-shift and permanent night nurses. *Int J Nurs Stud* 1990; **27**(3): 297–302.

214 Davies, R., Lacks, P., Storandt, M., Bertelson, A. Countercontrol treatment of sleep-maintenance insomnia in relation to age. *Psychol Aging* 1986; **1**(3): 233–8.

215 Fry, J., Pressman, M., DiPhillipo, M., Forst Paulus, M. Treatment of narcolepsy with codeine. *Sleep* 1986; **9**(1, Pt 2): 269–74.

216 Hoelscher, T., Edinger, J. Treatment of sleep-maintenance insomnia in older adults: sleep period reduction, sleep education, and modified stimulus control. *Psychol Aging* 1988; **3**(3): 258–63.

217 Meuleman, J., Nelson, R., Clark, R. J. Evaluation of temazepam and diphenhydramine as hypnotics in a nursing-home population. *Drug Intell Clin Pharm* 1987; **21**(9): 716–20.

218 Minors, D., Rabbitt, P., Worthington, H., Waterhouse, J. Variation in meals and sleep-activity patterns in aged subjects; its relevance to circadian rhythm studies. *Chronobiol Int* 1989; **6**(2): 139–46.

219 Moller, H., Blank, R., Steinmeyer, E. Single-case evaluation of sleep-deprivation effects by means of nonparametric time-series analysis (according to the HTAKA model). *Eur Arch Psychiat Neurol Sci* 1989; **239**(2): 133–9.

220 Morin, C., Kowatch, R., Wade, J. Behavioral management of sleep disturbances secondary to chronic pain. *J Behav Ther Exp Psychiat* 1989; **20**(4): 295–302.

221 Otsuka, K., Watanabe, H. Experimental and clinical chronocardiology. *Chronobiologia* 1990; **17**(2): 135–63.

222 Renfrew, J., Pettigrew, K., Rapoport, S. Motor activity and sleep duration as a function of age in healthy men. *Physiol Behav* 1987; **41**(6): 627–34.

223 Stanton, H. Hypnotic relaxation and the reduction of sleep onset insomnia. *Int J Psychosom* 1989; **36**(1–4): 64–8.

224 Weissman, D., Janjan, N., Byhardt, R. Assessment of pain during head and neck irradiation. *J Pain Symptom Manage* 1989; **4**(2): 90–5.

225 Winer, L., Shaw, M., Baumann, G. Basal plasma growth hormone levels in man: new evidence for rhythmicity of growth hormone secretion. *J Clin Endocrinol Metab* 1990; **70**(6): 1678–86.

226 Buckley, B. R., Maughan, R., Clarkson, P., Bleiler, T., Whiting, P. Serum creatine kinase activity after isometric exercise in premenopausal and postmenopausal women. *Exp Aging Res* 1989; **15**(3–4): 195–8.

227 Smith, S., Rinehart, J., Ruddock, V., Schiff, I. Treatment of premenstrual syndrome with alprazolam: results of a double-blind,

placebo-controlled, randomized crossover clinical trial. *Obstet Gynecol* 1987; **70**(1): 37–43.

228 Bhatia, S. Contraceptive users in rural Bangladesh: a time trend analysis. *Stud Fam Plann* 1983; **14**(1): 20–8.

229 Braun-Fahrlander, C., Ackermann-Liebrich, U., Wanner, H., Rutishauser, M., Gnehm, H., Minder, C. Effects of air pollutants on the respiratory system in young children. *Schweiz Med Wochenschr* 1989; **119**(41): 1424–33.

230 Clovis, J., Hargreaves, J. Fluoride intake from beverage consumption. *Commun Dent Oral Epidemiol* 1988; **16**(1): 11–15.

231 Condon, W. Multiple response to sound in dysfunctional children. *J Autism Child Schizophr* 1975; **5**: 37–56.

232 Cunningham-Burley, S., Irvine, S. 'And have you done anything so far?' An examination of lay treatment of children's symptoms. *Br Med J Clin Res* 1987; **295**(6600): 700–2.

233 Gold, D., Weiss, S., Tager, I., Segal, M., Speizer, F. Comparison of questionnaire and diary methods in acute childhood respiratory illness surveillance. *Am Rev Respir Dis* 1989; **139**(3): 847–9.

234 Groothuis, J., Berman, S., Chapman, J. Effect of carbohydrate ingested on outcome in infants with mild gastroenteritis. *J Pediatr* 1986; **108**(6): 903–6.

235 Hindmarsh, P., Matthews, D., Brook, C. Growth hormone secretion in children determined by time series analysis. *Clin Endocrinol Oxf* 1988; **29**(1): 35–44.

236 Morrongiello, B., Trehub, S., Thorpe, L., Podilupo, S. Children's perception of melodies: The role of contour, frequency and rate of presentation. *J Exp Child Psychol* 1985; **40**: 279–92.

237 Rush, D., Kurzon, M., Seaver, W., Shanklin, D. The National WIC Evaluation: evaluation of the Special Supplemental Food Program for Women, Infants, and Children. VII. Study of food expenditures. *Am J Clin Nutr* 1988; **48**(2 Suppl): 512–19.

238 Samet, J. Nitrogen dioxide and respiratory infection: pilot investigations. *Am Rev Respir Dis* 1989; **139**(5): 1073–4.

239 Schnore, S., Sangster, J., Gerace, T., Bass, M. Are antihistamine-decongestants of value in the treatment of acute otitis media in children? *J Fam Pract* 1986; **22**(1): 39–43.

240 Sorensen, E. Using children's diaries as a research instrument. *J Pediatr Nurs* 1989; **4**(6): 427–31.

241 Stone, P., Nicolson, N. Infrequently occurring activities and contexts in time use data. *J Nerv Ment Dis* 1987; **175**(9): 519–25.

242 Street, R. J., Cappella, J. Social and linguistic factors influencing adaptation in children's speech. *J Psycholinguist Res* 1989; **18**(5): 497–519.

243 Zaidi, A., Schnell, D., Reynolds, G. Time series analysis of symphilis surveillance data. *Stat Med* 1989; **8**(3): 353–62; discussion 363.

244 Copp, L. Pain diaries, journals, and logs. *Orthop Nurs* 1990; **9**(2): 37–9.

245 Oettle, G., Heaton, K. Is there a relationship between symptoms of the irritable bowel syndrome and objective measurements of large bowel function? A longitudinal study. *Gut* 1987; **28**(2): 146–9.

246 Van Egeren, L., Madarasmi, S. A computer-assisted diary (CAD) for ambulatory blood pressure monitoring. *Am J Hypertens* 1988; **1**(3): 179S–185S.

247 de Castro, J. Social facilitation of duration and size but not rate of the spontaneous meal intake of humans. *Physiol Behav* 1990; **47**(6): 1129–35.

248 de Shalit, N., Fattal, B. The health diary as a source of information on kibbutz morbidity. *Isr J Med Sci* 1990; **26**(2): 80–7.

249 Liebl, N., Butler, L. A chiropractic approach to the treatment of dysmenorrhea. *J Manip Physiol Ther* 1990; **13**(2): 101–6.

250 Mulligan, K., Butterfield, G. Discrepancies between energy intake and expenditure in physically active women. *Br J Nutr* 1990; **64**(1): 23–36.

251 Sandvik, L. Single case studies from a statistician's point of view. *Scand J Gastroenterol Suppl* 1988; **147**: 38–9.

252 Gordon, K. The multi-state Kalman Filter in medical monitoring. *Comput Methods Programs Biomed* 1986; **23**(2): 147–54.

253 Sjoden, P. Single case studies in psychology and psychiatry. *Scand J Gastroenterol Suppl* 1988; **147**: 11–21.

254 Berman, I. Musical functioning, speech lateralization and the amusias. *S African Med J* 1981; **59**: 78–81.

255 Lentz, M. Time-series analysis – cosinor analysis: a special case. *West J Nurs Res* 1990; **12**(3): 408–12.

256 Minors, D., Waterhouse, J. Mathematical and statistical analysis of circadian rhythms. *Psychoneuroendocrinology* 1988; **13**(6): 443–64.

257 Taylor, D. Time-series analysis. Use of autocorrelation as an analytic strategy for describing pattern and change. *West J Nurs Res* 1990; **12**(2): 254–61.

258 Teicher, M., Barber, N. COSIFIT: an interactive program for simultaneous multioscillator cosinor analysis of time-series data. *Comput Biomed Res* 1990; **23**(3): 283–95.

259 Fersini, C., Manfredini, R., Manfredini, F., Balboni, G., Fersini, G. Chronobiologic aspects of recurrent transient ischemic attack. *Prog Clin Biol Res* 1987; **227**: 167–71.

260 Graupe, D., Salahi, J., Zhang, D. Stochastic analysis of myoelectric

temporal signatures for multifunctional single-site activation of prostheses and orthoses. *J Biomed Eng* 1985; **7**(1): 18–29.

261 Moss, R., Wedding, D., Sanders, S. The comparative efficacy of relaxation training and masseter EMG feedback in the treatment of TMJ dysfunction. *J Oral Rehabil* 1983; **10**(1): 9–17.

262 Sigge, W., Basar Eroglu, C., Schutt, A., Basar, E. Pacemakers of the upper urinary tract using power spectral analysis of spontaneous activity. *Z Kinderchir* 1988; **43**(3): 147–9.

263 Togo, M., Togo, T. Initiation time of adolescent growth spurt estimated by a certain trough in time-series analysis of monthly anthropometric and urinalysis data in five siblings. *Hum Biol* 1988; **60**(2): 223–35.

264 Asplin, C., Faria, A., Carlsen, E., Vaccaro, V., Barr, R., Iranmanesch, A., Lee, M., Veldhuis, J., Evans, W. Alterations in the pulsatile mode of growth hormone release in men and women with insulin-dependent diabetes mellitus. *J Clin Endocrinol Metab* 1989; **69**(2): 239–45.

265 Hartman, M., Veldhuis, J., Vance, M., Faria, A., Furlanetto, R., Thorner, M. Somatotropin pulse frequency and basal concentrations are increased in acromegaly and are reduced by successful therapy. *J Clin Endocrinol Metab* 1990; **70**(5): 1375–84.

266 Moran, G., Fonagy, P. Psychoanalysis of diabetic control: a single-case study. *Br J Med Psychol* 1987; **60**(Pt 4): 357–72.

267 O'Rahilly, S., Turner, R., Matthews, D. Impaired pulsatile secretion of insulin in relatives of patients with non-insulin-dependent diabetes. *New Eng J Med* 1988; **318**(19): 1225–30.

268 Wheatley, T., Clark, P., Clark, J., Holder, R., Raggatt, P., Evans, D. Abnormalities of thyrotrophin (TSH) evening rise and pulsatile release in haemodialysis patients: evidence for hypothalamic-pituitary changes in chronic renal failure. *Clin Endocrinol Oxf* 1989; **31**(1): 39–50.

269 Vance, M., Thorner, M. Fasting alters pulsatile and rhythmic cortisol release in normal man. *J Clin Endocrinol Metab* 1989; **68**(6): 1013–18.

270 Desoye, G., Schweditsch, M., Pfeiffer, K., Zechner, R., Kostner, G. Correlation of hormones with lipid and lipoprotein levels during normal pregnancy and postpartum. *J Clin Endocrinol Metab* 1987; **64**(4): 704–12.

271 Aldridge, D. Goal setting: the patient's assessment of outcome and recognition of therapeutic change. *Comp Med Res* 1988; **3**: 89–97.

272 Lindberg, G. Single case studies in clinical trials. *Scand J Gastroenterol Suppl* 1988; **147**: 30–2.

273 Farmer, J., Kauffman, S., Packard, N., Perelson, A. Adaptive dynamic networks as models for the immune system and autocatalytic sets. *Ann N Y Acad Sci* 1987; **504**: 118–31.

13 The use of health diaries in the field of psychiatric illness in general practice

Joanna Murray

Summary

The individual's response to the occurrence of symptoms is conditioned by a variety of non-medical factors, of both an enduring (e.g. personality attributes) and a changing nature (e.g. social support). The health diary provides a particularly appropriate method of studying the daily variations in health and illness behaviour which make up so much of the clinical content of general practice.

Introduction

In a 1982 collection of social studies in medical care, Mechanic suggested that the main task for behavioural scientists working in this field is to understand why people with similar complaints behave so differently.[1] The term 'illness behaviour' was originated by Mechanic to characterize the considerable variation in the ways in which people perceive, evaluate and respond to physical and psychological discomfort.[2] The type of behaviour could not be regarded as a direct consequence of the nature and severity of the symptoms; many other non-medical factors appear to shape the response.

Large-scale health surveys provide some opportunity to compare in retrospect the behaviour of individuals who report similar complaints. It would appear that self-reported symptoms in the general population are so commonplace that few of us are symptom-free for long.[3,4] In the latter study, 91% of adults reported symptoms during the two weeks prior to interview, although only 16% had consulted a doctor during that time. Studies such as these clearly demonstrate the inadequacy of measuring either the incidence or the prevalence of illness through medical records. Only the tip of the iceberg of ill health is seen in the consulting room, and little is known of the nature of the treatment afforded to the vast majority of symptom episodes.

It does not seem to be the case that only the more serious complaints are brought to the doctor's attention. Zola[5] points out the curious paradox that in community surveys quite serious illnesses are found which have not received medical attention and yet the bulk of medical practice seems to be concerned with minor disorders. Since he finds little to distinguish medically attended disorders from ones which are ignored or treated at home, Zola proposes the following empirical picture of illness episodes. While people suffer from an array of discomforts almost daily and there is little in the nature of the symptoms which seems to determine which do and do not get professional treatment, something 'critical' must happen to turn a person into a patient. He postulated a number of non-medical reasons (or triggers) for consulting at a specific point in the illness: an interpersonal crisis, for instance, or perceived interference of the symptoms with daily activities. The type of cue to action seemed to depend on the cultural background of the patient.

While there remains much to explore in the diverse behaviour of individuals of similar health status, a greater research challenge is posed by the intra-personal variations in illness behaviour. Why is it that in the same individual a complaint which arouses little concern on one occasion may lead to great discomfort, anxiety and a medical consultation at some other time? Is it possible to account for the development of an illness and the subsequent actions of the sufferer by exploring the events preceding the report of symptoms? Can a greater understanding of illness behaviour be achieved from a detailed prospective monitoring of the health of individuals than from retrospective accounts? Such detailed monitoring calls for methodological approaches more familiar in clinical and pharmacological trials than in sociomedical studies. While methods of successive, controlled observation have been used to evaluate the efficacy of treatments, they have rarely been used to study individuals, who are neither patients nor experimental subjects.

Single case design

The method of intensive single case research, with the subject making his own health assessments and acting as his own 'control', was pioneered by Hogben and Sim.[6] Their objective was to determine whether the subject's symptoms of fatigue and muscular weakness ('low grade morbidity') were those of myasthenia gravis or whether they were functional. Three drugs were to be administered blind for diagnostic purposes and the subject was to make detailed self-reports at predetermined times of day. They argued that rigorous control of physiological, anatomical, genetic and social variables would result from the subject acting as his own control when successive observations were to be made. Changes in somatic and psychological functioning reported by the subject could more readily be attributed to the effects of the different drug treatments. Self-recording, on predetermined indices, was the most appropriate method, since an external observer would be impossibly intrusive and would influence the very behaviour under scrutiny.

The development of single case research occurred largely in the field of experimental psychology and, more specifically, operant conditioning[7] with an experimenter present to control the stimuli and to record the response. Behaviour (or overt performance) measures were narrowly defined to enable the precise measurement of responses to controlled stimuli. However, there is no apparent reason why single case design need be limited to experimental settings or to the performance of narrowly specified behaviour.[8] Since the main procedural requirement is continuous assessment, other methods such as self-report and psychophysiological measures can be used.[9]

Most single case designs in the field of applied clinical research have involved interventions controlled by an experimenter or a therapist.[10] However, if we adopt this design to study the natural history of an illness episode, the independent variables (such as stressful events, accidents, contact with sources of infection) cannot be controlled, and the 'experimenter' is replaced by the 'observer'. This chapter is concerned with intensive single case design where no experimental conditions are imposed. The 'observations' are obtained in the subjects' natural environment and are recorded by the subjects themselves. No controlled stimuli or treatments are administered to the subject and the dependent variables are idiosyncratic, in that they form part of the subject's normal repertoire of behaviour. The term 'descriptive' has been applied to this type of single case investigation.[9]

Several reviews of single case research provide support for widening the scope of this methodology.[11,8] Conditions once regarded as *sine qua non* are increasingly seen as optional, and the operational necessity to reduce the components of human behaviour to unrealistic simplicity before they can be measured need not apply in all disciplines. Naturalistic observation has become more acceptable and behavioural scientists seem less inclined to borrow from the laws of classical physics in postulating theories of human behaviour. Herbst[12] suggests that it is pointless to seek for the invariance in phenomena which a scientific law demands, since 'every person and every group has the characteristics of a behavioural universe which evolves its own laws and measurement scales'. However, this does not rule out attempts to apply these personal 'laws' to other individuals, provided that the parameters and functional relationships of the variables are clearly defined.

The pilot study of general practice patients, to be described later in this chapter, owes much of its design rationale to the pioneering work of Hogben and Sim.[6] The method selected to record the repeated measures was the self-report health diary, since it came closest to meeting the criteria for a non-intrusive method of monitoring the natural history of illness episodes. Using a single case design also eliminated the need to control for known sociocultural influences on illness behaviour, such as social class,[13] ethnic origin[14,5] and age.[15] It must be acknowledged that a generally applicable model of illness behaviour can only be tested on grouped results from large samples to take account of these sociocultural variations. This is beyond the scope of this chapter.

The health diary method

Given the frequency and transience of most symptom episodes and the very limited extent to which medical intervention is sought by most of the population,[3,4,16,17] health records and retrospective interviews cannot provide sufficient or precise data to study the events which precede and follow the onset of illness. The disparity between the experience of symptoms and medical attendance is dramatically revealed in health diaries. While Horder and Horder[16] and White *et al.*[17] in retrospective surveys estimated a ratio of 3–4 non-attended symptoms to every symptom for which medical help was sought, a health diary study of women registered with a South London practice showed that only one in 37 symptom episodes was treated by a doctor,[18] and a similar, though smaller, diary study[19] found that only one in 40 symptoms was likely to be treated medically. It should be emphasized that this low ratio of consultations to symptoms was recorded by young women, a group with high rates of general practice attendance despite generally good physical health. Health diary studies of men might reveal even greater proportions of unattended illness.

Allen *et al.*[20] made one of the earliest methodological comparisons of retrospective interviews with health diaries. They found much higher prevalence rates using the latter method, with interesting variations by type of symptom. Gastrointestinal disturbances were almost five times as likely to be recorded in diaries than recalled at interview for the previous month, whereas infective or parasitic diseases were equally recalled in both methods. The diary excelled most significantly in obtaining reports of mental disorders (including 'nervousness' and 'headaches'), for which the disparity was six to one. Even when illness episodes had been medically attended, they were still more likely to be recorded in the diary than the interview covering the previous month. However, a serious flaw in the design of this study was that the respondent acted as proxy for all members of the household in recording illness episodes, both at interview and in the diary. Presumably the prospective nature of the diary allowed the respondent to obtain more accurate daily health reports from other members of the household.

Verbrugge[21] has reviewed the benefits and drawbacks of health diaries and reached the firm conclusion that the diary is superior to the single extensive interview in:

1 reducing recall error and producing higher levels of reporting, which yield higher incidence rates, both for accurate conditions and for chronic conditions which are symptomatic during the diary period;

2 counts of diffuse conditions, for which people do not know the underlying medical condition, and for non-disabling and non-attended illnesses;

3 providing a more comprehensive view of people's health and illness behaviour.

Verbrugge suggested that the main drawback of the method lies in the very wealth of material it generates: the amount of detail strains the capacity of analytical and statistical techniques. Another challenge posed by sequentially repeated measures is the analysis of time series data, since it would be an oversimplification to treat each day's events as independent of preceding days. Methods of time series analysis discussed by Kratochwill[22] and Chassan[11] may offer some solutions. Data from each case can be examined for trend over time by plotting measurements against time (the day). A trend line can then be fitted to the plotted data and a significance test applied.[11] However, the number of consecutive days on which data would need to be recorded for statistical analysis may be greater than the majority of respondents are prepared to tolerate.[23]

Verbrugge considered 19 health diary studies carried out between 1940 and 1980. Only seven used diaries as a primary data source; the others used them as a methodological check on other health measures, or as an *aide mémoire* for subsequent interviews. Between four and six weeks seems to be the maximum period for which people will maintain an accurate diary: beyond this the drop-out rate rises and the volume of recorded data drops through respondent 'fatigue'.[21] Most studies require respondents to provide information only for those days on which symptoms occur, with the risk that some minor complaints will be dismissed as not worth recording, and that illness behaviour occurring on these days will also go unreported. Conversely, subjects may become so sensitized to their own health by the daily self-assessments that changes occur in their illness behaviour. They may begin to discuss their health more often with family and friends; they may become alarmed by the frequency of a symptom of which they had been hardly aware.

As a check on the influence of diary-keeping on subjects' behaviour, detailed background data on their recent state of health and illness behaviour should be collected during an extensive interview. Measures have been developed to assess individual 'predisposition' to various forms of illness behaviour, such as dependence on the doctor[4] and perceived locus of control of health.[24] The diary should not be treated as an independent source of longitudinal data on illness behaviour; various predisposing factors have been shown to have a contributory effect, particularly on physician utilization.[25,26,27,28]

The diary in general practice research

Health diaries seem to be particularly suited to observing the 'unique clinical content of general practice',[19] with its variety of presenting complaints, psychosocial problems, and underlying pathology. Indeed, it is in this setting that most diary studies have taken place, with respondents selected from a practice or health centre register.

Most studies have been designed to establish the prevalence of health problems among those with access to a health facility and so data on the family unit rather than the individual have been recorded.[28,29,30,31] In most cases women have been recruited as diary-keepers, presumably for their greater awareness of the health of all the family members and for their decisive role in the illness behaviour of their children. The studies of most relevance to this chapter are those which use personal rather than family diaries, in particular those of women.[32,33,19] Only with individual-level data is it possible to adopt single case methods, and to measure the predisposing variables contributing to the individual's illness behaviour.

Previous health diary studies have explored to some extent the relationship between background, predisposing or mediating variables, daily events (both external and internal) and illness behaviour. The common elements which underly these studies are represented in Figure 13.1. The nature of relationships between A and B variables and their influence on behaviour remain to be more fully elaborated. Although diary data has drawn attention to the lack of consistent

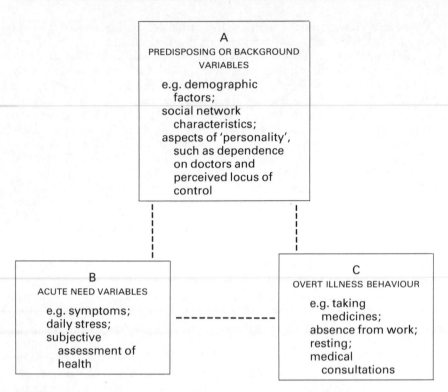

Fig. 13.1 Common elements in previous studies using health diaries.

response within a sample to the occurrence of similar symptoms, there is little explanation for intra-subject variability. The present author is engaged in a general practice study designed to explicate this variability. The pilot stage described below demonstrates the methodology and some of its pitfalls.

Background and objectives

The aim of the pilot study was to explore both predisposing (social and personality) variables and daily stresses or need variables (internal and external events) which might have the strongest associations with illness behaviour. More precise definitions of these two types of variables needed to be developed for the main study. There was also an important methodological objective:

1 to test the feasibility of applying the method of self-controlled daily self-report among general practice patients using a simple health diary;

2 to demonstrate, by means of simple graphical presentation, covariations in daily symptom reports, self-assessments of health and self-reported illness behaviour in a series of general practice patients with identified psychiatric morbidity;

3 by collecting extensive background information through personal interview, to construct measures of 'predisposing vari-

ables' for use in combination with the daily self-reports ('need' variables) in a model of illness behaviour.

Method

Design and sample

The single case design is the most appropriate method to explore intra-subject variation over time. The need to monitor the impact of small variations in health and the occurrence of events calls for the use of daily recording; self-report on a structured and predetermined set of indices is the only feasible method to apply with a non-institutional sample.

The respondents were recruited from among a group of patients with a high rate of general practice consultations: women with emotional or psychological problems. The enhanced rate of consultations by women, particularly in the age group 20–45, is well established.[25,34] After controlling for demographic, attitudinal and health status variables, a positive relationship has been found to exist between psychological distress and the use of primary care services.[35] As noted earlier, stress has been implicated indirectly in the greater use of medical care facilities via its impact upon illness[36] and in heightened sensitivity to symptoms.[37] Whatever the role of stress in illness behaviour, it is commonly held that psychologically distressed individuals use medical services disproportionately.[29,38,39,40]

Two general practitioners, in partnership within a large health centre in South West London, agreed to take part in the pilot study. The recruitment method agreed with the doctors was for them to identify women consulters between the ages of 20 and 60 years, whom they believed to be suffering from minor affective disorder, irrespective of presenting complaint. After explaining to potential respondents that a survey of everyday health and illness was underway at the surgery, those eligible were invited to take part in a brief interview with the research worker.

Assuming that the broad age band and expected frequency of consultation would bring in at least one potential respondent at each surgery, the author was at first present at the health centre during surgery hours. The rate of recruitment proved to be too low for this method to continue, so that it was agreed that the GPs would telephone the research worker during a consultation with a potential respondent. An arrangement was then made with the patient for an interview within a day or two.

At the interview, respondents first completed the 30-item General Health Questionnaire (GHQ),[41,42] a self-completion questionnaire designed to screen for likely cases of psychiatric morbidity in the general population. Those with a score of four or more (probable cases) were then asked to take part in the extensive interview. This interview included the administration of the Clinical Interview Schedule,[43] the second stage of the screening procedure designed to validate the GHQ and to provide opportunities for rating the severity of ten pre-selected psychological symptoms and 12 abnormalities manifest at interview. Respondents were also asked to rate their present health, and to describe any health problems and actions taken, recent consumption of medications, medical consultations, health behaviour (including smoking and alcohol consumption, diet and exercise). They were asked whether they had experienced any of 21 listed symptoms or complaints (derived from Dunnell and Cartwright)[4] in the past seven days. Detailed questions on relationships within the family and household were asked. If relevant, the respondent's attitudes to her marriage were discussed. Questions on friends and confidants included details of those with whom they discussed health and personal problems. Finally, details were recorded on problems in housing, finance, employment and any other areas of individual concern. Each respondent was asked whether she would be willing to complete a 28-day health diary, which was explained to her in detail.

The diary

The first item was an assessment of the respondent's day in general, along a five-point scale running from very good to very poor. They were then asked whether they had been able to carry out all their normal activities that day. A five-point self-assessment of health followed comparable with those used in a variety of other studies on subjective wellbeing.[44] There was then space to write in any symptoms or health problems they had experienced in the past 24 hours, together with any action taken for each problem. Details of any medications consumed were recorded. The final item on the first side of the page was a note of anything which had bothered or upset them that day.

The second side comprised a list of 21 symptoms or complaints, with a choice of three boxes for each item to denote whether the respondent had experienced the problem severely, slightly or not at all. The items, taken mainly from the list of 'everyday complaints' used in their community health survey by Dunnell and Cartwright,[4] include both somatic (e.g. feeling sick or vomiting, sore throat, headache, constipation or diarrhoea) and psychological complaints (e.g. feeling irritable or bad-tempered, feeling sad or depressed, feeling nervous or jittery, having difficulty getting to sleep).

Respondents were contacted by the research worker towards the end of the 28-day recording period and an appointment was made for collection of the diary and a brief follow-up interview. At the follow-up, the respondent again completed the GHQ and the research worker enquired about any changes in circumstances or health since the last visit.

Results

Twenty-four female patients were referred to the research worker by the general practitioners. Contact was made with 22 of these, of whom 18 were interviewed at length and agreed to complete the health diary (the remaining four were excluded because three had a negative GHQ score at the time of interview, and one respondent's command of English was too poor for her to take part).

Table 13.1   Some characteristics of the diarists

Age-group		*Marital status*	
25–29 years	5	Single	1
30–39 years	2	Married/cohabiting	10
40–49 years	3	Divorced/separated	2
50–60 years	4	Widowed	1
Children at home		*Employment outside the home*	
Under 5 years	4	Full-time	3
5–16 years	8	Part-time	5
Over 16 years	7	None	6
None	3	*Occupation of head of household*	
Housing tenure		Skilled non-manual	4
Owner-occupier	4	Skilled manual	2
Public sector	10	Unskilled manual	4
		Full-time housewife	3
		Unemployed/seeking work	1

Of the 18 who began the health diary, 14 completed and returned the document; one was too depressed after one week to continue, and the remaining three failed to respond to letters requesting a second visit by the research worker or were out when visited on a number of occasions.

Some of the characteristics of the 14 diarists are shown in Tables 13.1 and 13.2. Although daily reports from the 14 diaries are to be considered as individual-level data, details collected at the initial interviews show a variety of demographic characteristics, and a substantial degree of chronic ill health and social problems. All were found to have affective symptoms on the Clinical Interview Schedule, ranging from mild to severe.

Table 13.2   Health and social problems

Somatic conditions	
Chronic cardiovascular diseases	5
Chronic respiratory diseases	4
Recurrent urinary tract disorders	4
Chronic menstrual symptoms	3
None	3
Psychological disorders	
Chronic recurrent affective disorders	7
Acute affective disorder	7
Social problems	
Chronic marital problems	8
Childcare difficulties	4
Problems with adult children	4
Housing problems	5
Financial problems	6
Employment problems	4
None	1

Diary data

Ten respondents had no symptom-free days during the month of recording; the others recorded only one, two, seven and eight days without symptoms. Clearly, the number, nature and the severity of these complaints will vary from one individual to another and from one day to another in the same individual. Results will now be treated on a single case basis as a means of illustrating themes emerging from the pilot study, with a brief vignette of the respondent.

Predisposing and acute need variables and illness behaviour

The association between a high level of acute distress and a high rate of consultation is clearly demonstrated by the diary of Mrs D (see Figure 13.2). A mother of three in her late 20s, she assessed *none* of her 28 days as good, either in health or in general terms. On all but day 15, her assessment of her health and of the day in general were the same (thus only one white area appears on this histogram). A frequent attender at the surgery (ten times in the twelve months preceding the diary), she was suffering from severe anxiety symptoms, including dizziness and panic attacks, which seemed to be the culmination of chronic marital and financial problems and a rare venous condition which she believed threatened her life. In caring for three children under six years of age she had little support; although a local girl with a close relationship with her elderly mother, she considered herself to have no one in whom she could confide. Her illness behaviour during the month was at an exceptionally high level: she consulted her GP five times, tried and rejected a number of prescribed medications, and reported herself unable to carry out her normal activities on 19 days because of her health. Her diary shows the unremitting pattern of her symptoms: faintness and dizziness were rated as severe on 27/28 days; irritability as severe on 24 days; exhaustion, nervousness, sleep problems and headache were constant throughout the four weeks and frequently rated as severe. The only one of the 21 listed symptoms she did not experience was sore throat. Mrs D was referred by her GP for psychiatric consultation and during the last week of the diary she was awaiting an appointment. Her health, and in particular her psychological symptoms, deteriorated during the course of the diary. The fact that Mrs D rated her health below average on only 16 days, despite her severe symptoms, demonstrates the value of the single case approach: Mrs D's self-rated 'average' health would be rated as 'very poor' by most other women of her age.

The relationships between some of the diary variables are presented graphically in Figure 13.2*.

---

* The ratings (0–2) of each symptom have been added to give a daily 'symptom severity score' together with the number of symptoms recorded that day. For example, if a respondent recorded three symptoms and rated all as 'severe' her severity score would be 6; if she rated two as slight and one as severe her severity score would be 4 for that day.

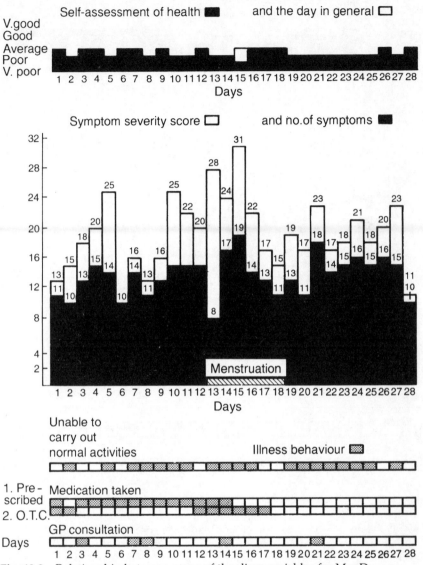

Fig. 13.2 Relationship between some of the diary variables for Mrs D.

As a contrast to the diary of Mrs D, Mrs C showed an improvement in health and a reduction in illness behaviour as the month progressed (see Figure 13.3). Mrs C is 25 years old, married with a six-year-old child. Her marriage to a man from a very different cultural background has been unhappy for some time and she has often sought the advice of the general practitioner during times of marital stress. She feels that her divorced parents burden her with their problems, and she sees herself as isolated, often lonely and unsupported emotionally. She had consulted her GP 14 times in the previous twelve months, and had been treated for depression. Unlike the other diarists, Mrs C reported nine symptom-free days, and no single complaint was recorded on more than

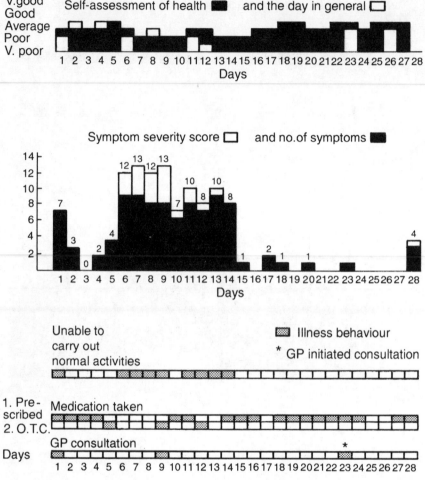

Fig. 13.3 Relationship between some of the diary variables for Mrs C.

twelve days. There was one clear episode of depressed mood lasting for about nine days, immediately preceding a menstrual period. During this time she reported herself unable to carry out her normal activities, and also recorded serious family rows (one with her father ending in physical violence). She took a prescribed antidepressant drug on 13 days, although only twice during the nine-day episode of acute depression. On the other eleven days on which she took this drug, she reported few, if any, complaints. She described herself as being 'very up and down' in mood, a description borne out by her diary. Like Mrs D, her problems seemed to be exacerbated by the absence of a supportive social network and, in particular, of a close confiding relationship. Marital and other family relationships were closely associated with Mrs C's illness.

In the next two cases, health problems had become chronic and the patterns of illness behaviour so well established that the diaries failed to show change.

Mrs K and Mrs L were both aged around 50 years with long-term marital problems. Both had problems with their older children, involving criminal behaviour, and both reported having no one in whom they could confide or from whom they received any support. They had consulted the general practitioner 10–16 times in the past twelve months. Their prevailing psychological symptoms of depression, anxiety, sleep disturbance and aches and pains did not vary sufficiently for any associations to be found with illness behaviour. Indeed, both respondents took prescribed medication each day and seldom assessed their health or the day in general as below average.

However, in the case of Mrs A, the diary does show the influence of an acute illness episode against a background of chronic symptoms. A mother of six young children, Mrs A regarded herself as friendless and isolated, with no practical or emotional support from her husband. With a family history of severe coronary disease, Mrs A herself had suffered recurrent deep vein thromboses during her pregnancies, and was currently in rather poor health. She had consulted her GP ten times in the previous twelve months with a variety of complaints. Two months before interview she had been involved in a road accident and had residual head and leg pains for which she was taking prescribed analgesics. Mrs A recorded no symptom-free days, and at some stage reported herself as suffering from 18 of the 21 listed symptoms. Exhaustion, headache, nervousness, irritability, pain in limbs, sleep disturbance and depression were her most frequently reported symptoms. Against this background of chronic psychological complaints, Mrs A reported an episode of acute gastrointestinal symptoms lasting for four days and leading to the one medical consultation during the month. During this episode, she evaluated both her health and the day in general as 'very poor', while for the remainder of the month her self-assessments were either 'good' or 'average', despite her chronic symptoms.

Other cases illustrate the relationship of 'new' symptoms with illness behaviour. When a respondent is already suffering from severe self-assessed psychological symptoms, a new complaint, of an apparently less disabling nature, can lead to medical consultation. Mrs G, aged 27 and with three children under four years of age, had been suffering from post-natal depression for four months, declining both medication and specialist psychiatric treatment. She reported experiencing 16 of the 21 listed symptoms at some time during the month, with exhaustion and depression on all but the last day. On 16 days she reported herself unable to carry out her normal activities.

She consulted a doctor twice during the month: once for a stiff neck, and on the second occasion for a sore throat while away from home on a family holiday. She received antibiotic medication for the second complaint which she took as prescribed. Her daily reports during the holiday suggest a time of increased stress, with marital disharmony and irritability with the children. This respondent, a trained nurse, was prepared to seek medical intervention in the form of drugs for her physical symptoms but not for her self-acknowledged depression.

Discussion

Fourteen case studies, involving an extensive exploratory interview, the administration of the Clinical Interview Schedule and the completion of a 28-day self-report diary, were conducted as a pilot study. The discussion of these cases will take the form of a methodological critique and an appraisal of the nature of predisposing and daily need variables included in the pilot study.

Study design

A fundamental problem of the design lay in sample selection. The majority of patients referred by the general practitioners were suffering from chronic and unremitting symptoms which showed little variation in severity from day to day. The expected covariation of illness behaviour with daily symptom changes could not be found in such cases. Not surprisingly, the doctors referred to the sample those patients who were well known to them because of their frequent attendances and who were known to have psychosocial problems. For the main study, respondents with more acute psychological symptoms will be recruited, since daily variations in symptoms would be more likely. Those with less chronic ill health are less likely to have become set in particular patterns of illness behaviour, such as the daily consumption of medication or regular medical consultation.

Two of the cases cited in this paper (Mrs A and Mrs G) show the influence on illness behaviour of an acute symptom episode, of whatever degree of severity, against a background of chronic psychosocial problems. The association in both these cases between the onset of new physical symptoms and a visit to the doctor suggests either that the additional health problems proved too much to cope with unsupported, or that the respondents considered physical illness more appropriate to medical intervention.

The occasion for selection of respondents, during a consultation with the general practitioner, probably served to reduce the amount of self-initiated illness behaviour during the diary period. All had received diagnosis, reassurance, prescription for medication, results of tests or a letter of referral to a hospital consultant. Their illnesses had thus been 'sanctioned' by the doctor and, to some degree, all respondents had been confirmed in the 'sick role'[45] and probably considered themselves entitled to take extra rest, to down rate their health or in other ways to take their symptoms more seriously. The keeping of a health diary may have become part of their sick role behaviour simply because *the doctor* had asked them to take part in the study at a time when they had presented themselves as sick. Some respondents seemed to believe that the diary was part of their therapy: 'Dr X thinks it might help me if I take part in this survey'. In the main study, efforts will be made to dissociate the diary study from the sick role: respondents will not be recruited at the time of consultation, but instead on the basis of self-completion postal questionnaires sent at random to patients on the practice list. It is hoped that this new emphasis on acute variations in health will improve the diary completion rate. The drop-out rate from the pilot stage may have resulted from the 'fatigue' engendered by the daily recording of chronic psychosocial problems. Several respondents did comment on the feeling of despondency created by their daily symptom reports.

The diary

It became apparent that offering respondents only three possible categories for daily symptom ratings (absent, slight and severe) resulted in insensitive measurement; two levels of severity cannot adequately reflect the daily variations in the experience of symptoms. A respondent who chose the rating 'severe' for a headache, for instance, was unable to increase the severity rating next day when the headache had become more troublesome. In analysing the data it is impossible to judge whether a 'severe' symptom remained unchanged throughout the month or became progressively worse. To resolve this problem, a visual analogue scale of 10 cm will be used for the self-ratings in the main study. The rating is made by placing a vertical line along the scale to denote the relative 'strength' of each symptom. The method provides much greater sensitivity and allows a variety of 'scoring' methods for the research worker – for example, the number of centimetres may be measured with a ruler to derive each symptom score; or each visual analogue scale may be divided into five equal sectors after completion and the subject's rating placed on a scale from 0 to 5.[46]

A second problem in the daily self-ratings arises from the difficulty in defining 'severity'. Each symptom will have a number of dimensions which may change in intensity from day to day – for example, frequency, duration, variability, painfulness, disruptiveness. In requiring a rating of severity we are expecting the respondent to make a multi-dimensional assessment. The literature on pain research[47] provides sufficient evidence of the linguistic dangers in trying to measure phenomena which are essentially subjective: 'Pain is a private matter'[48] which exists only because the sufferer considers it to be a problem. Since we cannot measure the strength or nature of the stimulus, we can only record the subjective response to it; in other words, we can ask only 'How bothered is the subject by what it is he is experiencing?'. The implication of the pain research literature is that attempts to measure severity should be avoided. In the main study, respondents will be asked to express how bothered they are by each symptom, using the visual analogue scales. Since single case analysis is to be used, it poses no problems that one individual's experience of discomfort cannot be compared with another's. We shall be comparing today's discomfort with tomorrow's in the same subject. Opportunity will be provided for each respondent to add her own additional symptoms to the pre-selected list, and to rate them on a visual analogue scale.

It was decided to retain the pre-selected list of symptoms for the main study rather than to attempt to construct ideographic symptom profiles. These were first introduced by Shapiro,[49] who constructed individual symptom profiles to evaluate treatment over time. This method would prove far too cumbersome for a self-completion health diary, since the incidence of new symptoms would require amending the diary during the period of completion. It is a method suited to clinical research among inpatients, not among members of the community at large.

The General Household Survey experience[50] has been that respondents record more symptoms when provided with a checklist. When asked to list their own symptoms, many are inhibited by their unfamiliarity with medical terminology. They may be reluctant to express in their own words some of the more 'personal' health problems.

The dependent variables, illness behaviour, will also be measured as a pre-selected list to include time off work, drug consumption, bed rest, resting more than usual, making an appointment to see the doctor, consulting another health worker, lay consultations, and purchasing medications. It is hoped that this will increase the rate of recording beyond that of asking the respondent what they did about their symptoms.

Predisposing and acute need variables

A small-scale pilot study such as this can only suggest the inclusion of variables for measurement in the main study. Among the 14 cases there was evidence of the factors thought to predispose to psychological symptoms and to illness behaviour. The most apparent was the lack of a close confidant in at least ten cases, a factor of significance in the development of depression[51] and in the severity of psychological symptoms.[52] Indeed, Lin *et al.*,[53] in a community study of the relationships between social support, stressful life events and the incidence of psychiatric symptoms, found that the contribution of social support to the prediction of symptoms was greater than that of life events.

It is beyond the scope of this chapter to enter the debate on the nature of the relationship between stressors, social support and the development of illness. Thoits[54] provides an extensive review of the evidence for the role of social support as a buffer against stressful events, concluding that the majority of studies suggest that a combination of low social support with one or more life events significantly increases symptoms of physical or psychological distress. However, she remains critical of the failure to formulate a precise, conceptual definition of social support and of the failure of most studies to develop valid or reliable indicators of the concept. In the main stage of the present study a standardized Social Problems Questionnaire (the SPQ), which has been developed and tested for reliability among general practice populations,[55,56] will be used to assess the level of social support, of both an intimate and more casual kind, in addition to measuring the extent of problems in housing, income, childcare, marriage, relatives, employment, leisure and social contacts. The multiple social problems reported by some respondents, in particular severe marital disharmony, suggests the importance of these factors in prolonging psychological illness. Since most respondents had symptoms of long duration, it was not possible to explore the association between social problems or life events and the incidence of symptoms.

Cobb,[57] in emphasizing that social support is an important component of the therapeutic process, believes the key factor to be its protective value. He explores the biological and social pathways to these effects, showing, for example, that lack of support often leads the patient to drop out of treatment or in other ways to fail to comply with therapeutic regimens.[58] This is one possible factor in prolonging the chronic episodes of depression evident in some of the pilot cases. The conceptual model of daily variations in health and illness behaviour will be applied in the design of the main study in much the same form as it was in the pilot study. Predisposing factors, such as the aspects of personality listed earlier and chronic health and social problems, interact with daily need variables to produce illness behaviour. At some point (perhaps the term 'threshold' might be applied), the balance of forces made up of predisposing and daily need factors no longer remains in equilibrium and the individual seeks external help for the discomfort. Zola's[5] conceptualization of an 'accommodation both physical, personal and social' to health problems is most appropriate. When this breaks down, because some new event or symptom has occurred to challenge the individual's ability to cope, help is sought.

Conclusion

The experience of this small-scale pilot study confirms the view that the self-controlled self-report health diary is an appropriate method for the study of psychiatric morbidity in general practice patients. Definitions of both independent and dependent variables have been refined by the findings of the pilot study, and the extensive background interview will include reliable and validated measures of both social problems and relevant personality attributes, or predisposing factors.

References

1 Mechanic, D. *Symptoms, Illness Behaviour and Help-seeking*. New York: Prodist, 1982.

2 Mechanic, D. The concept of illness behaviour. *J Chron Dis* 1962; **15**: 189–94.

3 Logan, W. P. D., Brooke, E. M. *The Survey of Sickness 1943–1952*. General Register Office Studies in Medical and Population Subjects No. 12. London: HMSO, 1957.

4 Dunnell, K., Cartwright, A. *Medicine Takers, Prescribers and Hoarders*. London: Routledge and Kegan Paul, 1972.

5 Zola, I. K. Pathways to the doctor: from person to patient. *Soc Sci Med* 1973; **7**: 677–89.

6 Hogben, L., Sim, M. The self-controlled and self-recorded clinical trial for low-grade morbidity. *Br J Prev Soc Med* 1953; **7**: 163–79.

7 Skinner, B. F. *The Behaviour of Organisms*. New York: Appleton-Century-Crofts, 1938.

[8] Kazdin, A. E. *Single-Case Research Designs. Methods for Clinical and Applied Settings.* Oxford: Oxford University Paperbacks, 1982.

[9] Shapiro, M. B. The single case in clinical-psychological research. *J Gen Psychol* 1966; **74**: 3–23.

[10] Barlow, D. H., Hersen, M. Single-case experimental designs: users in applied clinical research. *Arch Gen Psychiat* 1973; **29**: 319–25.

[11] Chassan, J. B. *Research Design in Clinical Psychology and Psychiatry.* 2nd ed. New York: Irvington, 1979.

[12] Herbst, P. G. *Behavioural Worlds: The Study of Single Cases.* London: Tavistock, 1970.

[13] Koos, E. L. *The Health of Regionville.* New York: Columbia University Press, 1954.

[14] Zborowski, M. Cultural components in response to pain. *J Soc Issues* 1952; **8**: 16–30.

[15] Maddox, G. Self-assessment of health status. *J Chron Dis* 1964; **17**: 449–60.

[16] Horder, J., Horder, E. Illness in general practice. *Practitioner* 1954; **173**: 177–85.

[17] White, K. L., Williams, T. F., Greenberg, B. G. The ecology of medical care. *New Eng J Med* 1961; **265**: 885–92.

[18] Banks, M. H., Beresford, S. A. A., Morrell, D. C., Waller, J. J., Watkins, C. J. Factors influencing demand for primary medical care in women aged 20–44 years: a preliminary report. *Int J Epidemiol* 1975; **4**: 189–95.

[19] Freer, C. B. Self-care: a health diary study. *Med Care* 1980; **18**: 853–61.

[20] Allen, G. I., Breslow, L., Weissman, A., Nisselson, H. Interviewing versus diary keeping in eliciting information in a morbidity survey. *Am J Pub Health* 1954; **44**: 919–27.

[21] Verbrugge, L. M. Health diaries. *Med Care* 1980; **18**: 73–95.

[22] Kratochwill, T. R. (ed.) *Single Subject Research: Strategies for Evaluating Change.* New York: Academic Press, 1978.

[23] Whitton, J. L. Periodicities in self-reports of health, sleep and mood variables. *J Psychosom Res* 1977; **22**: 111–15.

[24] Wallston, K. A., Wallston, B. S. Development of the Multidimensional Health Locus of Control (MHLC) Scales. *Health Educ Monographs* 1978; **6**: 160–70.

[25] Gurin, G., Veroff, J., Field, S. C. *Americans View Their Mental Health.* New York: Basic Books, 1960.

[26] Andersen, A. S., Laake, P. A causal model for physician utilization: analysis of Norwegian data. *Med Care* 1983; **21**: 276–8.

[27] Dean, K. J., Holst, E., Wagner, M. G. Self-care of common illness in Denmark. *Med Care* 1983; **21**: 1012–32.

28 Gortmaker, S. L., Eckenrode, J., Gore, S. Stress and the utilization of health services: a time series and cross-sectional analysis. *J Health Soc Behav* 1982; **23**: 25–38.

29 Roghmann, K. J., Haggerty, R. J. The diary as a research instrument in the study of health and illness behaviour: experiences with a random sample of young families. *Med Care* 1972; **10**: 143–63.

30 Alpert, J. J., Kosa, J., Haggerty, R. J. A month of illness and health care among low-income families. *Pub Health Rep* 1964; **82**: 705–13.

31 Robinson, D. *The Process of Becoming Ill.* London: Routledge and Kegan Paul, 1971.

32 Beresford, S. A. A., Waller, J. J., Banks, M. H., Wale, C. J. Why do women consult doctors? Social factors and the use of the general practitioner. *Br J Prev Soc Med* 1977; **31**: 220–6.

33 Scambler, A., Scambler, G., Craig, D. Kinship and friendship networks and women's demand for primary care. *J Roy Coll Gen Pract* 1981; **31**: 746–50.

34 Morrell, D. C., Wale, C. J. Symptoms perceived and recorded by patients. *J Roy Coll Gen Pract* 1976; **26**: 398–403.

35 Tessler, R., Mechanic, D., Dimond, M. The effect of psychological distress on physician utilization: a prospective study. *J Health Soc Behav* 1976; **17**: 353–64.

36 Meyer, R. J., Haggerty, R. J. Streptococcal infections in families. *Pediatrics* 1962; **29**: 539–49.

37 McKinlay, J. B., Dutton, D. B. Social-psychological factors affecting health service utilization. In: Mushkin, S. (ed.) *Consumer Incentives for Health Care.* New York: Prodist, 1974.

38 Cooper, B. The epidemiological approach to psychosomatic medicine. *J Psychosom Res* 1964; **8**: 9–15.

39 Kellner, R. *Family Ill Health: An Investigation in General Practice.* London: Tavistock, 1963.

40 Shepherd, M., Cooper, B., Brown, A. C., Kalton, G. W. *Psychiatric Illness in General Practice.* London: OUP, 1966.

41 Goldberg, D. P. *The Detection of Psychiatric Illness by Questionnaire.* Maudsley Monographs No. 21. London: OUP, 1972.

42 Goldberg, D. P. *Manual of the General Health Questionnaire.* Windsor: NFER, 1978.

43 Goldberg, D. P., Cooper, B., Eastwood, M., Kedward, H. B., Shepherd, M. A standardised interview for use in community surveys. *Br J Prev Soc Med* 1970; **24**: 18–23.

44 Murray, J., Dunn, G., Tarnopolsky, A. Self-assessment of health: an exploration of the effects of physical and psychological symptoms. *Psychol Med* 1982; **12**: 371–8.

[45] Parsons, T. Definitions of health and illness in the light of American values and social structure. In: Jaco, E. G. (ed.) *Patients, Physicians and Illness*. Glencoe, Illinois: The Free Press, 1958.

[46] Huskisson, E. C. Visual analogue scales. In: Melzack, R. (ed.) *Pain Measurement and Assessment*. New York: Raven Press, 1983.

[47] Melzack, R. (ed.) *Pain Measurement and Assessment*. New York: Raven Press, 1983.

[48] Fordyce, W. E. The validity of pain behaviour measurement. In: Melzack, R. (ed.) *Pain Measurement and Assessment*. New York: Raven Press, 1983.

[49] Shapiro, M. B. *The Personal Questionnaire: A Method of Measuring Change in the Symptoms of an Individual Psychiatric Patient*. London: Institute of Psychiatry, 1961.

[50] Cartwright, A. *Health Surveys in Practice and in Potential*. London: King Edward's Hospital Fund, 1983.

[51] Brown, G. W., Harris, T. *Social Origins of Depression: A Study of Psychiatric Disorder in Women*. London: Tavistock, 1978.

[52] Miller, P., Ingham, J. G. Friends, confidants and symptoms. *Soc Psychiat* 1976; **11**: 51–8.

[53] Lin, N., Ensel, W. M., Simeone, R. S., Kuo, W. Social support, stressful life events and illness: a model and an empirical test. *J Health Soc Behav* 1979; **20**: 108–19.

[54] Thoits, P. Conceptual, methodological and theoretical problems in studying social support as a buffer against life stress. *J Health Soc Behav* 1982; **23**: 145–59.

[55] Corney, R. H., Clare, A. W., Fry, J. The development of a self-report questionnaire to identify social problems – a pilot study. *Psychol Med* 1982; **12**: 903–9.

[56] Corney, R. H., Clare, A. W. The construction, development and testing of a self-report questionnaire to identify social problems. *Psychol Med* 1985; **15**: 637–49.

[57] Cobb, S. Social support as a moderator of life stress. *Psychol Med* 1976; **38**: 300–14.

[58] Sackett, D. L., Haynes, B. *Compliance with Therapeutic Regimens*. Baltimore: Johns Hopkins University Press, 1976.

14 The multivariate structure of treatment practices in complementary medicine

Lorraine Nanke and David Canter

Summary

The current study was designed to determine whether a meaningful order could be identified in the empirical relationships between treatments used by complementary practitioners. Results indicate that there is an underlying order which can be accounted for in terms of two interacting facets, mode of clinical intervention and degree of specialization. These findings provide some support for the existence of a reliable order between specialist approaches, and a genuinely holistic core of treatments which can be drawn on by practitioners. The contribution of these findings to cross-disciplinary dialogue and the development of clinically relevant research is discussed.

Introduction

Earlier research[1] has shown that many patients take advantage of the variety of complementary practitioners available to them by consulting more than one practitioner for their current complaint. It is also clear from examination of lists of registered practitioners that many are qualified in more than one discipline. Furthermore, informal discussion and observation of complementary practitioners reveals that many utilize a mixture of therapeutic practices in any one consultation.

This diversity and eclecticism poses special problems for the scientific study of the effectiveness of therapies in use. What are the actual constituents of treatment used by a practitioner? This problem is compounded by the finding that in the domain of psychotherapy, practitioners may be more effective with one therapy than they are with another. A primary research question, then, is whether there do exist any identifiable relationships between the variety of treatments used by practitioners, thereby giving rise to types of practitioners who use particular subsets of treatments, or whether there is a virtually random *ad hoc* use of treatments depending on the interests or idiosyncracies of particular practitioners. If the former is the case then research on efficacy can explore the differences between types of practitioner. If the latter is the case, then the task for the student of the power of complementary medicine is difficult indeed.

In view of these other differences, West has claimed that 'complementary medicine' is a general term encompassing approaches of varied type and worth[2] (p. 342). She has proposed a two-way classification system for complementary medical treatments (CMT) in the UK. Firstly, CMTs can be distinguished on the basis of a primarily physical, psychological or paranormal orientation (the latter being a judgemental term derivative from natural science). Secondly, CMTs can be categorized into those which require a high degree of professional training and those which are basically a variation on first aid, do-it-yourself, and self care techniques. She suggests osteopathy, chiropractic, medical herbalism, homoeopathy, naturopathy and acupuncture would fit the first category (as well as biomedicine), and everything else except a few psychotherapies would fit the second.

A distinction between the internalizing and externalizing systems of treatment has been proposed by Young.[3] Externalizing systems look outside the body for explanation of cause of suffering (e.g. paranormal belief that something injurious or evil entered the body from outside). By contrast internalizing systems look inside the body for explanations, and generally require a great deal of formal training.

These suggestions can be seen as 'meta theories' within which similarities and differences between CMTs can be described and compared. A meta theory is a robust logical framework which must be value-free in the sense that it is theoretically neutral, and does not simply translate one system into the language of another (e.g. translating homoeopathy into biomedical terms). The role of meta theory in facilitating cumulative research and its importance for the developing field of CMT has been described at greater length by Canter.[4] It is worth restating that the Facet Approach to scientific theory development is based on exploring the correspondence between theoretical classifications (e.g. internalizing and externalizing treatment approaches) and empirical observations, and providing a rationale for this correspondence.[5] As such, the Facet Approach could prove a useful tool for establishing an empirical basis for any proposed classification system or meta theory.

This account could prove useful in communication with critics who attribute the therapeutic efficacy of CMT to 'placebo factors' such as time and touch, and seem to take little account of the differences between treatment approaches. An account of the structure underlying CMT may help focus the debate on more productive questions such as what type of role psychological and other factors play in different types of treatment, including orthodox treatments.

Without such a meta theory there is a real danger that the term 'complementary medicine' lends a spurious coherence to a miscellaneous assortment of treatments, each with their own associated research programmes, theoretical explanations and clinical practices. It would be ironic if approaches which are united against fragmentation of the patient become themselves fragmented into separate and unconnected disciplines.

In brief, despite some similarities, there are many important differences between treatment approaches included under the heading 'complementary medicine', and the domain of their shared concern gives little indication of how they connect with each other. Though the NHS may be criticized for compartmentalizing the patient into a series of body parts or functions corresponding to different disciplines, this does constitute an implicit meta theory about the nature of treatments, and the relationships between them. By contrast, little is known about whether, how and to what extent complementary practices actually interface in patient treatment. The development of a meta theory of treatments would go a long way to addressing these problems, and the Facet Approach may be a useful tool contributing to the development of such a meta theory.

The current study

The current study is part of a series being carried out at Surrey University. The central aim of the research is to identify patterns of association between patient beliefs about their illness and treatment, presenting condition, treatment received and treatment outcome. The main focus of interest in this series is with homoeopathy, though data has also been collected from a range of practitioners where a particular study, such as the one reported here, is of general relevance to complementary medical practice.

This chapter describes one module of this series, which is designed to determine whether and what kind of order underlies CMTs. This is an important prerequisite to carrying out theoretically meaningful comparisons between different types of treatments. The main strategy adopted was to find out what complementary medical practitioners actually do with their patients. The relationship between treatments practised was chosen as a potentially fruitful approach to developing an empirically based classification system because, within the field of complementary medicine, many practitioners include a range of treatments in their repertoire.

The current study is based on the hypothesis that an examination of the treatments actually used by complementary medicine practitioners will reveal whether there is a coherent structure underlying the diversity of treatments collectively referred to as 'complementary medicine', and whether such a structure provides empirical corroboration for existing classification systems, or requires new hypotheses to account for observed variations.

Method

The questionnaire on which the current study is based is part of a battery which was distributed to three groups of complementary practitioners. The first group included all practitioners listed in the Register of Homoeopaths. The second group included all practitioners who attended the Research Council for Complementary Medicine's conference on research at Keble College, Oxford in April 1989. The third group included practitioners whose names had been included on returned questionnaires from the first two groups, in response to a question asking whether the participant had any colleagues who may be willing to participate in the research.

The sample is clearly biased towards practitioners who have an active interest in research, and homoeopaths. As such it is not representative of the range of complementary therapists in practice. However, the focus of concern here is with the relationship between CMTs practised, and there is little or no evidence linking practitioner discipline directly to treatment repertoire, so the sample is adequate to provide an initial account of the structure of relationships in this area.

The majority of practitioners in the current sample work exclusively in private practice (84.4%). Some work both privately and in the NHS (11.1%) and a small number exclusively in the NHS (2.2%).

In terms of qualifications, 31% did not list any qualification directly related to the practice of complementary medicine, and 43% listed qualification in more than one discipline. 11% of the sample were qualified medical practitioners.

Table 14.2 shows that the median length of clinical experience is 6–10 years, though it is noteworthy that over one-fifth have more than 20 years' experience.

Participating practitioners were asked to include their name and address, so the study was not anonymous. Despite assurances that names would not be entered on the computer, or used for purposes other than the current study, this perhaps reduces the overall responses. In total, approximately 500 questionnaires and Freepost envelopes were distributed, and 118 have been returned and included in the current study, a return rate of 24%.

Questionnaire development

A list of treatments was constructed on the basis of approaches which are well known, or referred to in the complementary medical literature. For the sake of brevity, the list was not comprehensive, but included a representative range of treatment approaches. In view of the importance attributed to 'time and touch', several items referring to advice and physical examination were included even though they do not constitute recognized treatments in their own right.

Practitioners were asked to rate each treatment for frequency of use with patients on a five point Likert-type scale, ranging from 'never' to 'always'.

Table 14.1 Demographic characteristics of respondents

Age	Sex	
	Male	Female
Under 25	1.5%	0.7%
26–40	17.0%	22.2%
41–60	20.7%	23.7%
Over 60	4.4%	5.2%
Missing data	4.3%	

Table 14.2   Clinical experience

Years of clinical experience	
Less than 2	13.3
2–5	23.0
6–10	28.9
11–20	10.4
More than 20	21.5
Missing data	3.0

Results

Frequencies of treatment use

As a first stage in the data analysis, the mean ratings for use of each treatment were calculated. Table 14.3 shows the rank ordered means for treatment use. Higher mean ratings correspond to increased frequency of use.

Table 14.3 provides some support for the suggestion that time and touch play an important role in CMT, as advice and physical examination are most frequently used. These are followed by homoeopathy (which reflects the questionnaire distribution), counselling, dietary advice and manipulative treatments.

The relatively high frequency with which dietary advice is used by practitioners in this sample is consistent with previous results showing this approach to be most useful in differentiating between GP and complementary treatment.[6] Specific CMTs which have been developed fairly recently, or represent novel clinical applications of particular objects or processes such as Kirlian aura diagnosis, biofeedback, music therapy, hypnotherapy and gem therapy, are the least frequently used by practitioners in this sample.

These mean ratings provide an indication of the types of treatment used by practitioners in the current sample. In order to examine the relationships between treatments practised, the data was subject to Smallest Space Analysis, a statistical procedure which merits some explanation.

Smallest Space Analysis of treatments matrix

Smallest Space Analysis (SSA)[7] is a non-metric multidimensional scaling procedure, based on the assumption that the underlying structure, or system of treatments, will be most clearly apparent if the relationship between every treatment and every other treatment is examined. As the raw mathematical relationships between all variables would be difficult to interpret, a geometric visual representation of these relationships is produced.

Table 14.3   Rank order of treatment use

Treatment	Item no.	Mean
General advice	(35)	3.3
Advice about health	(33)	3.2
Physical examination	(21)	3.1
Advice about illness	(34)	3.0
Homoeopathic remedies	(22)	2.8
Counselling	(36)	2.8
Recommended diet	(31)	2.6
Physical manipulation Massage	(20) (14)	2.1
Osteopathy Herbal remedies Stress management Relaxation training	(9) (24) (11) (19)	2.0
Vitamins/minerals	(27)	1.9
Naturopathic remedies Meditation Exercises/yoga	(23) (13) (12)	1.8
Spiritual healing	(3)	1.7
Psychotherapy Acupuncture	(37) (2)	1.6
Cranial osteopathy	(17)	1.5
Orthodox medication Particular oils	(25) (32)	1.4
Heat treatment Hydrotherapy	(10) (6)	1.3
Iridology Reflexology Colour therapy Chiropractic Radionics Injections	(28) (5) (4) (8) (29) (30)	1.2
Minor surgery Gem therapy Hypnotherapy Music therapy Biofeedback	(26) (7) (1) (15) (18)	1.1
Kirlian aura diagnosis	(16)	1.0

The SSA programme computes correlation coefficients between all variables, in this case treatments used by complementary medical practitioners, then rank orders these correlations. The original rectangular raw data matrix is transformed into a triangular matrix consisting of correlation coefficients for every variable with every other variable. These correlation coefficients are used to form a spatial representation of items, with points representing variables. The rank order of the distances between points is inversely related to the rank order of correlations, so that the closer two points are in the space, the more highly they are correlated. Iterations are performed comparing the rank order assigned to the correlations with the rank order of the distance while adjustments are made to the geometric representation. The closer the two rank orders, and the better the 'fit' between the geometric representation and the original correlation matrix, as it is technically termed, the lower the 'stress'. The iterations continue until the minimum stress possible is achieved, within the predesignated number of iterations and dimensions. A measure of stress called the coefficient of alienation[8] is used within the computing algorithm as the criterion to use in bringing the iterative procedure to an end. It can therefore be used as a general indication of the degree to which the variables' intercorrelations are represented by their corresponding spatial distances. The smaller the coefficients of alienation, the better the fit of the spatial plot to the original correlation matrix. However, as Borg and Lingoes emphasize, there is no simple answer to the question of how 'good' or 'bad' the representation is. This will depend on a complex combination of the number of variables, the amount of error in the data, and the logical strength of the interpretation framework.

To summarize, in the SSA configuration, the more highly correlated two variables are, the closer will be the points representing those variables in the SSA space. As the configuration is developed in respect to the relationships among variables and not from their relationship to some given dimension or axis, the orientation in space of the axes of the resulting geometric representation are arbitrary, even though the relationships between points are replicably determined. Therefore, the pattern of points (regions) can be examined directly without the need to assume underlying orthogonal dimensions.

An approach to research known as Facet Theory is used to test the evidence for ways of classifying variables on the basis of the regional structure of an SSA. The 'facets' are the overall classification of the types of variables. The spatial contiguity of the points representing them provides a test of the major underlying differences amongst these variables as revealed through their co-occurrence in questionnaire responses, and is therefore a test as to whether the facets are empirically supported. The SSA representation therefore offers a basis for testing and developing hypotheses about the structure of relationships between complementary medical treatments.

Facets can be developed as hypotheses which define the research questions of a particular study, and tested by assessing their correspondence to contiguous regions in the SSA plot, or generated on the basis of regional structures in the SSA plot as in the present case. The reliability of facets can be determined by the usual processes of scientific replication.

The mean ratings obtained for use of each treatment do not bear any inevitable relationship to the SSA plot, which is based on correlation coefficients rather than overall frequencies. Any relationship which is found is therefore not a statistical artefact but an empirical finding open to substantive interpretation.

Results of SSA

The SSA-1 was carried out on triangular matrix of Pearsons product moment correlation coefficients. Ideally, a coefficient of alienation of 0.15 or below is preferable with clear data sets which have a low error factor. The four-dimensional solution of the current SSA has a Guttman-Lingoes coefficient of alienation of 0.13 in 43 iterations, which is within these limits. However, as similar regional structures are identifiable in the two-, three- and four-dimensional solutions, the two-dimensional solution, with a coefficient of alienation of .29 in eleven iterations, is presented here for the sake of simplicity.

Figure 14.1 shows one projection of the two-dimensional SSA configuration. The numbers correspond to treatments listed on the original questionnaire, and can be individually identified from Table 14.3. The closer any two points are, the more likely are the treatments they represent to co-occur in the treatment repertoire of practitioners in the current sample. Conversely, the farther apart two points are, the less likely they are to co-occur in an individual's treatment repertoire. The SSA allows a test of all relationships between the 37 treatments included in the study. The two-dimensional SSA of treatments used is shown in Figure 14.1.

This plot provides some support for the hypothesis that there is an interpretable structure underlying use of CMTs. Two major facets can be identified in the SSA space.

Facet 1: mode of intervention

Distributed around the periphery of the plot are six conceptually distinct regions which can be seen as ordered categories of a facet representing mode, or locus, of clinical intervention. These six regions have been labelled on the basis of items contained within them, and lines have been drawn onto the plot to indicate the approximate boundaries of each region.

Table 14.4 lists the name of each region and the elements contained within it. Mean ratings obtained for each region have been included to provide a general profile of treatment practices in terms of this facet.

There are two main points to be made about these results. Firstly, in virtually all projections these regions are organized in the same circular order suggesting that this is a reliable pattern of relationships open to substantive interpretation. At the most basic level, this order does

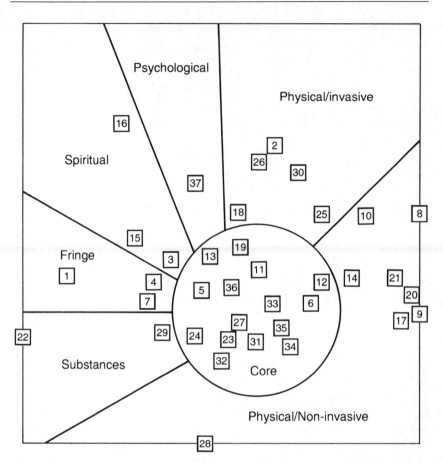

Fig. 14.1   Relationships between treatments used.

support West's[2] qualitative distinction between physical, psychological and paranormal treatments as these are consistently identifiable in separate regions around the periphery of the plot. However, the SSA plot suggests that within the domain of physical CMTs, clear distinctions can be drawn between the types of treatment described in regions 1 to 4 in Table 14.4.

Secondly, this order of relationships can be seen as reflecting a holistic model of the person, with different types of treatment located at adjacent levels from within the body, to body surface, to substances, to other objects and processes, to spiritual forces, to psychology which is adjacent to within the body.

This finding provides some grounds for the hypothesis that each level of intervention represents a different degree of invasiveness of each treatment type for the patient. The region which has been labelled physical invasive, including orthodox medical treatments and acupuncture, includes the most internal or invasive forms of treatment, and

Table 14.4   Modes of intervention: regional means

Region	Treatments included	Mean
1 Physical, invasive	Minor surgery, acupuncture, injections, orthodox medication	1.4
2 Physical, non-invasive	Heat treatment, massage, physical manipulation, physical examination, chiropractic, osteopathy, exercise, cranial osteopathy, hydrotherapy	1.8
3 Substances	Homoeopathy, naturopathy, diet, vitamins, oils, herbal remedies	2.1
4 Other objects or processes	Radionics, gem therapy, colour therapy, reflexology, hypnotherapy, iridology, music therapy	1.1
5 Spiritual	Spiritual healing, meditation	1.6
6 Psychological	Psychotherapy, relaxation, counselling, stress management, advice	2.5

homoeopathy at the opposite end of the plot represents the least invasive for the patient.

The circular order indicates that treatments are not differentiated simply on a linear continuum from more to less invasive types of treatment, but are qualitatively differentiated in terms of the nature as well as the degree of invasiveness. On this hypothesis, psychotherapy to one side of the physically invasive region, and osteopathy to the other side, represent similar degrees but different types of invasiveness.

This hypothesis is similar to Young's[3] distinction between internalizing and externalizing systems, though the current pattern of results seems to be better accounted for by internality of level of intervention rather than level of explanation associated with each treatment type. For example, hypnotherapy, vitamins and cranial osteopathy are all based on internal explanations of the patient's condition, but appear widely distributed across the plot. This distribution can be accounted for in terms of their differing points of intervention.

Though this category system is necessarily broad and coarse-grained, it does show that in general terms CMTs are differentiated into groups on the basis of level of clinical intervention with patients.

Facet 2: degree of specialization

The second facet from the centre to the periphery of the plot can be interpreted as degree of specialism. A circular line has been drawn onto the SSA plot to show the approximate boundaries of each region.

Treatments included within the central region are relatively highly correlated, and include treatments from all specialties described by facet 1 (mode of intervention) except the physically invasive region. The notional centre of this region involves giving general advice, and advice about health and illness. Treatments distributed around advice within this circle include oils and vitamins from the substances region, reflexology from the 'fringe' region, meditation from the 'spiritual' region, counselling, stress management and relaxation from the psychological region, and exercises and massage from the physically non-invasive region.

This central region includes treatments from all modes of intervention except the physically invasive, and is roughly equidistant from the specialties distributed around the peripheral circle. This finding provides support for the suggestion of a core of treatments which are genuinely holistic, in the sense that all levels of clinical intervention with patients except the physically invasive are represented. These treatments can be seen as the conceptual core of CMT, which may be drawn on to differing degrees by practitioners associated with the peripheral specialties.

The matrix of correlations between representative treatments from this core region are shown in Table 14.5.

In West's terms, this central region represents treatments most nearly associated with self-help or 'time and touch' which may, but do not necessarily, involve extensive professional training.

Items in the peripheral circle represent distinct specialisms within the domain of CMT which discriminate well between practitioners. These treatments have the lowest intercorrelations, and include most of the well-established and highly elaborated disciplines within the field of CMT which are normally associated with extensive professional training. The term 'specialist' in this context is not used to denote degree of professionalism or training associated with any particular treatment, but the extent to which a treatment is used independently of other particular treatments. For example, herbal medicine is located within the core region despite the fact that it is a well-established professional treatment, whereas homoeopathy emerges as a particularly specialized treatment on the periphery of the space. This is only partially accounted for by the large number of homoeopaths in the current sample: it suggests that use of homoeopathy is relatively independent of use of any other treatment. By contrast, use of herbal medicine is more closely associated with the central core of treatments and related specialisms such as naturopathy. The correlations between these specialist treatments are shown in Table 14.6.

Comparison between the correlation matrices in Tables 14.5 and 14.6 shows the relatively high positive association between core treatments, and the relatively low or negative association between specialist treatments, which are graphically represented in the SSA plot (Figure 14.1).

In summary, the SSA plot of treatment use can be interpreted in terms of two interacting facets: mode of intervention and degree of specialization.

Table 14.5 Correlations between core treatments

	General Advice	Advice on Health	Stress Management	Counselling	Diet	Vitamins	Exercise	Massage	Naturopathy
General Advice	★								
Advice on Health	.67	★							
Stress Management	.43	.50	★						
Counselling	.62	.61	.52	★					
Diet	.50	.68	.40	.37	★				
Vitamins	.40	.46	.38	.31	.57	★			
Exercise	.28	.33	.43	.26	.33	.44	★		
Massage	.35	.42	.34	.22	.28	.28	.52	★	
Naturopathy	.39	.42	.35	.23	.58	.71	.35	.14	★

Table 14.6   Correlations between specialist treatments

	Psycho-therapy	Spiritual Healing	Homoe-opathy	Oste-opathy	Acu-puncture	Orthodox Medicine
Psychotherapy	★					
Spiritual Healing	.23	★				
Homoeopathy	−.22	−.07	★			
Osteopathy	−.02	−.15	−.31	★		
Acupuncture	.21	.05	−.20	.09	★	
Orthodox Medicine	.14	.09	−.06	.27	.09	★

Discussion

The results obtained by the current study indicate that there is a coherent and interpretable structure underlying practitioner use of CMTs. The distribution of treatments used can be accounted for in terms of two interacting facets which have been described here as mode of intervention and degree of specialization. Mode of intervention seems to reflect a holistic model of the person, with different types of treatment being characterized by clinical intervention at different levels of the person. Degree of specialization refers to a distinction between core treatments from all levels of intervention except the physically invasive which are relatively highly correlated. These can be seen as a set of approaches which may be drawn on by different types of practitioner, by contrast with the well-differentiated range of specialisms which are relatively independent of use of any other particular treatments. These facets resemble West's classification of CMTs on the basis of physical, psychological and spiritual orientation, and degree of training required, and to this extent provide empirical corroboration for her proposal.

The current findings cast a new light on the concept of 'holism' and suggest that the philosophy of CMT may be reflected in the pattern of relationships between treatments used in two ways. Firstly, the order of specialisms reflects a holistic model of the person, with different treatment types characterized by different levels of intervention with the patient. The only level within this structure which has no analogue within the NHS is spiritual: this provides some support for Campbell's[9] suggestion that it is the implicitly and sometimes explicitly spiritual view of human nature which makes CMT holistic, and differentiates it from orthodox medicine (p. 143).

Secondly, it is often assumed that the holistic approach is clinically associated with increased 'time and touch'. However, as Campbell[9] has pointed out, good practitioners, whether orthodox or complementary, do take the wider aspects of patients' problems into account so this may be a pseudo-distinction between the two systems. Conversely, in the context of traditional healing, Press[10] has provided considerable evidence that the stereotypical healer offering long consultations to unravel complex individual problems is based more on myth than on fact. The current results suggest that it may be possible to differentiate between practitioners across both orthodox and complementary disciplines in terms of the extent to which they do utilize 'time and touch' and self-help based treatments from this core region.

There is also an analogy between these results and findings in psychotherapy outcome research which demonstrate the importance of core therapist qualities, namely warmth, genuineness, and accurate empathy, in the many different types of psychotherapeutic treatment.[11] Within psychotherapy, there is a considerable degree of consensus that these core qualities play an important role in producing therapeutic change. There is far less agreement about whether they are sufficient for therapeutic change. In broad terms, humanistic or client centred practitioners tend to see core conditions as sufficient to produce change, whereas cognitive, behavioural and psychodynamic practitioners tend to believe that particular techniques are also required.[12] There is some research evidence that the core conditions interact with therapist orientation, type of patient, and type of treatment.[13]

The results of the current study suggest corresponding questions can usefully be asked in the domain of CMT, e.g. what contribution do the core of 'time and touch' and self-help related treatments make to treatment outcome in particular patient populations, with particular practitioner orientations, and particular treatments? On one hand, both sceptics who attribute the clinical efficacy of CMT to 'placebo factors' and CMT practitioners who stress the role of treatment in facilitating the body's own self-healing may be claiming that these are sufficient conditions for therapeutic change. On the other hand, many CMT practitioners, like psychoanalysts and behavioural psychologists, believe that it is the appropriate use of particular treatments which accounts for therapeutic outcome.

The identification of a coherent and differentiated structure underlying CMT considerably detracts from the force of arguments which dismiss these approaches en masse, and provides a broad framework for the generation and testing of specific hypotheses about the relation between different types of treatment and their contribution to treatment outcome.

References

1. Canter, D., Booker, K. Multiple consultations as a basis for classifying patients' use of conventional and unconventional medical practice. *Comp Med Res* 1987; **2**(2): 141–60.

2. West, R. Alternative medicine: prospects and speculations. In: Black, B., Boswell, D., Gray, A., Murphy, S., Popay, J. (eds.) *Health and Disease*. Milton Keynes: Open University Press, 1984; p. 342.

3. Young, A. Internalising and externalising medical belief systems: an Ethiopian example. In: Currer, C., Stacey, M. (eds.) *Concepts of Health, Illness and Disease: A Comparative Perspective*. Leamington Spa: Berg, 1986.

[4] Canter, D. A research agenda for holistic therapy. *Comp Med Res* 1987; **2**(1): 104–16.

[5] Canter, D. (ed.) *Facet Theory*. New York: Springer Verlag, 1985.

[6] Fulder, S. *The Handbook of Complementary Medicine*. 2nd ed. Oxford: OUP, 1988.

[7] Lingoes, J. C. *The Guttman-Lingoes Nonmetric Program Series*. Ann Arbor: Mathesis, 1973.

[8] Borg, I., Lingoes, J. C. *Multidimensional Similarity Analysis*. New York: Springer Verlag, 1987.

[9] Campbell, A. *The Two Faces of Homoeopathy*. London: Robert Hale, 1984.

[10] Press, I. The urban curandero. *Am Anthropol* 1971; **73**: 741–56.

[11] Truax, C. B., Mitchell, K. M. Research on certain therapist interpersonal skills in relation to process and outcome. In: Bergin, A. E., Garfield, S. L. (eds.) *Handbook of Psychotherapy and Behavior Change*. New York: Wiley, 1971.

[12] Walrond-Skinner, S. *A Dictionary of Psychotherapy*. London: Routledge, 1986.

[13] Mitchell, K. M. *et al.* A reappraisal of accurate empathy, non possessive warmth and genuineness in effective psychotherapy. In: Gurman, A. S., Razin, A. M. (eds.) *Psychotherapy*. New York: Pergamon, 1977.

15 The use of alternative treatments in the Finnish adult population

Tuula Vaskilampi, Pirkko Meriläinen and Sirkka Sinkkonen

Introduction

The historical roots of the health care system in Finland

The official health care system of Finland belongs to the long Scandinavian tradition according to which local communities own and run health services. Health is not mentioned in the Finnish Constitution but its spirit and applied practice make it clear that every citizen is entitled to health care and that society, i.e. public authorities, is responsible for organizing it.[1] Public responsibility and control have increased since the Second World War when the modern welfare state was formed. However, the industrialization process was late and rapid in Finland compared to other European countries.

The fast pace of economic growth and industrialization is illuminated by the following data. While Britain's average real per capita income surpassed that of Finland by 200% between 1925 and 1935, in 1977 it was 30% smaller than that of Finland.[1,2,3] As late as the 1950s, agriculture and forestry employed 46% of the population, which figure dropped down to 9% by 1980.[1] Finland can be considered young as a European welfare state.

The welfare state has been closely associated with scientific Western medicine which has received the mandate to provide services. These services only are legally recognized and are covered by subsidized fundings. Indeed, with the development of the modern welfare state priority and legitimacy has been given to one healing model based on natural scientific paradigms, while other healing traditions and new models have become informal, hidden and often illegal.[4,5,6,7,8,9,10] In Finland this means that they are outside health care personnel education and they are not eligible for public support (social security).

In the history of Finnish health care, public midwives were appointed in the eighteenth century and district medical officers at the end of the nineteenth century. The 1950s and 1960s saw the creation of a hospital network, and since the Primary Health Care Act (1972) made provision for community care, Finland has been chosen as one of the European reporting countries of the WHO Programme of Health for All by the Year 2000.[1,11] The modern health care system of Finland is comprehensive, covering primary and secondary care as well as curative and preventive care. One of the basic principles of Finnish health policy has been to increase equality by breaking down economic and geographical barriers to care.

The health services and health status of the population in Finland

The availability of health services has increased remarkably during the past 20 years, and the differences in services between rural and urban communities have decreased.[11,12] The patient–doctor ratio has increased from 1100 inhabitants per doctor at the end of the 1960s to a ratio of 450 inhabitants per doctor in the 1980s. In spite of the development of primary health care, the proportional number of hospital beds is still high, being 15.2 hospital beds per 1000 inhabitants. The entire population is covered by health insurance, which includes compensation for lost earnings and treatment expenses for public and private health services. The average visit rates to a doctor have been 2–4 times per year in recent years.[1]

The health of the Finns has been characterized by exceptionally high mortality among men and very low infant mortality (5.8 per thousand in 1982). There are also differences between male and female health status. The life expectancy of Finnish women is almost 80 years while that of the men was approximately 70 years in the 1980s. Cardiovascular diseases, suicides and lung cancer stand out in male mortality rates. Also, disability pension rates have been high in Finland. Cardiovascular, musculoskeletal and mental health problems have been the main causes of early retirement.[1,11,12,13]

The emergence of alternative medicine in Finland

In spite of the modern and comprehensive official health care system, which holds a strong position in Finland, there exists alongside scientific medicine an unofficial system based on different healing traditions.[6,14] In health service research, this unofficial sector was largely neglected in Finland as it was in other Western countries until the 1970s. The scope, role and function of unorthodox medicine in the Western welfare states are poorly described and understood because of lack of empirical studies and theoretical discussion. Alternative medicine has been seen as regressive,[15,16] and bound to disappear as soon as rationally and effectively organized scientific services were fully developed. The main concern of the Finnish health policy was to increase access to official health care, which was regarded as the right of every citizen. Health care and education systems were to create social equality and integration. The basic barriers were seen to be economic and cultural, which were expected to disappear with social security.[4,17] The contents and the process of health care were overlooked.

The fully established welfare state has faced criticism, which is expressed by citizens and political parties on the left and right. This, together with post-industrialism, has brought reactions such as counter-cultural social movements, privatization and different development projects inside welfare services. The basic dissatisfaction is with the efficiency, effectiveness and legitimacy of welfare services. Separate issues have emerged; the freedom of citizens, the control of the state penetrating into the private life, and the side effects of mass production. The urban middle class has been especially active in searching for solutions and new lifestyles.[18,19]

Health services represent this general criticism. There is dissatisfaction expressed with biomedical paradigms and organizational structures.[20,21,22] In this context alternative medicine has become popular – it is forming its own field. It offers different discourses varying from rational to irrational and from empirical to religious and mythological ways of thinking. It operates beyond the natural sciences in the universe of symbols and meanings, where holistic, natural and ecological ideas are emphasized.[14,23,24,25,26,27]

In Finland, this unofficial field became visible in the 1970s and 1980s. The interest in Finnish folk medicine has increased as well as in foreign and modern treatments outside scientific medicine. There are increasing numbers of health shops, different physical, body-building centres, seminars, training courses and healing sessions. Finnish traditional healers work individually in face-to-face treatment situations. There are cuppers still using knives and horns in saunas,[6] 'blood-stoppers' who treat patients with secret words,[28] bone-setters and traditional masseurs.[27] In their practices, they are the bearers of traditional wisdom and skills.

In the modern alternative field, some charismatic religious and spiritual healers have become famous, running collective healing sessions. There are several modern therapists who mainly work individually, too. They have received their training through different courses.[29]

It is typical of Finnish alternative medicine that it is unorganized, not legally recognized and operates in private markets outside public support.[29]

The use of alternative medicine in Europe

In Sweden, 3.8% of the adult population (16–74 years of age) had used herbal remedies and 2.1% had visited an alternative therapist in the last two weeks in 1980 and 1981. The most commonly used therapies were homoeopathy, including traditional herbal medicine, and 'chiropathy' including traditional bone-setting.[30]

In 1981, J. van Hecke estimated that 10–12% of the Belgian population made use of alternative health care for different health problems.[31] In the UK, studies estimating the level of utilization in population surveys suggest that anything up to 14% of the population may have used unorthodox health care in the beginning of the 1980s.[32] In Norway, 14% of the people are said to have used traditional medicine at some time.[33]

Different European surveys have shown that women use alternative medicine more commonly than men. They show also that the use of alternative medicine is greatest among people of working age. Relatively more people from the middle and upper social classes use alternative medicine. This is not, however, as clear a determinant as age and sex.[34] For instance, in Sweden unorthodox medicine was typically used by the farming population[30] and in Switzerland the use rate was evenly distributed. Paranormal healing has a different determinational structure from other alternative therapies.[34]

Finnish pilot surveys suggest that the use of alternative medicine is related to sex. Women use alternative medical resources more frequently than men.[14,27,30,31] In the 1970s, modern alternative treatments seemed to be typical of urban health culture among the middle class and female population and traditional folk treatments typical of rural health culture in Finland.[14,27,34,38,42,43,44]

The study by Meriläinen[27] has also suggested that there exist different traditional health cultures on a regional basis in Finland. Massage and manipulation of vertebrae (bone-setters) are traditional folk treatments of Western Finland, whereas cupping is typical of Eastern Finland and visits to other traditional healers are common in Northern Finland.

It was seen as important to have a survey of the entire Finnish population covering both the official and unofficial systems, since the earlier surveys had been conducted with selected samples and limited treatments.

The aims of the study

Based on earlier empirical studies and theoretical discussions about the crisis of the welfare state, the aim of the study was to discover the scope and use rate of alternative medicine. It was tentatively suggested that use is determined by sex, health status, health behaviour, social class and place of residence.

In this study, Finland is taken as a typical example of the modern welfare state which has undergone rapid changes, the state having become a firmly established provider of public services. It might be illustrative of the same general trends taking place in other welfare states.

Material and methods

The empirical data was collected by telephone interviews. The study was part of a wider health education study undertaken by the National Board of Health. It was conducted by the Central Statistical Office of Finland during 1982.

The study group was formed by stratified sampling from a Finnish adult population between 15 and 64 years of age. The sample was random, extracted from the entire population of this age group in the Census Bureau. The first stage of the sample consisted of 2008 people, and the final sample of 1755 people formed the study group. The total response rate was 92.2%. There were, however, variations in the response rate for different questions; that is why the total number (N) varies.

The study group can be considered representative of the entire Finnish adult population when compared with basic sociodemographic factors (Table 15.2). The data was analysed by using cross-tabulations and linear discriminant analysis, whenever distributions allowed it. Variables were selected for the model stepwise and the selection was based on Rao's v test statistics. The variables are shown in Appendix 1.

Table 15.1 The response rate of the final sample and reasons for non-participation

	N	%
Reasons for non-participation		
– Did not answer	56	3.2
– Permanent or temporary disability	26	1.5
– Was not available	55	3.1
Response rate	1618	92.2
The size of the final sample	1755	100.0

Table 15.2 The basic background variables of the interviewed study group and the Finnish adult population (15–64 years of age) in 1982

	Study group % (N = 1613)	*Whole population** % (N = 3,269,789)
Age (years)		
15–24	23	24
25–44	46	45
Sex		
Male	49	50
Female	51	50
Marital status		
Unmarried	33	35
Married	57	57
Widow, separated, divorced	10	10
Education		
Primary school or less (7 years or less)	54	56
Less than secondary school (8–11 years)	23	23
Secondary school or more (12 years or more)	20	21
Occupational status		
Entrepreneurs, directors and higher officers	49	46
Lower officers and employees	35	35
Retired and unskilled workers	16	18
Place of residence		
Urban community	61	61
Rural community	39	39

**Source*: Statistical Central Office 1983

In this study the term 'alternative medicine' was taken to include health promotion, preventive or curative treatments outside the official health care system based on scientific medicine. Alternative medicine refers to the alternative paradigms of natural science. The operational definition takes the training of medical and health care personnel and the national social security system into account as 'gate keepers'. All treatments which are not in the medical curriculum or not recognized in the social security system are regarded as alternative. Alternative medicine is divided into two main categories: 1) old Finnish traditional medicine; 2) modern alternative medicine which is diffused by innovations from other cultures. Most of the latter products are commercial mass-production items.

The main items of alternative medicine for the study were chosen on the basis of earlier pilot studies. It was seen as important to cover the whole variation of treatments and that is why official treatments were also included.

The health status was measured by different questions: subjective health status was based on the feelings of the respondents; objective health status was measured by diagnosed chronic diseases and experienced symptoms measured by psychosomatic index CMI (Cornell Medical Index). Health behaviour was operationalized by using the questions on smoking. The social class was measured by the income and education (Appendix 1).

Large population surveys require clearcut and commonly used concepts. Thus, only treatments generally known could be mentioned by name. Also, to appear in the analysis, each therapy must have a high rate of usage.

Results

Use of different treatments

Nearly 70% of the studied individuals had consulted a doctor in 1982 and nearly 60% had used drugs prescribed by a doctor. Table 15.3 displays that scientific medicine was used more frequently than alternative medicine. Women used both official and unofficial medicine more frequently than men.

The most popular traditional treatment was massage, which was used by 11% of the study group. Health products were the most frequently used form of modern alternative medicine. Over half of the interviewees had used them during the past six months. However, this reflects eating habits and a health-conscious lifestyle rather than illness-related behaviour, whereas herbal (natural) remedies were used for curing illnesses by 17% of the interviewees (Table 15.3).

Modern alternative health care and its determinants

Natural products and other forms of modern alternative medicine were analysed separately as they were used for different purposes.

Natural products
Health (natural) products were known to most of the interviewees. 97% of the women and 93% of the men had heard or read about them. Nearly

Table 15.3 The percentage rates of the use of scientific and alternative medicine among Finnish population, 15–64 years of age, with respect to sex in 1982

	Male % (N = 783)	Female % (N = 830)	All % (N = 1613)	Used some time in past
Scientific medicine				
Visits to doctor	62	74	69	
Prescribed drugs	51	65	59	
Non-prescribed drugs	59	69	64	
Alternative medicine				
Finnish folk medicine				
Massage*	10	12	11	28
Vertebrae treatment				
(bone-setting)	3	5	4	17
Cupping/blood-letting	0.5	0.5	0.5	4
Other folk healers	0.5	1	1	2
Modern alternative medicine				
Health products†	48	59	54	
– natural food	27	30	28	
– special products‡	21	29	26	
Natural remedies‡	10	24	17	
Physiotherapeutic				
treatments	10	14	12	
Relaxing treatments	5	6	5	
Acupuncture§	1	2	2	
Hypnosis	0.5	0.5	0.5	

* Traditional massage excluding treatments given by physiotherapists.
† Natural products (commercial health products): the use rate during six months in 1982.
‡ The categories 'special products' and 'natural remedies' are based on official registration. Special products include, for instance, tonics, herbal teas, food supplements.
§ Acupuncture is practised within the framework of official health care and treatments are given by physicians in Finland.

half of the interviewees (43%) found these products effective for health promotion and prevention of disease and 17% for purely curative use, whereas 25% maintained they were useful both as preventive and curative treatments. However, 15% felt they could not recommend these products for any use. Men twice as often as women felt they could not recommend the products for any useful purposes.

Health (natural) products included health food, special products and natural cosmetics. Using this model in discriminant analysis 840 persons were interviewed, out of whom 397 had used natural products (Table 15.4) belonging to one or more categories of health products over a period of six months in 1982. The variables for the model were selected stepwise and the selection was based on Rao's v test statistics. The determining factors were sex, high income level, psychosomatic symptoms, chronic disease diagnosed by doctor and positive subjective health status (Appendix 1). To form a symptom index, in the interview the Cornell Medical Index of Psychosomatic Symptoms was used quantitatively. Subjective health status was represented by the opinion of the person being interviewed.

Since sex was significantly related to the use of health products, discriminant analysis was undertaken separately for men and women to find out whether their explanation model is different.

This discriminant analysis explained 53% of the variation. The variables were selected stepwise using Rao's v test (Appendix 1). This analysis included 434 men, of whom 168 had used natural products. Among men the use of health products was related to a high income level, the amount of psychosomatic symptoms, a positive subjective health status,

Table 15.4 Statistics and the most discriminating factors in linear discriminant analysis of the use of health products

Variable*	Standardized canonical discriminant function coefficients	Test statistic Rao's v	Significance of changes in Rao's v $p<$
Sex	0.97	27.14	0.000
Income	0.48	34.25	0.008
Symptom index	0.45	42.24	0.005
Subjective health status	−0.29	43.83	0.208
Chronic disease	−0.26	46.47	0.104

* See Appendix 1.
Coefficient of determination – 53%. Total percentage of cases correctly classified by discriminant function – 59%.

Table 15.5 Statistics and the most discriminating factors in linear discriminant analysis of the use of health products among males

Variable	Standardized canonical discriminant function coefficients	Test statistic Rao's v	Significance of changes in Rao's v $p<$
Income	0.65	7.51	0.006
Symptom index	0.62	12.86	0.021
Subjective health status	−0.56	19.66	0.009
Smoking	−0.32	22.02	0.125
Education	−0.25	23.45	0.231

Coefficient of determination – 53%. Total percentage of cases correctly classified by discriminant function – 56%.

non-smoking and a low education level, i.e. men who were well off, did not receive higher education and expressed several psychosomatic symptoms but felt themselves to be healthy and health-conscious used health products more frequently.

With women, the explanation model is different from that of men. The discriminant analysis (Table 15.6) has been concluded in a similar way as that for men.

The explanation of variation in this group model was 14%. Among the respondents there were 406 women, out of whom 229 had used health products. The most important single factor was chronic disease. Education showed an inverse relation among the sexes, as less educated men used health products more frequently, whereas among women it was the better educated who used them more frequently. Psychosomatic symptoms were related to the consumption rate with both sexes.

The modern alternative treatments
The selected modern alternative medicine included natural remedies, homoeopathic remedies, hypnosis, acupuncture, physiotherapeutic treatments and relaxing treatments. The most commonly used ones were natural remedies (17%), physiotherapy (12%) and relaxing treatments (5%). The other treatments were used only by 2% or less. Physiotherapeutic treatments cover both official and unofficial treatments. However, they were included in modern alternative treatments here. Their position in the Finnish health care system can be considered to be still marginal.

Women used herbal remedies more often than men and this same trend is apparent in all stratified groups in the background variable, the absolute and percentage figures, however, being so small that statistical analyses are only tentative (Appendix 2). This table shows that the highest consumptions were found among women who had chronic disease (20%), had felt ill (21%) and whose household is small (20%). This trend can be noticed among regular users, whereas the pattern is different among irregular users.

The use of physiotherapeutic treatments was very significantly related

Table 15.6 Statistics and the most discriminating factors in linear discriminant analysis of the use of health products among females

Variable	Standardized canonical discriminant function coefficients	Test statistic Rao's v	Significance of changes in Rao's v $p<$
Chronic disease	−0.69	2.89	0.089
Education	0.57	4.966	0.150
Symptom index	0.47	6.25	0.258

Coefficient of determination – 14%. Total percentage of cases correctly classified by discriminant function – 54%.

to age (Appendix 3). The elderly were more frequent users than the young.

The analysis of the use of modern alternative medicine was done by discriminant analysis in the same fashion as with health products. The cumulative index was formed from herbal remedies, homoeopathic drugs, physiotherapy, relaxation treatments, hypnosis and acupuncture. The interviewed persons were classified as users of modern alternative medicine if they had exploited one or several different treatment categories.

There were 878 people interviewed, out of whom 243 (27%) had used one or several forms of modern alternative medicine. The model applied explained 72% of the variation. The use of modern innovations in alternative medicine was related to sex, age and health status, being more frequently used by women and young people. There were subjective feelings of ill health and chronic disease diagnosed by doctor as well as a number of psychosomatic symptoms in the explanation model. Thus it was typical of the users to feel ill and to experience illness as well as to have had a diagnosis of chronic disease by a doctor. The use of modern alternative medicine was related to non-smoking which suggests there were attempts to live a healthy lifestyle (Table 15.7). The fact that sex was significantly related to the use of modern alternative medicine may show that there are different determinants for sex groups. However, the analysis based on sex categories cannot be done owing to an uneven distribution of usage rates among men.

Traditional folk medicine

Traditional medicine was well known; 62% of the studied individuals mentioned one or several Finnish traditional folk treatments. They mentioned cupping, bone-setting, massage, herbs, health spas. Out of those who knew old Finnish folk treatments, 31% had used them

Table 15.7 Statistics and the most discriminating factors in linear discriminant analysis of the use of modern alternative treatments

Variable	Standardized canonical discriminant function coefficients	Test statistic Rao's v	Significance of changes in Rao's v $p<$
Sex	0.50	54.42	0.000
Chronic disease	−0.44	30.47	0.000
Age	−0.31	63.97	0.002
Smoking	−0.29	76.99	0.0006
Symptom index	0.28	71.53	0.019
Subjective health status	0.15	78.41	0.233

Coefficient of determination – 72%. Total percentage of cases correctly classified by discriminant function – 62%.

irregularly and 5% claimed to have used them regularly. The most popular folk treatment was massage, used by 11% in 1982.

Cross-tabulation (Appendix 4) shows that 14% of the study group had used one or several traditional treatments. The use of traditional folk medicine is significantly related to old age, unmarried status, rural dwelling place and ill health.

Discriminant analysis was tested for the entire study group and separately for both sexes. However, uneven distribution was too high to allow the separative use of the analysis within sex groups. It included massage, bone-setting, cupping and visits to a folk healer. Any person who had used one or several treatments was classified as a consumer. The explanation model was set up in the same fashion as the earlier analysis of this study.

The discriminant analysis of the entire group explained 44% of the variation in the use of folk medicine. The analysis encompassed 878 people, out of whom 132 had used one or more folk treatments.

The use of folk medicine (Table 15.8) is explained by the health status of clients, strong feeling of illness (i.e. they have symptoms, feel ill and have a disease diagnosed by a doctor) and sex, as well as old age. Discriminant analyses did not take unmarried status and rural dwelling place into the explanation model, as cross-tabulation did due to their intercorrelation.

Cumulative use of alternative medicine

Scientific Western medicine was the largest single treatment category; 60% of the respondents had used only official medicine. Of a group who used a mixture of medical approaches (32%), 22% had used both some scientific and some alternative treatments, as well as heavy consumers

Table 15.8 Statistics and the most discriminating factors in linear discriminant analysis of the use rate of folk medicine*

Variable	Standardized canonical discriminant function coefficients	Test statistic Rao's v	Significance of changes in Rao's v $p<$
Symptom index	0.44	9.65	0.002
Chronic disease	−0.36	14.48	0.000
Sex	0.33	5.28	0.022
Age	0.29	4.26	0.039
Smoking	−0.27	2.37	0.124
Subjective health status	0.23	1.72	0.189

* Massage, bone-setting, cupping/blood-letting, visit to folk healer included.

Coefficient of determination – 44%. Total percentage of cases correctly classified by discriminant function – 63%.

(10%) who had used all the different categories: doctor visits, prescribed drugs, non-prescribed drugs, modern alternative medicine and folk medicine. Seven percent of the study group had not used any treatments in 1982 and 1% were 'pure types', using only alternative medicine. Cumulative use is very significantly related to sex. It is typical for women to use a mixture of health care resources, while men more frequently than women were 'pure types' of users (Figures 15.1, 15.2 and Appendix 5).

The heavy consumption group was analysed further and found to be significantly related to age and sex. The women, and the elderly in both sexes were more frequently heavy consumers than the others (Table 15.9).

Table 15.9 The percentage distribution of mass consumption* with respect to age and sex

	Sex				Altogether	
	Male		Female			
	%	N	%	N	%	N
Age (years)						
15–24	12	7	2	2	6	9
25–44	38	23	49	49	45	72
45–64	50	30	49	49	49	79

Chi-square 7.185, $p < .05$
* excluding health products

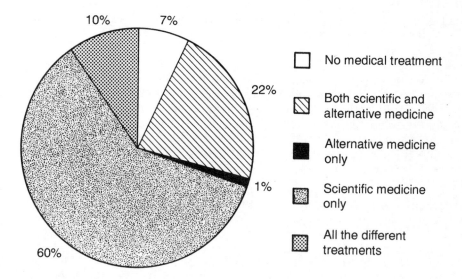

Fig. 15.1 The cumulative use of scientific and alternative medicine excluding natural products.

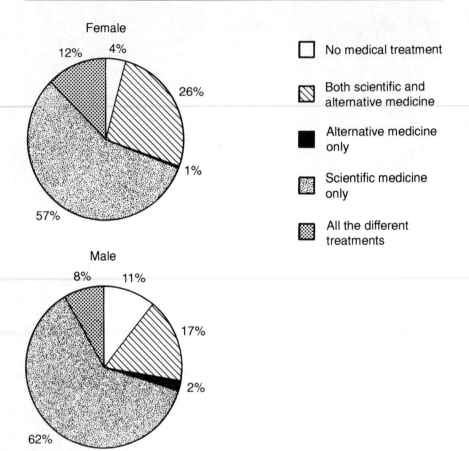

Fig. 15.2 The cumulative use of scientific and alternative medicine excluding natural products with respect to sex.

In addition, chronic disease diagnosed by a doctor together with the amount of psychosomatic symptoms and subjective health status were very significantly related to mass consumption. However, this association disappeared when sex was taken into account. It might be due to the complicated pattern of tolerance level of pain and illness behaviour among the sexes. The other background variables were not associated with mass consumption.

Mass consumption covers different use patterns. Folk medicine was taken as one specific form of heavy consuming. Out of a group of heavy consumers, 58 people used all the various types of folk medicine. Table 15.10 shows that mass consumption of folk medicine is determined by rural place of residence, single marital status, low income level and educational level as well as presence of a chronic disease. The same variables also appeared in the cross-tabulation of the use of one or several types of folk medicine but were not independent explanation factors.

Table 15.10 Statistics and most discriminating factors in linear discriminant analysis of consumption of traditional folk medicine in the high consuming group

Variable	Standardized canonical discriminant function coefficients	Test statistic Rao's v	Significance of changes in Rao's v $p<$
Place of residence	0.72	12.45	0.000
Marital status	0.46	20.25	0.138
Income	−0.39	23.19	0.087
Education	−0.35	18.05	0.124
Chronic disease	−0.30	15.70	0.071

Coefficient of determination – 14%. Total percentage of cases correctly classified by discriminant function – 63%.

The study suggests that traditional folk medicine with its high consumption rate is a remnant of rural health culture.

Conclusions

Alternative medicine usage, both modern and folk, was determined by female sex, ill health (taking into account subjective feeling), and disease as diagnosed by a doctor, as well as perceived symptoms. The modern alternative medicine was used more frequently by the younger population while traditional folk medicine was more typical for the elderly.

Alternative medicine is commonly used. Physical, manual treatments and herbal drugs as self-medication are the most common treatments; psychological and parapsychological treatments, especially spiritual and religious, are rare. The most popular treatments can be considered to be in the domain of a rational and empirical worldview emerging both from the folk experience and cultural innovation.[48]

It can be argued that in Finland there has been an increase in the total use of modern alternative medicine, while folk medicine has not changed since the 1970s.[36,38] The use of alternative medicine was typically associated with the use of scientific medicine; the use pattern is complementary rather than alternative.

In the study, Finland has been taken as an example of a Western welfare state, which has undergone rapid changes. Its growing economy and new urban lifestyle have broken traditional social systems and networks. The health care system is facing new demands and expectations from the people.

Discussion

The study suggests that there are at least two different health cultures; a) modern alternative medicine common to the young or middle-aged well-educated women, and health conscious well-off men; and b) folk medicine practised among the elderly population. Heavy consumers of folk medicine typically come from low social classes and rural areas. Both folk and modern alternative medicine is related in several ways to ill health.

Women are active in official and unofficial health care as well as in mass consumption form. They also combine different types of care more frequently than men. This can be seen as a cultural phenomenon, which might represent women's active general participation in everyday life and in alternative social movements.[49]

The results are not directly comparable to other studies due to different types of samples, concepts and study period.

After our survey, one comprehensive study was done on the use rates in Europe: a Danish population survey in 1987. It shows that 10% of the adult population had used one or more treatments during one year. This suggests that the Finns use unorthodox treatments more frequently than the Danish.[45] The Dutch Health Interview Survey showed that in 1987, 11.8% of the population had visited an alternative practitioner. This figure also suggests that the Finns are heavy users of unorthodox medicine.[46] In France[47] and in Belgium[31] surveys were conducted to measure contact with alternative medicine during a person's whole lifetime; results showed that, in France, 49% of the adult population and in Belgium, 39.1% of the Flemish families, had used alternative medicine.

The Finnish and Danish profiles of treatments are exceptional. While in Finland, the most frequently used treatments were herbal remedies, massage and other physical manipulations, and in Denmark reflexology, in other European countries homoeopathy and acupuncture were the most popular treatments.[34]

The response rate of the study can be regarded as high and the questions were answered seriously by the study group. The comparable results were similar with the earlier pilot studies, which suggest, that they are reliable. The figures of this study probably underestimate the whole use rates. Social acceptability influences responses in that people tell of their use of 'accepted' treatments but hide those which are not commonly known and accepted. Thus treatments based on empirical knowledge might be reported more accurately than treatments based on mystical or religious explanations. However, it can be argued that the study gives a valid overview of use and its general determinants. The survey method does not give directly the meanings and symbolic ideas shared in subcultures; for that, qualitative studies are needed.

The study suggests that the official health care system based on scientific medicine alone has not been able to satisfy demand. Outside public support and dominant culture, there exists alternative medicine. In towns, modern alternative medicine can be seen as part of a more cosmopolitan lifestyle and it gives an opportunity for the new middle class to find new solutions, whereas among old people and in the countryside, folk medicine is part of their own culture.

Alternative medicine has different functions in modern society depending on subgroups and the form of treatments. Among old and less educated people, it offers coping systems by keeping the integration of traditional social ties; in modern urbanized structure, it offers new definitions.

People are capable of using several different treatments simultaneously and of using different worldviews (paradigms) in explaining their ill health. There does not appear to be direct conflict towards scientific medicine, but behaviour and belief systems are fragmented and multi-dimensional. A pluralistic system has emerged to replace the domination of the biomedical model.[50,51]

We live in a pluralistic health care system. The social and cultural changes of post-industrial societies have faced new demands and challenges. We might ask ourselves how health care represents wider social changes, and what role it should have in society? To answer this question requires more comprehensive and comparable studies to give us basic information on the current situation.[51]

Appendix 1

Variables in discriminant analysis

Sex	Men	1
	Women	2
Age (years)		15–24
		25–44
		45–64
Marital status	Married	1
	Single	2
Income		2500 Fmk
		2501–3500 Fmk
		3501–4500 Fmk
		4501–5500 Fmk
		5500 Fmk
Education	Primary school or less (7 years or less)	0
	Secondary school or more (8 years or more)	1
Place of residence	Town	0
	Countryside	1
Smoking	Non-smoker	0
	Smoker	1
Subjective health status	Very well or well	0
	Fairly well	1
	Ill or very ill	2
Psychosomatic symptoms	None or only a few	0
	Some	1
	Several	2
Chronic disease diagnosed by physician	Yes	0
	No	1

Appendix 2

Percentage distribution of regular and irregular use of herbal remedies in relation to background variables

Background variables	The use of natural remedies						Absolute figures in groups on which percentages are based		
	Regularly			Irregularly					
	Male %	Female %	All %	Male %	Female %	All %	Male N	Female N	All N
Age (years)									
15–24	4	6	4	5	11	8	183	168	351
24–44	3	11	7	8	11	9	370	368	738
45–65									
Marital status									
Married	5	13	9	7	10	8	458	490	948
Unmarried, single, separated, widowed	3	18	8	6	12	9	325	340	665
Education									
Primary school	5	15	19	5	11	8	424	492	916
Secondary school or more	3	9	6	8	12	10	359	338	697
Socioeconomic status									
Entrepreneurs, directors, employees	5	9	8	8	11	9	332	488	821
Skilled workers	3	16	8	5	10	7	348	203	551
Retired, others	6	19	13	6	14	11	102	139	241
Place of residence									
Town	6	13	10	6	11	9	74	93	167
Countryside	2	12	7	7	11	9	330	303	636

Appendix 2 – *cont.*

Background variables	The use of natural remedies						Absolute figures in groups on which percentages are based		
	Regularly			Irregularly					
	Male %	Female %	All %	Male %	Female %	All %	Male N	Female N	All N
Size of household									
One person	4	20	13	7	13	10	74	93	167
Two persons or more	4	12	8	6	11	9	709	737	1446
Smoking									
Non-smokers	4	14	10	8	10	9	477	632	1109
Smokers	3	8	5	4	13	8	306	198	504
Subjective health status									
Very well or well	5	8	6	6	11	9	485	500	985
Fairly well	3	17	11	8	10	9	248	274	516
Ill or very ill	6	21	14	6	14	10	50	56	106
Chronic disease (diagnosed)									
Yes	7	20	14	9	13	9	217	262	479
No	3	9	5	6	10	8	566	568	1134
Psychosomatic symptoms index									
No symptoms or very few	3	8	5	5	9	5	388	282	670
Some symptoms	5	12	9	7	10	9	195	232	427
Several symptoms	5	17	12	9	14	12	200	316	516
Total	4	13	8	6	11	9	783	830	1613

Appendix 3

The percentage of the use of physiotherapeutic treatments and age

The use of physiotherapy	Age						Altogether	
	15–24		25–44		45–64			
	%	N	%	N	%	N	%	N
None	97	(342)	89	(660)	80	(418)	88	(1420)
1–2 times a year	1	(4)	6	(44)	11	(55)	6	(103)
Once a month	1	(2)	19	(3)	6	(30)	3	(51)
Once a week	1	(3)	2	(13)	4	(20)	2	(36)
Once a day	0		0	(1)	0		0	
Does not know	0		0	(1)	0		0	

Chi-square 67.535, $p < .001$

Appendix 4

Percentage distribution of the use of traditional folk medicine related to background variables

Variable	The use of traditional folk medicine	
	%	N
Age (years)		
15–24	6	351
25–44	14	738
45–64	20	524
	***	
Sex		
Male	13	783
Female	15	830
	ns.	
Marital status		
Married	17	988
Single (widowed, separated)	11	665
	***	
Education		
Primary school or less	15	869
Secondary school or more	13	697
	ns.	
Place of residence		
Urban area	12	977
Rural area	16	636
	*	
Size of household		
One person	17	167
Two persons or more	14	1447
	ns.	
Subjective health status		
Very well or well	11	985
Fairly well	18	522
Ill or very ill	24	106
	***	
Chronic disease diagnosed by physician		
Yes	21	479
No	11	1134
	***	

Appendix 4 – *cont.*

Variable	The use of traditional folk medicine	
	%	N
Psychosomatic symptoms		
None at all or very few	14	1559
Some	31	421
Several	17	121
	***	
Total	14	1613

[1] A cumulative index is used, which includes cupping, blood-letting, bone-setting, massage, visits to other folk healers. The usage rates include one or several treatments used by the interviewees.

[2] $* p < .05$, $** p < .01$, $*** p < .001$
Chi-square
ns = non-significant

Appendix 5

The percentage distribution of the cumulative use of scientific and alternative medicine, excluding natural products, with respect to sex

Use of different treatments	Sex				Altogether	
	Male		Female			
	%	N	%	N	%	N
No medical treatment	11	88	4	33	7	121
Both scientific and alternative medicine	17	136	26	214	22	350
Alternative medicine only	2	13	1	11	1	24
Scientific medicine only	62	487	57	474	60	961
All different treatments (heavy consumption)	8	59	12	98	10	157
Total					100	1613

Chi-square 51.0872, $p < 0.001$

References

[1] Ministry of Social Affairs and Health. *Health Policy Report by the Government to Parliament*. Helsinki, May 1985.

[2] World Bank. *World Development Report 1979*. Washington DC, 1979.

[3] Senghaas, D. *The European Experience: A Historical Critique of Development Theory*. Leamington: Berg Publishers, 1985.

[4] Titmuss, R. *Essays on the Welfare State*. London: Unwin University Books, 1963.

[5] Vaskilampi, T. Terveydenhuollon yhteiskuntapoliittiset näkökohdat. In: Koskiaho, B., Roos, J. P., Salavuo, K., Sipilä, J., Walls, G. (eds.)* Jyväskylä: Jyväskylän yliopisto, 1981.

[6] Vaskilampi, T., Hänninen, P. Cupping as an indigenous treatment of pain syndromes in the Finnish cultural and social context. *Soc Sci Med* 1982; **16**: 1893–1901.

[7] Berliner, H. S., Salmon, J. W. The holistic alternative to scientific medicine: history and analysis. *Int J Health Serv* 1980; **10**: 133–48.

[8] Goldstein, M. S., Jeffe, D. R., Sutherland, C., Wilson, J. Holistic physician: implications for the study of the medical profession. *J Health Soc Behav* 1987; **28**: 103–19.

[9] Gordon, J. S. The paradigm of holistic medicine. In: Hastings, A. G., Fadiman, J., Gordon, J. S. (eds.) *Health for the Whole Person*. Boulder, Colorado: Westview, 1980.

[10] Salmon, J. W. *Alternative Medicines: Popular and Policy Perspectives*. London: Tavistock, 1984.

* Tutkimus yhteiskuntapolitiikan viitoittajana.

11 Ministry of Social Affairs and Health, National Board of Health. *Health Care in Finland.* Helsinki, 1986.

12 Nyman, K. Terveyspalvelusten käyttöön vaikuttaneet tekijät vuosina 1964, 1968 ja 1976. *Sosiaalivakuutus* 1980; **5–6:** 152–63.

13 Terveydenhuolto. *Lääkintöhallituksen Vuosikirja 1983–1984. Suomen virallinen tilasto 11: 81.* Helsinki, 1985.

14 Meriläinen, P., Vaskilampi, T., Sinkkonen, S. A pilot study on the use of alternative treatments in Eastern Finland. In: Vaskilampi, T., MacCormack, C. (eds.) *Folk Medicine and Health Culture: Role of Folk Medicine in Modern Health Care.* Kuopio, Finland: University of Kuopio, 1982.

15 King, S. H. *Perceptions of Illness and Medical Practice.* New York: Russell Sage Foundation, 1962.

16 Koos, E. L. *The Health of Regionville.* New York: Columbia University Press, 1954.

17 OECD. *Public Expenditure on Health. OECD Studies in Resource Allocation No. 4.* Paris: OECD, 1977.

18 Mishra, R. *The Welfare State in Crisis.* Brighton: Harvester Press, 1986.

19 Jordan, B. *Rethinking Welfare.* Oxford: Blackwell, 1987.

20 Freidson, E. *Profession of Medicine.* New York: Dodd Mead, 1970.

21 Illich, I. *Medical Nemesis.* London: Calder and Boyars, 1975.

22 Zola, I. In the name of health and illness: on some sociopolitical consequences of medical influence. *Soc Sci Med* 1975; **9:** 83–7.

23 Report of the Commission for Alternative Systems of Medicine. *Alternative Medicine in the Netherlands.* The Hague, 1981.

24 Fulder, S., Munro, R. *The Status of Complementary Medicine in the United Kingdom.* London: Threshold Foundation, 1982.

25 Statistiska Centralbyrån. *Levnadsförhållanden. Rapport no 1. Hälso-och sjukvårdskonsumption 1974.* Stockholm: Liber, 1978.

26 Naturheilmittel. *Trendanalyse 1970–1975.* Allensbach: Institut für Demonskopie, 1975.

27 Meriläinen, P. *Väestön terveydenhoidon kokonaisuus: itsehoito, virallisten ja epävirallisten terveyspalvelujen käyttö sekä niitä määräävät tekijät. Kuopion yliopiston julkaisuja. Yhteiskuntatieteet, alkuperäistutkimukset 1/1986.* Kuopio, 1986.

28 Räsänen, O. Hanna the healer. A case study of a Finnish spiritual healer. *Etnol Scand* 1983; **5:** 65–78.

29 Vaskilampi, T. The role of alternative medicine: the Finnish experience. *Comp Med Res* 1990; **4:** 23–7.

30 Socialdepartmentet. *Fakta och röster om alternativ medicin. En delrapport från alternativmedicinkommittén.* Stockholm: Almänna Förlaget, 1987.

[31] Sermeus, G. Alternative health care in Belgium: an explanation of various social aspects. *Comp Med Res* 1990; **4**: 9–13.

[32] Thomas, K. Non-orthodox health care in the UK. *Comp Med Res* 1990; **4**: 32–4.

[33] Efskind, L., Johansen, A. T. Folkmedisin og overnaturlig helgredelse. *Tidskrift norske laegeforenig* 1976; **96**: 1382–6.

[34] Sermeus, G. *Alternative Medicine in Europe: A Quantitative Comparison of the Use and Knowledge of Alternative Medicine and Patient Profiles in Nine European Countries.* Brussels: Belgian Consumers' Association, 1987.

[35] Bruusgaard, A., Efskind, L. Befolkningens syn på bruk av folkmedisine. *Tidskrift norske laegeforening* 1977; **97**: 1385–8.

[36] Vaskilampi, T., Meriläinen, P., Sinkkonen, S. *Suomalaisen aikuisväestön luontaistuotteiden ja kansanomaisten hoitomuotojen käyttö ja tutkimus. Lääkintöhallituksen monistesarja. Aikuisväestön terveyskasvatustutkimus II, Syksy-79.* Helsinki, 1980.

[37] Meriläinen, P., Vaskilampi, T., Sinkkonen, S. Kysely vaihtoehtoisten hoitomuotojen tutkimuksessa – esitutkimus vaihtoehtoisten hoitomuotojen käytöstä Kuopion ja Maaningan aikuisväestölle vuosina 1979 ja 1982. In: Vaskilampi, T. (ed.) *Vaihtoehtoisten hoitomuotojen tutkimuksen problematiikkaa.* Jyräskylä: Institute of Social Policy, University of Jyväskylä. Research Report No. 45, 1986.

[38] Meriläinen, P., Sinkkonen, S., Vaskilampi, T. Suomalaisen aikuisväestön virallisten ja epävirallisten terveyspalvelujen käyttö vuonna 1982. *Sairaanhoidon Vuosikirja* 1985; **21**: 207–31.

[39] Arkko, P., Arkko, B., Kari-Koskinen, O., Taskinen, P. A survey of unproven cancer remedies and their users in an outpatient clinic for cancer therapy in Finland. *Soc Sci Med* 1980; **6**: 511–14.

[40] Ahlström, A., Räsänen, L., Loikkanen, S. Luontaistuotekaupan asiakkaista. *Sosiaalinen Aikakauskirja* 1983; **67**: 501–613.

[41] Meriläinen, P. The overall health care of populations: Self-care, utilization of official and unofficial health care services in Finland. Manuscript, 1987.

[42] Meriläinen, P., Vaskilampi, T. Aikuisväestön kansanomaisten hoitomuotojen käyttö Suomessa. In: Laaksonen, P., Piela, U. (eds.) *Kansa parantaa.* Kalevalaseuran Vuosikirja 63/83: 78–84, SKS, Helsinki, 1983.

[43] Prättälä, R. Vegetarismin ja luontaistuotteiden käytön tutkiminen – esimerkkejä erilaisista lähestymistavoista. In: Vaskilampi, T. (ed.) *Vaihtoehtoisten hoitomuotojen tutkimuksen proglematiikkaa.* Jyväskylä: Institute of Social Policy, University of Jyväskylä. Research Report No. 45, 1986.

[44] Jacobson, N. *Naturläkemedel och okonventionella behandlings metoder.* Stockholm: Civil Tryck Ab, 1979.

45 Rasmussen, N., Morgall, J. M. The use of alternative treatments in the Danish adult population. *Comp Med Res* 1990; **4**: 16–22.

46 Visser, J. Alternative medicine in the Netherlands. *Comp Med Res* 1990; **4**: 28–31.

47 Bouchayer, F. Alternative medicines: a general approach to the French situation. *Comp Med Res* 1990; **4**: 4–8.

48 Leslie, C. M. Pluralism and integration in the Indian and Healing. In: Landy, D. (ed.) *Studies in Medical Anthropology*. London: Macmillan, 1998; pp. 511–17.

49 Peterson, A. Naiset yhteiskunnallisissa liikkeissä. In: Saarinen, A., Hänninen-Salmelin, E., Keränen, M. (eds) *Naiset ja Valta*. Gummerus Oy, Jyväskylä: Tutkijaliitto, 1987.

50 Vaskilampi, T. Culture and folk medicine. In: Vaskilampi, T., MacCormack, C. (eds.) *Folk Medicine and Health Culture: Role of Folk Medicine in Modern Health Care*. Kuopio, Finland: University of Kuopio, 1982.

51 Aldridge, D. Complementary medicine in Europe: some national perspectives. *Comp Med Res* 1990; **4**: 1–3.

16 Medical anthropology as clinical method: the body paradigm

Beatrix Pfleiderer

The Turkish worker Aslan pointed towards his liver when he described the weakness and unease that he felt. His GP listened with increasing helplessness. He had examined the patient's liver and had found nothing. The more detailed the description Aslan gave, the more doubtful the doctor felt. He finally referred him to the Heidelberg University Hospital of Internal Medicine. There the staff soon became as helpless as Aslan's GP. They could not understand an illness that arose each Friday afternoon from Aslan's liver, spread all over Aslan's body and finally declined on Monday morning when he started work in the factory.

Aslan called his symptom *uezuentue*. But the consulted Turkish doctor simply translated the term as 'sadness'. Although Aslan agreed to the lexical translation of his discomfort, the staff needed more. Not even a semantic translation was enough since Aslan's body showed signs that were not part of the culture-specific grammar of Western medicine. His body paradigm belongs to humoral medicine; he thinks in terms of vital flows, energy centres and energy loss. His body paradigm derives from the specific medical paradigm which is still prevalent in most Turkish rural and even urban communities. He ascribed his sadness to a loss of energy in the energy centre of his body, the liver. The German psychiatrist – Aslan's last resort in the German medical system – ascribed his sadness to his loneliness, since he had left his family behind in Turkey.

Medical anthropology as method

I would like to show with the material presented in this chapter that medical anthropology provides tools for evaluating everyday clinical practice and reality. As we have read in the above example, the patient's perception and his experience of his problem need to be understood in context. It is the task of the medical anthropologist to discover such meanings, and to remind conventional medicine that explanations exist other than its own, which are critical and valuable for patient care.

Cecil Helman,[1] as medical anthropologist and general practitioner, highlighted the practical value of this approach for clinical practice and research in his work with two groups of patients who had either respiratory or gastrointestinal, so-called 'psychosomatic', disorders. For years, physicians had suggested that patients with chronic diseases were themselves responsible for their own illness because of their lifestyles, emotions or personality styles. This personal responsibility for the cause of the disease was negotiated over time on the clinical encounter itself according to the prevailing medical view. Patients themselves had altogether differing explanatory models of their problems which centred around the natural symbols of respiration and digestion/excretion. By carefully semi-structured interviews lasting for 1 to $1\frac{1}{2}$ hours, Helman was able to discover the comparative themes common to each diagnostic category such that he could understand 'the ways that patients made sense of their physiological experiences, of the diagnostic label of "psychosomatic", and of their interactions with clinicians over the years'[1] (p. 7).

To illustrate these methods, I will use the body paradigm as a key to medical theory, development and practice, with an emphasis on eating/feeding as a natural symbol. The body (that is to say, our bodies) is the product of the culture we live in, the historical period we were born into and the ideology we choose to live with. I will show how social and political our bodies are and, also, how little individual influence we have on them ourselves. Not only fashions and styles of dress but also politics shape our bodies. Being a medical anthropologist, I will use examples that demonstrate how medicine, that is to say our mainstream medical culture, forces a body politic on us by telling us what is normal and what is not normal with our bodies, or what is right and what is wrong. I will conclude by showing that the body is a reflection of society: in capitalistic societies it has become an individual enterprise that is invested in, cared for, looked after and worked on, or rather laboured on, in order to be gratified in a culture-specific way. Medical anthropology can inform doctors working in clinical settings about the relativity of body concepts, their implication for illness behaviour and health-seeking processes. It can also instruct them about the underlying matrix that governs a patient's way of dealing with stress, symptoms and the relationship of his body with the outside world.

Before dealing with the European body paradigm, I will show how non-European cultures view and experience the body in space and time. I will present culture-specific ethnophysiologies and body grammars, and then proceed to the discussion of Western medical culture and the development of the present-day body politic for medical and clinical practice.

The body as a social event

While doing fieldwork in India, people told me that the body is made up of three vital fluids or *dosas*, that are responsible for all bodily processes, good or bad. And that, like the cosmos, the body has a male principle, *Purusha*, which is indivisible, atomic and immutable, and a female principle, *Prakriti*, that is subject to change. Again, when the foetus has come to life, the hard and enduring parts of the body are produced by the male, whereas the lighter and softer parts of the body come from the mother. They imagine the body not in terms of anatomy, but in terms of the flow of substances through channels and the transformations of the substances into one another. Physiology in Indian medical texts is concerned with purification of substances one from the other. The most purified element (and the most precious for that matter!) is semen, which is partless, 'like gold a thousand times purified'[2] (p. 937). Semen that is not used in procreation is stored in a man's head in order to increase his reasoning power, they say. Within semen, the texts tell us, we find consciousness which corresponds to the male principle, the soul. The soul is liberated with the death of the body in which the perishable parts, those that come from the mother, disappear, freeing the soul of the female substrate. The soul undergoing the karmic cycle of rebirths is thus the eternal element. This particular ethnophysiology is reflected in Hindu social organization. The child consists only of the man's genes. The female and her body, which actually produces the child, are just the carrier of the baby's body. This is why, the women told me in the village where I worked, men have to have control over the female's body in order not to jeopardize the continuation of the line. But the women also told me that they know how to control men, if absolutely necessary.

In this context, they taught me a version of the body not present in Indian medical texts. They said that when you leave behind the cosmic order and the social order governing your body, and live against the rules – walk in the wrong direction at the wrong time, go to bed with your husband at the wrong place and time, eat food that stirs up your *dosas* – then a demon is likely to possess you. Your body no longer belongs to you; it belongs to the demon who eventually terrorizes the whole family without your being able to prevent it.

Here the women describe a body expelled from the proper order, which creates disorder and an unorderly world. The body, in this case, is responsible for keeping up the proper cosmic and social order, for the benefit of the whole group the individual lives in. These Hindu women have a cosmocentric worldview as opposed to the sociocentric worldview of the Chinese or the Japanese, where the responsibility for the individual body equals the responsibility for the whole social group.

The chaste Hindu woman also adds to the fame of her husband's lineage when she is ready to commit *sati*, being burned alive after her husband's death. She sacrifices her individual body in this conjugal communication with death. As an incentive, this act makes her a deity, a *sati*, honoured by a memorial stone at the village entrance. Her living body has been transformed in order to fuel the social group with the divine, the sacred.

In other societies that practise human sacrifice, like the classical Mayas of Yucatan or the Aztecs of Mexico, the well-prepared, decorated and embellished body of the sacrifice is seen as the enacted communion with the metaphysical part of the cosmos, with God. The body of the human sacrifice becomes God and thus adds to the metaphysical power of the social group.

The body never represented itself in earlier and in present-day non-Western societies: it stood for society, the cosmos and the divine. The skin was not its boundary, neither was death. In these non-Western societies the body was – and is – a collection of symbols that do not depict the individual who owns the body. It announces the various strands of his embeddedness in the cosmos, in the sacred, and in his social standing.

In a society like the San (Kalahari Bushmen), the body embodies their cosmos. It is the carrier of their worldview. In weekly healing trance-dances, the members of the group become one. They share their common energy by singing the texts that control the body energy, as Richard Katz[3] describes in his widely read book, *Boiling Energy*. The energy rises and the dancers fall in trance and thus become one with their cosmos, with the sacred. 'They become like one organic being'[4] (p. 270). The Bororo tribe in South America understands the individual only as reflected in relationship to other people. The Cuna of Panama say they have eight selves, each associated with a different part of the body[5] (p. 15).

In other cultures we find the body to be the symbolic reflection of the land people live in. They build analogies between their landscape and their bodies. For example, the Qollahuayas of Bolivia, who understand their bodies in terms of the mountain, see the mountain in terms of their bodies' anatomy[5] (p. 20).

The Chinese view their bodies with a different metaphor. The anatomy of their bodies reflects the hydraulic landscape of China. As rivers flow through the land, so energy moves through the body in the meridians. The flow of water in the rivers has to be controlled, which society does with the help of dams. The individual has to control the flow through the meridians. Stagnation or blockage in the meridians signifies disease and death. With acupuncture needles the doctor restores the flow and heals the patient. If the river stagnates or a flood inundates the land, there can be catastrophes, hunger and perhaps even the end of the culture.[6]

Our Turkish patient, Aslan, experienced his body in terms of the ancient Galenic or humoral paradigm. His body grammar seemed to be total nonsense to the Western-trained clinical staff to whom he was exposed during his crisis.

European culture and the body politic

Now turning to Europe and so-called Western culture, let's explore the Government of the Body and the Case of the Diet.

Western culture doesn't exist, by the way: it is only a construct that includes cultures as diverse as the Americans, the Basques, the Bavarians, the Sicilians, the Finns. But since most people believe in this construct, let's not part with it in this chapter.

Western culture is unique in its views of the body, because it separates the body from the mind. One of those responsible for this view is Aristotle, who gave a biological view of the human soul in his text *De Anima*. Another Greek to whom we give credit for this view is Hippocrates, who in 400 BC warned the *iatros*, the physician, 'treat only what is observable and palpable'. Rene Descartes, who wrote around 1630 *Cogito, ergo sum* (I think, therefore I am), decided that the body is made up of a *res cogitans* and a *res extensa*. *Res cogitans* refers to the thinking part of the body and *res extensa* to its extension, the body machine.[5]

The present-day dilemma in biomedicine, the view of the body not as a mindful but as a mindless entity, is caused by this Cartesian legacy. Since Descartes, the development of medicine has no longer been part of the metaphysics of misery and evil. The key to the patient is no longer prayer and ritual, but rather seeing and examining what is wrong with the body machine and fixing those parts in need of repair. The English physician Sydenham described how 'narration-dependent' medicine disappeared in the seventeenth century and was replaced by an 'observation-dependent' medicine. Earlier, the signs a patient's body produced were the report for the physician. This report was *person-oriented*. Body signs and language were congruent. With the use of the stethoscope, auscultation and digital percussion, this was replaced by objective signs. The medicine of observation went beyond the boundaries of the body. With the intrusion of the physician's gaze into the patient's body, it became an object and the patient became silent. This was the beginning of the accumulation of 'objectified' medical knowledge. The body became a part of nature and hence dominated by the laws of nature. In the naturalistic worldview, reality consists of evidence, and this reality means that the more physical the evidence, the more real a subject is. The body was separated from the mind. The mindless body became the object of science. A disease is described in terms of material evidence.

There is another important strand in Western thought that came to influence the views on the body. The human body was a metaphor of political institutions in the Middle Ages. The king was the head of society, as the Pope was the head of the Church (in England, both the head of Church and State came to be embodied in the king). Both are social bodies. The king even had a double body: one that perished and decayed and the other symbolic one that stood for society. We still speak today of the social body, the head of state, the body of the Church, and of course, the corporation, a legal *corpus* or body.[7]

If we proceed along these lines, we may want to think of the organization of the body in terms of the government or, even better, of the control over the body; in short, the body politic. Let's do that by looking at the body, food, and the control of eating habits.

Modern European – and later Western – culture considers the body machine, the *res extensa*, something to be governed, to be controlled. It even has to be controlled by disciplines. The first discipline was the Greek medical regimen, the *diatia*, or in English, the diet. The diet was a mode of living set within a particular government of the body by medical practices. We can imagine such regimens occurring along a voluntary/involuntary continuum. Voluntary governments, writes Turner in his book *The Body and Society*,[7] involved a social contract between patient and doctor. In exchange for the medical fee, the patient contracted into a mode of living to restore his or her health. Like other political contracts, the medical regimen involved a certain loss of self-will: the regimen worked only if followed. Examples of involuntary regimens in past centuries are the enforced incarceration of the insane (in England, Germany, France) and in the late Middle Ages, the seclusion of lepers.[8] Regimens therefore imply an element of responsibility on the part of the patients. (We remember, in Indian and Chinese culture, responsibility to the body was responsibility to the cosmos and society.)

Eating can be conceived as a fundamental 'body technique'; that is, an activity which has a basic physiological function. But this activity is heavily mediated by culture. Eating patterns reflect hierarchy and control. Eating patterns reflect morality and discipline. Eating patterns reflect subordination and autonomy.

While feeding a child is an act of support and care, it is also the imposition of a mode of living (a regimen) on a subordinate. Gaining control over our own feeding patterns while we mature involves a growth in personal autonomy. Refusing to eat or engaging in forced vomiting is an act of rebellion.

Anorexia is an example of rebellion. It involves a power struggle within the family over food. The parents attempt to force their daughter to eat. The young woman refuses to become mature and (paradoxically!) to show her autonomy over her own body. Anorexia is a present-day epidemic, a culture-specific illness, a neurotic fast that reflects women's status in present-day society.

Anorexia was also the strategy of young women who became nuns and famous mystiques like Catherine of Siena or the even more famous Teresa of Avila, writes Bell[9] in his book *Holy Anorexia*. Their anorexia was rebellion against the family and escape from the family into the nunnery. The Pope acknowledged their anorexia as a holy disease, a body state that came from God. They were controlled by priests – not by doctors – who observed the young women's nutritional regimen.[9]

Religious fasting preceded our present-day dieting. In Europe, fasting was part of the monastic culture. With the rise of Protestantism, however, the family became the locus and rationalization of personal asceticism and fasting. The body is thus the location for the exercise of will over desire. The government of the body becomes, in Western culture, the government of citizens. Or, more specifically, the government of the body becomes the government of women. The *will-over-desire* dictum for women from the seventeenth century onward meant control of sexual desire, eating desire, and the desire for appropriate expression (as in art, music and literature).

The visible metaphor for the controlled female body is the corset. A constricted waistline achieved by tightlacing dominated fashion in Europe from the 1830s to the 1890s. The loose body reflected loose morals; hence it had to be tightlaced. These tightlaced corsets are the symbol for the woman's body as a property and commodity controlled by men[7] (p. 197–8). The corset is at the same time an affirmation of female beauty and a denial of female sexuality. Medical evidence indicates that corsets injured the cervix, often making coitus painful and thus reducing fertility[7] (p. 197).

The first women who expressed rebellion were not only anorexic women, but also hysterical women. These women expressed their rebellion through their bodies. The body of the hysterical woman who rebelled against a society that controlled her vital expressions spoke a silent language – and yet a loud one. The physicians of the time said of their hysterical female patients: 'They are creatures without backbone, their limbs refused to serve them, as did their ears and their tongues. They are treacherous, you cannot trust them, because whatever they do is staged, is a lie'. In other words they are 'not responsible', they do not fulfil the contract. Since they were acting, Charcot, the founder of modern psychiatry, gave them a stage in his hospital in Paris in the 1880s.[10]

Freud, who invented psychoanalysis between 1895 and 1900, had a different approach: he reconstructed archaeologically the geography of the cultural wounds that these women had inscribed into their bodies. Their bodies produced symptoms that could be retranslated by psychoanalysis into a matrix of social causes.[10]

Present-day anorexia nervosa, however, belongs to the continuum of body practices which includes dieting, jogging, keeping fit and other forms of secular asceticism. But there is another reason for its occurrence. Women are notoriously under-represented in professional occupations. Thus there is a contradiction between the achievement orientation in middle-class homes and public restraint on female success outside. Women's bodies thus become symbolically occupied while remaining economically unoccupied. Given the low fertility of women in advanced capitalistic societies, especially in the middle classes, the imagery of the unoccupied womb and the occupied body is symbolically pertinent to the case of anorexic women. Their bodies and their body practices act out the paradox of their actual social and political situation and their hopelessness.

The relentless pursuit of thinness associated with fatness is not only the case with anorexic women. It is also associated with the modern form of asceticism. Subordinating the flesh, as in Christian asceticism, now reflects modern consumerism's aim of enhancing pleasures. As I have already said, our culture suggests that we think of our bodies as objects. We realize ourselves through labour on our bodies. And this labour on the body is social practice.

We labour over our bodies by eating, sleeping, cleaning, dieting, exercising. These labours that we call body practices are both individual and collective. The body is the site of enormous symbolic work and symbolic production. Such is the case of Western cosmetics (as opposed to traditional cosmetics that signified status and position) that has lost its rootedness in the sacred cosmos. Dieting, like exercising, is determined by commercialized fashion and by individualized sexuality. But wearing corsets and jogging are also part of the general medicalization of society whereby surveillance and discipline are now self-imposed by the individual. It also represents the sexualization of society.

By becoming desirable we also suppress desire. The asceticism of diet is harnessed to the hedonism of consumption; one of the contradictions of late capitalism. Today's slim woman is less likely to be looking for a marriage partner than her counterpart in the corset. Slimness is now, under the promotion of the food and drug industry, geared to the narcissistic ends of personal happiness, social success, social acceptability. The slim body is no longer the product of an ascetic drive for salvation or of the artificial aid of the corset. It is instead a specific feature of calculating pleasure as the ethic of late capitalism. Corsets, jogging and anorexia have one important medical side effect: they suppress menstruation. Thus, being desired and being fertile are in opposition.

At the same time, jogging and slimming reduce medical costs and thus serve the interest of the state. This is a rationalization of the body. And below is what I consider to be the core value of our culture regarding bodies:

> The new personality requires validation from audiences through successful performances of the self. The new self is a visible self. The new body, suitably decorated and presented, came to symbolize overtly the status of the personal self. Identity became embodied in external performances.[7] (p. 202)

In the last section of this chapter I would like to show how mainstream medicine exerts control over bodies by weight control which takes place at many levels and in many forms.

Morality and medicine: the case of fat people

The obese woman is not simply fat; she is also regarded as being out of control and a poor performer. Margaret MacKenzie, an anthropologist, quotes from interviews about the stigmatization of fat people in American culture in her 1980 study *Fear of Fat*.[11]

> 'I wouldn't hire a fat person, they are unreliable. If they can't get themselves together how could they be competent?', says one.
> 'I know there must be fat people who are intelligent, but I can't really believe it', says another.
> 'Fat is ugly. I'd never marry a fat person', says a third.

Fat people are the untouchables, the pariahs of Californian, of American, culture, writes MacKenzie. This is a new form of racism. And society, a society of rationalizing thin bodies, lets medicine enact the legitimized new forms of punishment. The fat body is medicalized. It becomes a victim of regimens such as weight-watching, which is not that different from Alcoholics Anonymous, rigorous dieting and surgery.

This food abuse or 'foodaholism' is an invention of American culture, in a country in which the food industry spends $1 billion a year on advertising. Vitamin sales total about $200 million per year. The medical profession has found a new object and a new pastime: it has medicalized the fat.

First came the moral: fat is ugly, fat signifies lack of success, etc. Then came the regimen. Those who are fat produce high risk factors. They die earlier of heart attacks, diabetes, cancer. And, what is most important, they violate the contract between the individual and society: they don't pay by jogging in order to enjoy the harvest by being desired, being attractive, being reliable, etc. They don't play the game of consumerism. Perhaps they are spoilsports, wet blankets, or even deviants and heretics. And heretics are dangerous in a collective society.

In American culture obesity has become a disease. Thirty-six percent of the adult population suffers light forms of obesity; 10% suffers from gross obesity. It is the most common 'illness'. Having proved that it is a disease, the medical profession went ahead and formed an association of specialists: the bariatricians (*baros* = weight in Greek, *iatros* = healer). The first order of business was, of course, to manufacture 'patients' that suffer from the 'disease' that is called obesity. This parallels the creation of the psychiatrist from the mad-doctor 150 years ago, who again created psychiatric diseases like hysteria or mania. People had to be talked into being mentally ill. Now people have to be talked into recognizing that they are overweight[12] (p. 105–21).

The 'obese' patient is already created. One of the promoters of bariatric medicine, Asher, already has a characterization of his ideal patient: 'Obese patients are difficult. They don't stay on diets; they lie to their doctors; they don't keep appointments'[10] (p. 110). How come this sounds like the doctors of hysterical women 100 years ago?

The 'enemy', food, is fought by surgery. Two Los Angeles surgeons, who began to use so-called intestinal by-pass operations, started this war in 1956. These two medical warriors wrote in the *American Journal of Surgery*, '. . . a high degree of cooperation is essential, a relationship of mutual respect. Trust . . . must be present between the physician and patient . . .'[11] (p. 118).

Medical anthropology informs us that fat people may enjoy more prestige in other cultures. In West Africa young girls are brought to bridal training huts for fattening procedures. In Polynesia a woman has to look strong and healthy lest she might not find a husband, and the same is true for a Bavarian farmer's wife. In many cultures people believe that fertility of women is proportionate to the amount of fat on their bodies. We cannot prove the opposite. Medical anthropology provides methods that allow us to look behind the scenes. The truth is not the act but rather is found backstage. In the case of fat people, medical anthropology can show that it is the interest of the state that designs morals and fashion. Both morality and fashion are used to control their victims, that is, fat people. Moral judgement becomes a medical judgement, a diagnosis. And the fat body, or the case of obesity, becomes medicalized. This is possible because, since Descartes, the body is subjugated to the laws of nature. Clinicians turn into the custodians/guardians of morality. If used properly and with care, medical anthropology could be the conscience that accompanies the development of medicine.

Suggestions for researchers and practitioners of medicine in a pluralistic and cosmopolitan world

As we can see from the material presented in this chapter, each culture produces specific body concepts, concepts related to illness and disease, and a variety of body regimens for the maintenance of health and the treatment of illness. A doctor or practitioner of complementary medicine has to be aware of this when dealing with patients either from his own or a foreign culture. With each patient, the researcher/practitioner will find a cultural substrate in their explanation of illness and illness behaviour. It is therefore advisable for a researcher/practitioner in a pluralistic society to be able to deal with the cultural aspects of patients' complaints. In order to do this he or she will have to conduct an ethnographic assessment of the patient's cultural construct of body paradigms, disease and illness, perhaps by simply adding a few more questions when taking a patient's history. A conventional case history in biomedicine consists of data about the physiological and anatomical aspects of the body. In psychosomatic medicine a second layer of socio-psychological data is added to the case history. The patient's social situation is explored and discussed. The nature of his communication patterns are examined. His biography is looked at in order to find patterns of expressions in the form of disease, catastrophes or social or psychological problems.

The picture a researcher/practitioner gets from the patient is only complete, however, when the practitioner has elicited cultural data on the patient's body. This third layer of data will give information on the patient's cultural background. As we have seen, a Turkish patient may carry traits of humoral medical culture and consider the liver as the body's centre of energy. A patient from traditional India may carry traits of the Ayurvedic medical paradigm. A European patient may believe in several paradigms, because he is influenced by his GP, who happens to practise homoeopathy, and his acupuncturist, who made him read a treatise on Chinese medicine, and his mother, who happens to be a faith healer. In order to get this data from a patient it is wise for the researcher/practitioner to become a medical anthropologist for only a few minutes, by asking the patient to describe the whole complex of the disease that causes the present complaints. The patient should describe how he himself explained the first signs of the disease, how he reacted to them and why he did so. Having done this, the practitioner is aware of the patient's explanatory model. An explanatory model is rarely a 'pure type'; it is usually a mix of several therapeutic cultures to which the patient was exposed recently. Medical anthropology has taught us in recent years that people like migrant workers rapidly adopt the illness theory of the practitioners of their host country.

After having elicited the explanatory model of the patient, the researcher/practitioner should proceed to collect some data on the patient's body paradigm. He or she should ask the patient how the present ailment influences the body's function and why this is so. Perhaps a small list could be drawn up of what is 'healthy' and what is 'unhealthy' for the patient, and why this is so.

These questions are already enough to involve the patient in a discussion about his cultural body paradigm and will render sufficient data for the researcher/practitioner. With this data he or she will be able to 'diagnose' and classify the patient's 'medical' culture. Only with this knowledge will the researcher/practitioner be able to communicate fully with the patient. In these times of extensive travel and migration, the researcher/practitioner should always keep in mind that a North European patient may adhere to an Asian medical paradigm, and a migrant worker may follow the paradigm of biomedicine. The researcher/practitioner should not exclude any 'maybes'.

References

1 Helman, C. Psyche, soma, and society: the social construction of psychosomatic disorders. *Culture, Med Soc* 1985; **9**: 1–26.

2 Egnor, M. T. Death and nurturance in Indian systems of healing. *Soc Sci Med* 1983; **17**(14): 935–45.

3 Katz, R. *Boiling Energy*. Cambridge, Mass.: Harvard University Press, 1982.

4 Marshall, L. The !Kun Bushmen in the Kalahari Desert. In: Gibbs, J. L. (ed.) *Peoples of Africa*. New York: Holt, Rinehart & Winston, 1985.

5 Scheper-Hughes, N., Lock, M. The mindful body. *Med Anthropol Quart* 1987; **1**(1): 6418.

6 Dann, G. Personal communication.

7 Turner, B. S. *The Body and Society*. London: Blackwell, 1984.

8 Foucault, M. *Madness and Civilization*. New York: Mentor Books, 1965.

9 Bell, R. *Holy Anorexia*. Chicago: University of Chicago Press: 1985.

10 Bernheimer, C., Kahane, C. (eds.) *In Dora's Case*. New York: Columbia University Press, 1985.

11 MacKenzie, M. *The Fear of Fat*. Unpublished manuscript, 1980.

12 Szasz, T. *Ceremonial Chemistry*. London: Routledge & Kegan Paul, 1975.

17 Observational methods: a search for methods in an ecosystemic paradigm

David Aldridge

Summary

Observational methods, common to the social sciences, are used to understand suicidal behaviour. Three stages of research are described: a preliminary stage of hypothesis generation and model-building using the published literature; a second stage where emerging hypotheses are tested in interactive contexts; and a third stage where hypotheses are refined and tested in a particular context. This research method stays close to clinical practice and is a useful tool for formulating clinical trials. It is also a useful conceptual tool for the clinical appraisal of chronic problems.

Introduction

The process of research relies upon careful observation. What we choose to observe and the way we make those observations are critical acts dependent upon theory and training. Not only is seeing believing, but in this sense believing is seeing; our belief systems guide us to what we accept as evidence. Our research observations hopefully challenge the way in which we see things, and give us the opportunity to formalize our observations such that other people can see them too.

The work presented here to illustrate the process of observation is an example taken from practical experience. The author was trying to understand the problem of suicidal behaviour and deliberate self-harm. At the time this study was made, suicidal behaviour was increasing in incidence in modern Western countries and proved to be intractable to both therapeutic interventions and preventive measures. Such behaviour had become the most common reason for acute medical admissions of women to hospital and posed a major challenge to the health services.[1]

From his clinical experiences the author began to have doubts about his own way of thinking about the problem, and the ways in which his colleagues were describing what was then considered to be 'a uniquely individual problem'. Limited excursions into a wider field of family therapy and social science literature led him to seek interactive understandings which would better fit what appeared in clinical practice; i.e. when people became suicidal they did so in a context of difficult personal and social relationships. People who become suicidal appear to be socially isolated. While they have become isolated from their families, they often have a network of support agencies. In attempting to begin the process of research, the researcher was faced with the lack of an acceptable model for understanding human behaviour as a complex of inter-related levels of understanding. In particular, there was no established methodology for family therapy research.[2,3]

What follows then is concerned with the development of an appropriate methodology for understanding a particular human behaviour (attempted suicide) in its complexity. The intention is to provide an ecosystemic framework for observational studies; i.e. how do observations from differing levels of human experience fit together to form an ecology of ideas? The aim of the research work was to provide clinical initiatives based on familial and relational understandings, and all the work was carried out in the context of community psychiatric practice. The results of these initiatives have been presented elsewhere,[4,5,6,7,8]

A thread which runs through this work is concerned with the understanding of personal meaning, and how those meanings are negotiated in relational contexts. The meanings presented here are those generated within the culture, within the professional literature, those which are developed within families where attempted suicide has occurred, and those given by the people who themselves have attempted suicide or deliberate self-harm.

There is a long tradition of research into suicidal behaviour. The intention of this research study was to build upon that research tradition and offer a complementary interpretation of previous research results. Therefore, any developing understandings and new observations could cast a new light on previous research. If links with previous understandings could be maintained then other clinicians from different traditions would find complementary explanations accessible. Rather than saying, 'Out with the old, in with the new', this approach attempted to ask how we can have multiple perspectives and use them to inform clinical practice such that previous understandings are re-interpreted and assimilated.

General considerations

The general stance of this work was ethnographic[9] and, therefore, descriptive. These descriptions were based upon carefully structured observations and participant observation methods common to the social sciences.[10] Investigations were carried out in natural settings as far as possible and those investigations were concerned with describing processes of interaction between people. The idea of 'equifinality' taken from systems theory, i.e. that there are many ways of reaching the same goal, was vital to this approach both in terms of methodology and for clinical understanding.

Another consideration was that of progressive focusing. In this way of working, generalized statements from the broad field of understandings were progressively refined by studying particular real-life situations. This progression was structured as a number of related stages. The progressive refinement of hypotheses by testing them in interaction was isomorphic with the principles of some family therapy schools. This isomorphism was intended. The hope was that research generated with a particular methodological form would influence therapy with that same form in an attempt to make the research clinically relevant.

Several methods were used in this study. Such a combination of methods is known as the technique of 'triangulation',[10] a term borrowed from navigation. When an explorer is investigating new territory it is possible for him or her to estimate his or her position from known navigational aids. Using a single navigational source will give an idea of what course is being taken, but no idea of distance. When two known sources are used, each separated by a known distance, then the position of the observer can be calculated by geometry. Using this analogy we can estimate our conceptual whereabouts using new data based upon previously known ideas.

Another interpretation of triangulation is that several sets of data used to describe the same phenomenon in differing situations can be compared one with another. In this study the meaning of suicidal behaviour was considered as it was reported in newspapers, by women who engaged in suicidal behaviour in hospital, from the letters of people who had attempted suicide, and by the relatives of people who described themselves as suicidal (see Figure 17.1).

Stage 1

The literature relating to suicidal behaviour was reviewed. This included descriptions of completed suicide and those behaviours variously labelled as 'attempted suicide', 'deliberate self-harm', or 'parasuicide'.

Seemingly similar behaviour is mapped differently according to the theoretical persuasion of the observer. In general, when theorists describe suicidal behaviour they take it for granted that episodes of such behaviour are sufficiently similar to group them together as if those episodes are identical. As will be demonstrated later, there are discrepancies between individual particular meanings, familial meanings and shared cultural meanings.[11,12,13]

In this work, a middle order description was attempted which rooted concrete descriptions of suicidal behaviour in a personal relational context, yet also referred to social meanings of the phenomenon.[14] Clifford Geertz[15] calls this stratified hierarchy of meanings a 'thick description'. The descriptive perspectives gleaned from the literature were historical, ecological, anthropological, ethnographical, motivational and personal.

> Suicidal threats . . . whether carried out successfully or unsuccessfully pervade our entire social structure. Our study has disclosed that the threat of suicide forces persons to marry, prevents marriage dissolutions, coerces companionships between persons despite their mutual infidelity, prevents marriages, forces parents to acquiesce in their offspring's vicious habits, precludes institutionalisation, is rewarded by escape from further military duty, is used to obtain favoured treatment over siblings, is employed as a device to avoid military induction. It should be significantly stated that these by no means represent an inventory of all factual situations embracing suicidal threats[16] (p. 45).

Generate hypotheses from the literature and clinical experience

	A psychiatric hospital setting	A general hospital ward	A psychiatric day hospital setting	Community sources
Stage 1	Find* cases and collect data from staff and patients	See* cases and develop means of collecting data	See** cases in differing contexts	Discover** cases from community/ public sources
Stage 2	Develop hypotheses from cases; follow up at time intervals	a) Collect data from post-episode discharge interviews using strategic assessment technique b) Organize follow-up	a) Collect data from special case interviews b) Collect data from family therapy video-taped interviews	a) Cultural data from newspapers b) Letter data via magazine article
Stage 3	Discover negative cases and reconsider hypotheses	Review data and develop hypotheses during and after follow-up	Review data and document videotaped material to test hypotheses; present hypotheses for further testing	a) Analyse newspaper data b) Analyse letters

* cases of suicidal behaviour as presented by the ward staff
** as referred by the general practitioner or consultant psychiatrist

Submit refined hypotheses for controlled investigation

Fig. 17.1   The process of research in the study as a whole.

While the influence of suicidal behaviour on others is a common description in the literature, this influence is invariably seen as a manipulative act on behalf of the patient. Few accounts acknowledge the reciprocal nature of the relationship between the identified patient and those with whom they live.

A historical perspective

Outbreaks of suicide throughout history, as today, were causes for concern. The causes ascribed to such behaviour were sickness of mind, intemperance, gluttony, duelling and foolhardiness.[17] However, by the eighteenth century, causal factors became related to the environment such as bad air, the seasonal temperature and idleness. This indicated a shift from a moral to a secular view of the behaviour. Suicidal behaviour then, as now, was considered a problem meriting national concern.

By the nineteenth century, two diverging descriptions developed: the statistical sociological view, and the medico-psychiatric. In both descriptions there were a number of causal factors[18]: (i) predisposing factors of heredity, temperament and climate; (ii) direct accidental factors of passions, domestic trouble and the like; (iii) indirect accidental factors of bodily pain and illness; and (iv) general factors of civilization, religious fanaticism and civil disorders. These views appeared to herald a multiple perspective account of suicidal behaviour wihich linked the personal with the relational in the context of the societal.

However, no such composite description emerged as the differing disciplines of medicine, psychology and sociology pursued their own versions of what they considered to be true. Suicide was generally seen as a consequence of societal changes where individual behaviour was located in a context of change and disorganization. What is interesting in this historical perspective is that the meaning of suicidal behaviour changes over time, and can have a plurality of meanings according to the stance taken by the observer.

An ecological perspective

The most prevalent sociological explanation of suicidal behaviour is that of Durkheim.[19] The process leading to suicide is centred on a failure by the person to accommodate the ecological niche he or she occupies. Individual wellbeing is reflected in the balance of individual and social forces. Should an imbalance exist then the forces oppose each other and pathology is created. As the pathology of society (or the individual) increases then the tendency to commit suicide will also increase. Both individual and social factors are seen as causative but only social factors are seen as being fundamentally important in explaining suicide rates.

A number of authors have developed this ecological under-standing.[20,21,22] In these descriptions an individual's ties with society are dissolved; particularly with those in the person's immediate social milieu (their niche). This loss is precipitated by rapid changes in social circumstance resulting in individual isolation and loss of social status.

This is the beginning of an understanding of the location of the individual within an intimate relational context within a broader context of social change.

An anthropological perspective

The anthropological descriptions emphasize both the interconnectedness of events and that culture communicates information to those who participate in those events.[23,24,25] As Bateson says,[26] the notion of a message is implicit in the context of the behaviour.

Symbolic meaning of behaviour is condensed into concrete actions by ritual occasions. These ritual occasions are concerned with movement across social boundaries from one social status to another (maiden to wife, sick to well, living to dead). The purpose of these rituals is to proclaim a change of status and to bring it about. Suicidal behaviour may then be a ritual form for achieving a change of status.

Rituals of bodily mutilation in other cultures are seen as rites of transition where bodily mutilation marks the entry into adult society. At a metaphorical level[27] these acts are described as acts of death where one status dies and another is born. Similarly, sacrificial offerings of life are often made to obtain benefits. Although the physical body of the sacrificial victim may be damaged, what matters is the expression of a reciprocal relationship.

In this perspective suicidal behaviour is concerned with symbolic rituals for recognizing and achieving transition from one social state to another. Implied within these meanings is the metaphoric death of one state within the context of a reciprocal relationship. To understand suicidal behaviour we may need to consider what transition is being attempted, and in what relational milieu, i.e. adolescent to adult in a family, physically ill patient to mentally ill patient in a hospital context.

An ethnographical approach

From a cultural standpoint suicidal behaviour is seen both as an acceptable means of coping with interpersonal stress,[28] and as an effective way of altering the behaviour and expectations of significant others.[29,30] However, other researchers[31,32] found that some communities regarded suicidal behaviour as a manifestation of mental illness, and as something which 'happens to' people rather than being an intentional act.

Yet other researchers propose that social experience informs community attitudes and personal behaviour.[33] The suicide rates of migrant groups in Australia are more like those of the countries of origin, no matter how long the migrants have lived there, although the methods used become closer to the Australian-born with time.[34] The change in methods used for suicidal behaviour is greater in cultures with a language similar to that of Australia. This appears to support the proposition that there are personal, familial and cultural repertoires of distress management.[5,6,12,13]

A motivational perspective

The explanations offered by those who practise suicidal behaviour have been neglected in research studies. Marital disharmony and relationship conflicts are present in two-thirds of suicidal patients, and suicidal behaviour is seen by these patients as an effort to re-establish a close dependent relationship with a loved one, or an attempt to change that person's behaviour.[11] The resolution of conflict with a key person by verbal means is seen by patients as a sensible but personally difficult solution to a problem which exists in a context of communicational difficulties or disrupted relationship.[35]

The actors themselves in this perspective are less concerned with large-scale social descriptions but more concerned with regulating changes in interpersonal contexts of relationship which may be conflictual.

A perspective of personal psychology

Psychological descriptions of suicidal behaviour reiterate the concept of conflict either intrapsychically[36,37,38] or relationally. Adler[39] considers suicidal behaviour as an attempt to win over a significant other. To this same end, Bateson[26] suggests that a runaway of such behaviour can occur up to a threshold which might be on the other side of death.

The idea of language of suicidal behaviour, where the behaviour is a cry for help, has been developed by several authors.[40,41] However, not all commentators see it in such a benign light and regard suicidal behaviour as rather perverse communicational strategies by which individuals manipulate others to gratify their own needs as emotional blackmail,[42] to obtain attention,[43] to influence social agencies,[44] to gain access to institutions or to modify the environment.[45,46,47] While admitting the relational nature of the problem the focus is always on the individual in these accounts and not the relationship.

George Kelly[48,49] suggests that instead of making the explanations of suicidal behaviour pathological or nonsensical, we should look at the act itself and see what it accomplishes for the person who performs it. His description emphasizes the position of the observer. As observers, we call certain actions suicidal because we predict our own category of consequences upon behaviours.

In this study the intention was to find out what the behaviour was intended to accomplish for the person engaged in that behaviour in their own terms (construing in a Kellyian sense), and what the behaviour accomplished in terms of their significant others. Kelly's theory of construing behaviour[49] is important in this understanding as it involves others in the validation, or legitimation, of personal behaviour.

A family interaction perspective

Changing circumstances and relational conflict were seen as important factors in the aetiology of suicidal behaviour in the previously mentioned literature. Suicidal behaviour appeared to be a strategy of controlling change and coping with stress in the literature concerned with family interaction.

The factors associated with families were:

(a) Marked family hostility with prohibition that one member does not respond with overt hostility. That member is not allowed to leave the field and there is a shifting coalition between that member and another family member against a third family member.[50,51,52]

(b) Role disturbances and role failure in every area of personal functioning[50,53,54] where 'failure' by one family member functions to stabilize conflict within the family. This is obtained at the price of estrangement and isolation from broader social contexts.

(c) A process of escalation where developmental changes occur in the management of life cycle transitions,[55] and these developmental changes have been managed by symptomatological behaviour to reduce conflict. In such families individual change is seen as disloyal.

(d) Partners are symbiotically attached and tolerate no strivings for autonomy on the part of either partner: intimacy and separation are mishandled.[56,57,58]

(e) Crises are not tolerated and are handled with hostility. The handling of crises is related to family organization and a family tradition of crisis management which develops over the years.[59,60]

(f) A pattern of communication which attempts to control the rate of personal and familial change.[5] This communication expresses the problem and states the solution; 'Treat this family as if it were a matter of life and death'.

Suicidal behaviour appeared to be present when some families attempted to manage developmental change. In these families there was a tradition of distress or conflict management by one member becoming symptomatic. While suicidal behaviour appeared to be deviant and negative from an understanding of personal behaviour, at a familial level the behaviour could be seen as positive in regulating change and maintaining coherence. At the cultural or community level the behaviour could be negatively construed. When this occurred a family with a deviant member became socially isolated, although that member may have maintained their coherence as a unity, albeit at the expense of the person's own life. This isolation also prevented any therapeutic intervention until an act of suicidal behaviour occurred. Then the behaviour appeared to external observers as impulsive, unpredictable or irrational. In our attempts to understand illness behaviour, particularly that which appears impulsive, we may need to survey the interpenetrating realms of personal, familial and communal construing.[12,24,61,62,63]

A model of the management of systemic distress

Several commentators had seen suicidal behaviour as unpredictable and impulsive.[35,44,64] It might be suggested here that when we as clinicians cannot understand behaviour then, rather than see this unpredictability as a characteristic of the patient, we may consider reviewing our own understanding of the phenomenon as being misguided or in-appropriate.

In an attempt to understand the process of becoming suicidal, a model was developed from the clinical and theoretical literature (see Figure 17.2). This model proposed a general understanding of the management of systemic distress which was isomorphic for different levels of organization; individual, familial or cultural.

A developmental crisis (a) is recognized by a system according to its own cognitions which in turn are located within and informed by a cultural context.[23] This is news of difference in a Batesonian sense[65] and is referred to as a life event in some literature. A life event in this sense can range from the invasion by a virus, the dysfunction of an organ, a marital row, the loss of a partner or the news of imminent redundancy.

Thresholds of distress (level x) (b) are threatened by homoeostatic adaptations to this crisis; e.g. blood sugar levels are elevated, pain is expressed, symptoms appear, someone complains more.

There then follows a strategic move (c) to reduce that distress according to the systemic repertoire of distress management. These are attempted solutions.

Distress is reduced (d), the repertoire of distress management is validated (e), and stability is maintained (f).

This is a simple homoeostatic loop.[66]

However, should distress not be reduced then an alternative strategy from the repertoire of distress management is used (g) and the system scrutinizes itself for evidence of distress (Is $x1 > x$?). If distress is reduced then this alternative strategy is validated as a legitimate means of reducing distress.

The current level of distress may be higher than at step (b) although within the thresholds of tolerable distress. In this way some families learn to live with allergy, stress, pain, anxiety, depression and delin-quency.

If distress continues to escalate (i) and systemic thresholds are threatened to excess, to a point where the viability of the system is threatened, then distress management strategies are generated from the next 'higher' level of systemic organization, i.e. organic to personal, personal to marital, marital to familial, familial to communal.

This strategy will depend upon the repertoires of distress management available at this next contextual level. These strategies will depend upon the traditions and epistemology of the systemic level[67] (biography, family history, ethnic culture or professional practice[68,69]), and may

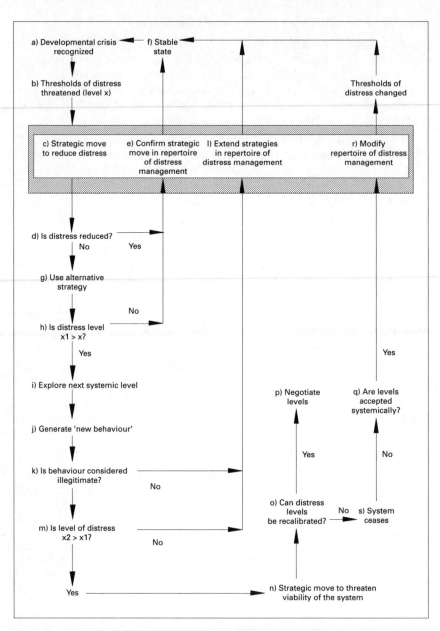

Fig. 17.2 A model of the systemic management of distress.

appear as 'new' behaviour (j) at the level in which it is currently expressed.

This new behaviour is then subjected to validation (k) within the context in which it occurs. In some cases this new behaviour may have temporal validation; e.g. it is acceptable for the patient to withdraw for a while. In other cases there may be conditional validation; e.g. the parents of an adolescent may tolerate withdrawal but the extended family may consider it to be strange behaviour.

If this behaviour is considered legitimate, or distress is reduced (l), then it effectively extends the repertoire of distress management[70] informed by the cultural matrix in which it is embedded. We see this in patients entering psychiatric hospitals who rapidly adopt a new set of behaviours.[7] This is often seen as evidence of a previously hidden pathology rather than a set of situationally legitimate behaviours for the expression of distress within the psychiatric ward culture.

Although the behaviour may be considered illegitimate, distress levels may be reduced. In this way 'deviant' strategies are included within the repertoire of distress management. We see this in the abuse of medication, the abuse of alcohol and self-mutilatory behaviour.

The current levels of distress may not be reduced (m) (Is $x2 > x1$?). The system then calibrates itself to accommodate a higher level of distress. When this occurs a family member who has become symptomatic to maintain the family stability may become a chronic patient, or necessarily symptomatic; e.g. diabetic, hypertensive, asthmatic, anorexic, depressed or delinquent.

If distress levels escalate further in the face of an unresolved developmental crisis (n), then the viability of the system is further threatened by an overt strategic move. This move will be sanctioned at a cultural level appropriate for the patient and based upon the systemic tradition of manifesting overt distress; e.g. blood sugar levels escalate to become diabetic coma, essential hypertension becomes elevated into a cardiovascular accident, or strategies of medication for symptomatic relief are escalated into episodes of self-poisoning.

Emergency measures are then introduced (o) to recalibrate the system. If not, the patient may die.

New efforts are made to recalibrate levels of systemic distress (p). This is the stage when specialist teams are called in and the problem is reviewed.

If the emergency is successfully negotiated (q) then systemic change may occur; e.g. blood pressure is stabilized, a man may change his lifestyle, retire from his job, his daughter may leave home and the marital relationship become closer.

Distress thresholds are recalibrated (r). For some patients this is a change to a new level of improved health, for others this is a new level of invalidity or disability. Stability returns (f).

If the emergency is not successfully negotiated and change does not occur then the system ceases (s); an organ is removed, a person dies, a couple may become divorced, an adolescent is expelled from school or a person leaves an organization.

These changes themselves may be interpreted reflexively as a 'crisis' and the loop continues (a).

Generation of hypotheses

From the common ground of interaction discovered in this suicidal behaviour literature, a tentative hypothesis was developed about the process of becoming suicidal. Suicidal behaviour appeared to involve a process of interaction between intimately involved people. This interaction contained an element of relational conflict which escalated over time, and this conflict was indicative of a change in status of that relationship. When conflict occurred in a relationship the mutual behaviour of those involved was invalidated and described as illegitimate in that context.

These emerging hypotheses based on the general literature concerning suicidal behaviour were then compared with ideas in the field of family interaction literature. The family interaction literature suggested that familial distress and conflict are managed by one family member becoming 'symptomatic'. When such distress management failed, in a context of unresolved 'crises' or failed attempted solutions,[52,55] then the familial distress escalated and the symptoms worsened. If the threshold for these symptoms was threatened to excess then the system was threatened with a loss of viability. Suicidal behaviour was an expression of this threatened loss of viability.

Using this theoretical knowledge from varying literature sources, hypotheses were generated for testing. These hypotheses were:

1 Suicidal behaviour is an attempt to bring about a coherent systemic resolution in the face of change.

2 Suicidal behaviour is a metaphoric communication of the threat to the viability of a relationship system (e.g. 'This family is about to die').

3 There is a family history of accommodating change by the use of the sick role as a means of reducing conflict at times of crisis.

Stage 2

The hypotheses were then tested out in differing settings for further refinement. Any negative cases were incorporated to modify the emerging hypotheses, i.e. cases or examples which did not support the emerging ideas were used to modify those ideas. Rather than rejecting that which does not fit, this approach urges the researcher to reconcile conflicting sets of information. Each differing level of observation (individual, familial, social) generated data appropriate to that level. From this data, it was possible to abstract commonalities from differing descriptions for comparison. The varying settings are presented below.

Cultural construings: newspaper data

Newspaper reports of suicidal behaviour were scrutinized for the years of the study in which data was collected and analysed for content. Whenever suicidal behaviour, or any deviant behaviour, is commented on publicly then cultural definitions of that behaviour are invoked which maintain the status quo and offer definitions by which that behaviour can be understood.[12,71,72,73] Newspaper reports present gross understandings of behaviours, some of which are not available for immediate experience. These reports often direct 'to' some understandings and 'away' from others.[74] As a number of authors suggest, facts do not speak for themselves; they are given meaning within a 'frame of reference'.[75,76,77]

The use of newspaper reports as a secondary source of research data falls under the general term 'archival record analysis'.[10] In this sense newspaper reports are public archival records, whereas personal letters are private archival records. Modern newspapers have published indexes which are available through municipal libraries and it is relatively easy to search through newspaper indexes using keywords to find the desired items. With electronic data forms of archiving this problem will be simplified further.

In this study, *The Times* newspaper was scrutinized for the years of the study. The intention was to elicit what general understandings were available at a cultural level to understand the behaviour in question. While such data could be analysed on a quantitative and comparative basis (i.e. how many column inches were given to reporting suicidal behaviour in comparison with other health-related issues), this study was interested in a qualitative analysis of the data to understand the themes and issues which were included when suicidal behaviour was reported publicly. Each report was then classified according to a common set of criteria; in this instance, age, gender, marital status, precipitating factor and method used.

Studying one newspaper alone is a biased sample if the researcher intends to study suicidal behaviour as it is reported in newspapers. Ideally several newspaper resources would be used which indicate a broader level of readership in terms of social class, political persuasion, geographical location and educational background. In this case the intention was not to make an exhaustive search, merely to probe into a general established medium for descriptions of suicidal behaviour.

The basic question during this stage was that of 'How do ordinary people (i.e. non-specialists) talk about, or write about, suicidal behaviour?'. The emphasis was not only on explanations and causes, but also on what information people regarded as necessary to include when they talked about a particular problem. Whereas medicine talks about problems in the abstract and objectively, the actors involved in suicidal behaviour present their behaviour and the reasons for it concretely and subjectively.[23] Newspaper reports are not necessarily concerned with upholding a medical status quo through the maintenance of objective knowledge about suicide, but there is a need to maintain a consensus view of what counts as deviant behaviour and how such behaviour is to be understood and discussed.

During the time that this study was being made Bobby Sands was starving himself to death in the Maze Prison, Belfast, Northern Ireland.[78] His death was seen as a political act to gain concession within a tradition of Irish martyrdom. His mental health was never questioned. His actions, although self-inflicted, were not seen as 'suicidal'; nor was it suggested that he was suffering from anorexia nervosa. Self-starvation leading to death was understood as a 'political' act if there was a clear understanding of the social and historical contexts in which it occurred. Such 'political understandings' of family organization, where symptoms have a historical and relational context, had been made by Laing[79] and Palazzoli[80] regarding self-starvation.

In studying the newspaper accounts, sudden death was deemed to be suicidal by considering the nature of the act itself (e.g. it was violent), the presence of criminality and if there was a further contextual element of mental disturbance (e.g. depression). To validate the judgement of suicide a causal train of deviance was invoked from the person's biography (e.g. this person drank a lot, was prone to swings of mood and became violent on occasions).

Suicidal behaviour in general was seen as legitimate in certain situations (see Figure 17.3): for men over 40 years, for political protesters or policemen, for those who were violent, depressed or psychiatrically disturbed and those who had lost a significant other. These factors reflected the suicidal risk factors which Tuckman and Youngman proposed.[81]

However, such legitimate status and understanding were denied to most women, men under 40, those who were not 'depressed' or 'undisturbed', the unemployed, or those who had primary relationships intact. Women who engaged in suicidal behaviour were given the status of irresponsible children.

The assessment of the legitimacy of personal behaviour appeared to be critical for the understanding of suicidal behaviour. While the death of a political martyr was understood in a social political context, the same understanding was not extended to any other deaths or attempted deaths. These were culturally construed as unique individual events.

Personal understandings: personal letters as a source of data

A number of studies presented the reasons people gave for taking overdoses,[64,82,83] but few had concentrated on finding what descriptions suicide attempters made of their own behaviour.[11,84] A short article was placed in a magazine asking for information by letter from respondents about what had helped them after an episode of suicidal behaviour. This was an attempt to discover how people talk about their experience, and what measures they believed had been of help. Diaries have been used as intimate journals of suicidal behaviour[14] and provide valuable insights into the reasons, circumstances and motivations which people give for doing what they do. Letters also provide a source of private archival record analysis. As George Kelly[49] writes about understanding biographical material:

> First of all, it may be seen as factual material out of which a person has to make some kind of sense at some time in his life. Second, it reveals something of what the person's con-

struction system must have been in order to account for his behaving in certain ways in the past; hence it suggests the kind of thinking and behavior to which he may have recourse if his present way of life suddenly becomes invalid or unpredictive. In the third place, it indicates the kind of social expectancies with which the person has been surrounded and hence the validators with which he has had to check his construct system (p. 752).

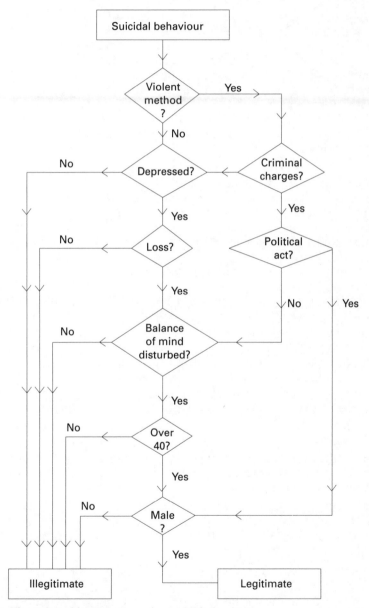

Fig. 17.3 The cultural legitimation of suicidal behaviour.

The contents of these letters generated by the magazine article were then analysed according to the types of information presented by the respondents; age, gender, marital status, number of children, reason for the attempt, personal relationships at the time of the attempt, method used for the attempted suicide, number of previous attempts, any regrets at surviving, was the respondent currently feeling suicidal, the nature of the support offered, the attitude of professional contacts, the attitude of significant others, and at what stage were the respondents in terms of their family life cycle.

From these letters a questionnaire was designed using the common descriptions offered by the respondents. The intention was to fill in missing data, in that not all the letters contained the data categories mentioned above. For example, not all respondents remarked upon their current feelings of suicidal ideation. These questionnaires were then sent to the respondents. Hawton[35] remarks that observers' descriptions differ from those of actors, and it is necessary to consider actors' descriptions of behaviour. The author's contention was that these actor descriptions were paramount for formulating future therapeutic interventions.

Descriptions gleaned in the clinical setting are often tinged with social desirability. In this part of the study social considerations were reduced, or at least changed, in that the researcher had no personal contact with the respondents in terms of a helping or therapeutic relationship. For these respondents the material was presented after the event and the researcher was not involved in their clinical programme or as a gateway to further treatment. The respondents were also treated as expert informants who had valuable insights to offer; their accounts were important as a significant source of research material, not in determining how sick or deviant they were. It became clear from this material that while the respondents clearly described their situation as one of personal distress this distress occurred in a context of escalating relational conflict.

The corollary to this form of neutral data collection using letters was that several women said how much they were helped by being given the chance to write down their experiences from their own point of view as a positive event; i.e. with the intention of helping others.

All the respondents in this part of the work were women. The intention was to collect descriptions of what helped after an episode of suicidal behaviour. What emerged from these accounts, apart from information about what had helped, were detailed biographical accounts by the women of their behaviour.

These individual accounts reinforced the need to understand interaction. The letters referred to how the women understood their own behaviour in relationship to the behaviour of significant others (see Figure 17.4). As Kelly[49] says:

> It is, of course, the comparison he sees or construes which affects his behavior. This much of social life is controlled by the comparisons he has come to see between himself and others[49] (p. 31).

This letter material offered a way of understanding how these women made sense of their lives, how they understood the past in terms of causal trains, and the social expectations of those with whom they lived. Most of the women presented individual problems which they located within a current problematical relational context (see Figure 17.4). Their current distress was seen as a process of escalation in conflict with a significant other, and the suicidal behaviour was often seen as a means of avoiding confrontation.

For example, one woman wrote:

> I am now 51 and currently divorced, and therein lies the key to my tranquillity . . . I was absolutely desperate . . . caused by lack of sleep. I had two daughters and a husband who went out every night. He would come in about 2 a.m. and berate me, calling me a slut and saying the house was a mess.

> I finally formed an association with a vet who wanted to go away with me but I could not leave my daughters. I became very ill and had constant vomiting if I attempted to eat.

> I never quite got fit. Gradually . . . a lethargy crept over me and all I wanted was peace and restful nights . . . I took about two-thirds of a jar of barbiturates and went to bed.

This woman's persistent problems were treated with medication throughout the time she was married. At no time did it appear that there was any attempt to resolve the marital conflict.

In their letters these women wrote of situational difficulties in an intimate relationship, yet the current medico-psychiatric literature still concentrated on seeking characteristics of personal disposition. These women also said that they were best helped by:

(a) someone objective to talk to who would listen to them and recognize their view of the problem;

(b) financial, practical, social support; and

(c) some concrete activity to engage themselves in.

The women in this sample who repeated suicidal behaviour were those who described their behaviour as their own problem, and that this problem was nothing to do with anyone else.

Fig. 17.4 The presentation of symptoms and problems in differing contexts as gathered from the correspondence data.

	Individual symptoms	Interactive problems	Total
Individual Context	15%	4%	19%
Interactive Context	64%	17%	81%

N = 53

Small group understandings: the psychiatric hospital ward

This was an attempt to understand the behaviour interactively in an extreme situation and to discover differing views of that behaviour within the same setting. It was hoped that understandings gleaned from this bounded setting of the psychiatric hospital ward could be extended to other settings such as the family.[78] If personal distress occurring in a situation of escalating relational conflict was a particular feature of suicidal behaviour, as the letters and literature suggested, then this pattern should have been replicated in the hospital ward.

The author had immediate access to the process of events in the role of research psychologist. In terms of methodology the approach was one of participant observer.[85] Participant observation is an eclectic tool using various methods and techniques some of which include formal and informal interviewing, formal and informal documentary sources and the acceptance of open-endedness in the direction which the study takes. The assumption was that by participating in the process of interaction, in this case the hospital ward, the observer had some idea of the dynamics of social situations and became privy to incidents which were not generally reported in case notes. While such situations were not conducive to hypothesis testing and measurement, they were conducive to observing episodes of behaviour which could be used for *generating* hypotheses, for reformulating the problem according to real-life situations as opposed to objective abstractions, and for understanding variables which were difficult to categorize. Data gathered in such a way is rich in detail yet lacks general validity. When combined with the observations from other data sources and situations, then the researcher is encouraged to find elements common to varying situations, as a process of abstraction, but remaining true to specific subjective situations.

The legitimation of behaviour became a central issue in understanding the interaction between staff and patients in a hospital ward.[7] Although the four women believed themselves to be legitimate in their interaction, the ward staff would only validate such behaviour if certain factors of age, biography, mental health status and relational circumstance were present. Eventually this validation of legitimacy was withdrawn from the women as their suicidal behaviour increased. They became construed by the staff as deviant, illegitimate in their demands and uncooperative. This negative connotation was mutual. The patients saw the staff as unsympathetic, uncaring and unable to help. The staff in return felt that their therapeutic skills were negated (see Figure 17.5).

This mutual negative connotation also occurred in a broader systemic context where staff factions were in covert disagreement. When ward distress escalated then an outbreak of suicidal behaviour would occur. In the tradition of psychiatric hospitals, suicidal behaviour is one option available from a cultural repertoire of distress management. From an interactional perspective there was no need to invoke past causal trains for explaining behaviour. Suicidal behaviour was an available strategy for maintaining systemic coherence, reducing conflict and clarifying the systemic hierarchy, albeit temporarily. The conflict resided in the

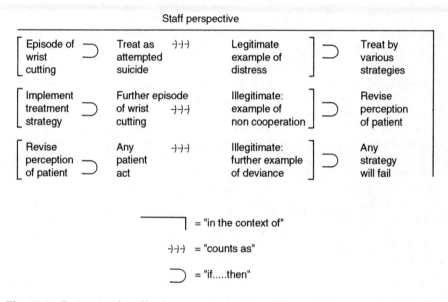

Fig. 17.5 Patient and staff rules in a psychiatric ward setting.

organization of the system rather than in any one individual or relationship. Once a person was labelled as illegitimate and deviant as a person, rather than a person exhibiting deviant behaviour, then systemic distress escalated. The escalation of such distress threatened the viability of such a system.

Evidence for this escalating distress and mutual claims of illegitimate demands from the actors involved were then sought in specific family contexts related to actual events of suicidal behaviour.

Familial understandings: the general hospital data

In attempting to develop a family systems approach it was necessary to see families immediately after an episode of suicidal behaviour. The main intention was to discover how individuals and families described what had happened to them, in the way that personal and situational understandings have been discovered previously. Field research strategies[10] as developed by the social sciences are a particularly valuable way of collecting data about episodes and series of events.

The major centres for research into suicidal behaviour had developed schedules for assessing suicidal behaviour based primarily on individual behaviour and secondarily on the individual in a social context. This approach was concerned to discover an understanding of the relational dynamics which preceded the episode of suicidal behaviour, and what that behaviour meant within a relational context. The assumption was that personal meanings gain validation within a group of significant others. At times of personal transition, such life cycle changes (child to adolescent, adolescent to adult, young adult to married adult living away from home, active worker becoming retired) require that personal meanings concerning identity and behaviour are negotiated anew.

Patients were seen with their families in the general hospital after an episode of deliberate self-harm. These structured interviews were made with a colleague who was the psychiatrist responsible for the management of the patient.[4] The ward sister invited the family or significant others to attend. The consent of the patient was always requested and always given. The assessment design for this part of the study was based on: (i) a family systems understanding which included the significant others (family, friends, close relatives) involved with the patient; (ii) an assessment of the problem which would discover the genesis of the behaviour, and how the current behaviour was maintained,[86] and (iii) the idea that the process of assessment would invoke answers from several realms of construing (personal, relational, familial).

The data collected during the structured interview consisted of general demographic data; the means of referral to the hospital (i.e. who discovered the patient); who was involved in the current family dynamics and information about current intimate relationships; what recent life events had occurred (according to the patient's, or family's, criteria of what counted as a life event); details of the episode of suicidal behaviour; the problem as presented by the patient, and their significant other(s); the ways in which they had previously tried to solve their problems; the changes that they expected from helping agencies; and the ways in which the significant others responded to the situation.

Patients who were admitted to a local general hospital after an episode of suicidal behaviour were seen with their families. They were assessed using a schedule developed from the principles of Brief Therapy.[4] This assessment method has been successfully used in another clinical setting.[87]

The life events which these families described appeared to represent four general categories:

1 events of transition; death, loss of a partner, leaving an institution or leaving home;

2 events of conflict; a row or series of rows, asking for divorce or the threat of violence;

3 social events; a court appearance, debt or threat of imprisonment;

4 events associated with behavioural problems; continuing pain, medical investigations, hospitalization and problems with episodes of drinking.

The problem presented after an episode of suicidal behaviour was rarely that the person felt suicidal. There was usually a clear description of a specific problem. The problem was often that of marital conflict or individual symptomatology. This individual symptomatology was located within a context of transitional life events and interpersonal problems. Significantly, all these people had been treated with medication for their symptoms despite raising the interpersonal nature of the problem with their medical practitioner.

It appeared that when people were given the chance to talk about their problems they located those problems in an ecology which included significant others. Even those persons who described their distress as purely an individual problem located this distress within a context of change related to key others; a feature which was reflected in the letters from the women who had attempted suicide (see Figure 17.4).

Clinical hypotheses

In addition to generating hypotheses necessary for the research study, it was also possible to generate three principal clinical hypotheses as a provisional guide for future therapeutic interventions.

1 **Systemic transition**: A family was faced with 'change' and the necessary adjustments to accommodate that 'change' were not made. Suicidal behaviour in these circumstances was a strategy of 'promotion'; i.e. the behaviour attempted to promote change. This hypothesis was based mainly on the life events data. The changes involved were usually concerned with entrances or exits to the family system. Any such changes demanded reorganization of the family system and the suicidal episode appeared to promote this.

2 **Rigid homoeostasis**: A family was faced with 'change' and this 'change' was accommodated by previously tried solutions. This strategy was part of a tradition where one member adopted the 'sick' status. Suicidal behaviour in such families was a strategy of 'restoration'; i.e. in the face of change the behaviour atempted to restore the status quo. This hypothesis was made when there were transitional life events which contextualized somatic or behavioural problems. These patients would often have thick files of hospital notes.

3 **Marital conflict**: Suicidal behaviour was a strategy in a pattern of escalating symmetrical or complementary behaviour. This strategy could be an attempt to promote conflict resolution or maintain that

conflict. In these families both the life events and the problems were stated in terms of marital conflict. Within the marital relationship both partners presented as hostile to each other yet depended on each other at times of crisis. There was a succession of rows which escalated in frequency and intensity. These rows were punctuated by attempts at conflict resolution. Sometimes these involved a medical practitioner who saw this relational distress in individual terms as 'anxiety', 'depression' or 'sleeplessness'. Medication was then prescribed for the individual, and it was often this medication which was used as the means for the attempted suicide.

Systemic transition and rigid homoeostasis are opposing poles of change management. One is an attempt to bring about developmental changes, the other is an attempt to inhibit changes and return to the status quo. Any interventions then must bear these change strategies in mind. It could be that pre-emptive change strategies in a situation where suicidal behaviour has already occurred will exacerbate the problem. However, therapeutic strategies can be implemented readily in situations where suicidal behaviour is indicating a need to change. In the author's work the neutral strategy of research meets these situations. For the situation of necessary change the family interview and the episode itself are all that is needed. For the situation of 'too much change' then research assessment rather than therapy offers no overt expectations of therapeutic change.

The refinement of hypotheses

From these previous descriptive personal, relational and familial studies it was possible to present hypotheses about the occurrence of suicidal behaviour in a personal and social context. This behaviour appeared to occur when:

1 there was an escalation of familial problems within a context of systemic transition;

2 there were overt expressions of hostility and an immediate threat to the viability of the system;

3 there was a negative connotation of the patient by a treatment or support agency with ascriptions of further deviancy;

4 any attempts at problem resolution were seen as evidence of further pathology.

Stage 3

The following work had been descriptive and yielded much naturalistic data about suicidal behaviour as it occurred in daily life. Clear guidelines emerged for practical assessment and therapy concerned with the recognition of the rate of familial change; (i) that asking systemic questions is sometimes a therapeutic activity; (ii) that the neutral stance of research is appropriate in a crisis; and (iii) that formulating and negotiating clear goals with the patient and family is beneficial.

However, these findings were still general. There are many situations of crisis where problems escalate at a time of change yet suicidal behaviour does not occur. Similarly, families are often threatened with disruption and death without anyone becoming suicidal.

The next stage was to study 20 families in the context of a first family therapy assessment session at a psychiatric day hospital[6] using the previously refined and developed hypotheses. These family sessions were videotaped. Each interview was concerned with a) gaining a relational view of the problem being presented, b) who was involved in the family management of the problem, c) what previous solutions had been attempted to resolve the problem, and d) what therapeutic goals could be negotiated. The intention was to discover the way in which certain families who were in crisis talked about their problem in terms of causes, reasons and relationships, with the intention of discovering if particular criteria distinguished 'suicidal' families. These videotapes were supported by formal case notes from the referring practitioners, and informal case notes made at the clinical meeting which accepted the referrals to the day hospital.

Ten families were to contain a person who was referred by the consultant psychiatrist as 'suicidal'; i.e. there had been an overt expression of suicidal intent or an episode of parasuicide or deliberate self-harm. Ten control families were to be in a situation of escalating distress, but 'non-suicidal'; a crisis intervention with no stated suicidal intent and no parasuicidal behaviour or deliberate self-harm. However, once the sessions were recorded on videotape, a problem arose. During the process of collecting background information from the notes, or while transcribing the videotape data, it was discovered that four of the ten non-suicidal families had a member present who had threatened suicide or that the same, or another, family member had previously attempted suicide. This meant that the videotaped material had to be treated as four groups: a recent suicide attempt, a previous threat of suicide, a discovered attempt in recent history and a group where no suicidal behaviour appeared to be present.

Analysis of the videotapes

The videotapes were analysed by developing a method proposed by Pearce and Cronen.[63] This method proposed that particular episodes of behaviour occur at different levels of interaction; personal, relational, familial. The intention was to discover individual construings of events, and how these were then punctuated into episodes of behaviour. Punctuation in this sense is how people decide what is the beginning of a sequence of events and what is the end of the sequence of events; e.g. 'You started it', 'No, I didn't, you started it'. These individual meanings and constructions of events were then compared with dyadic and familial construings as if there were rules for interaction within these families.

The basic premise was that meanings are organized systemically in communication. When families talk to each other, meanings are not simply organized aggregates of personal views but negotiated in interaction. These meanings are contextualized by what they constitute (reports) and how they are to be regulated (commands).[24] Family systems theory emphasizes that family interaction can be studied as a dynamic interplay of personal understandings within a relation context and this interaction appears to be rule governed (who says what, when, to whom).

These rules were codified as constitutive and regulative rules. *Constitutive* rules (see Figure 17.6) describe the assignment of meaning to events; they specify how sensory input counts as meaning, or how personal behaviour can count as meaning at a familial level. For example; in the context of friendship a kiss constitutes a greeting, in the context of lovers a kiss constitutes an invitation (so the author is informed), and in the context of discipleship a kiss can constitute betrayal. The same behaviour gains different meaning according to a constitutive role in context.

A *regulative rule* (see Figure 17.7) is concerned with social action within a particular context. Given certain conditions of constitution it is necessary, prohibited, obligatory to act in a certain way. For example; if a

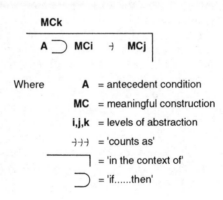

MCk

A ⊃ MCi ⫞ MCj

Where   **A**   = antecedent condition

          MC = meaningful construction

          i,j,k = levels of abstraction

          ⫞⫞⫞ = 'counts as'

          ⎤ = 'in the context of'

          ⊃ = 'if......then'

Example: Constitutive rule for greeting

Close friendship (**MCk**, the context)

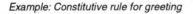

Person enters	⊃	kiss	⫞⫞⫞	greeting
(**A**, the antecedent condition)		(**MCi**)		(**MCj**)

Adapted from Pearce and Cronen, 1980

Fig. 17.6 Constitutive rules.

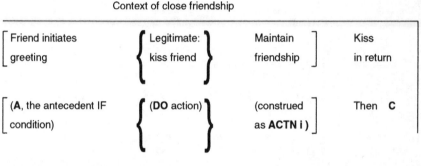

Example: Regulative rule for greeting

Context of close friendship

| Friend initiates greeting | Legitimate: kiss friend | Maintain friendship | Kiss in return |
| (**A**, the antecedent IF condition) | (**DO** action) | (construed as **ACTN i**) | Then **C** |

Adapted from Pearce and Cronen, 1980

Fig. 17.7 Regulative rules.

person cried when asked a simple question in the context of a particular family in this study, this constituted manipulation in their understanding and should be ignored (regulation).

The videotapes were transcribed by the author and scrutinized for sequences of interaction about particular assessment themes; the constitution of the problem, the genesis of the problem and the regulation of the problem. These problems were usually talked about by the families in terms of particular episodes of behaviour. When the tapes were transcribed and analysed into circular sequences of interaction, general familial characteristics were written down and the families compared. For example; the same interaction sequence would be analysed from the position of the patient and from the position of the parents of the patient (see Figure 17.8a), or as a process of mutual influence (see Figure 17.8b).

Results of the videotape data

From the analysis of the videotapes it was possible to generate three categories which differentiated those families where suicidal behaviour was present from those families where suicidal behaviour was absent

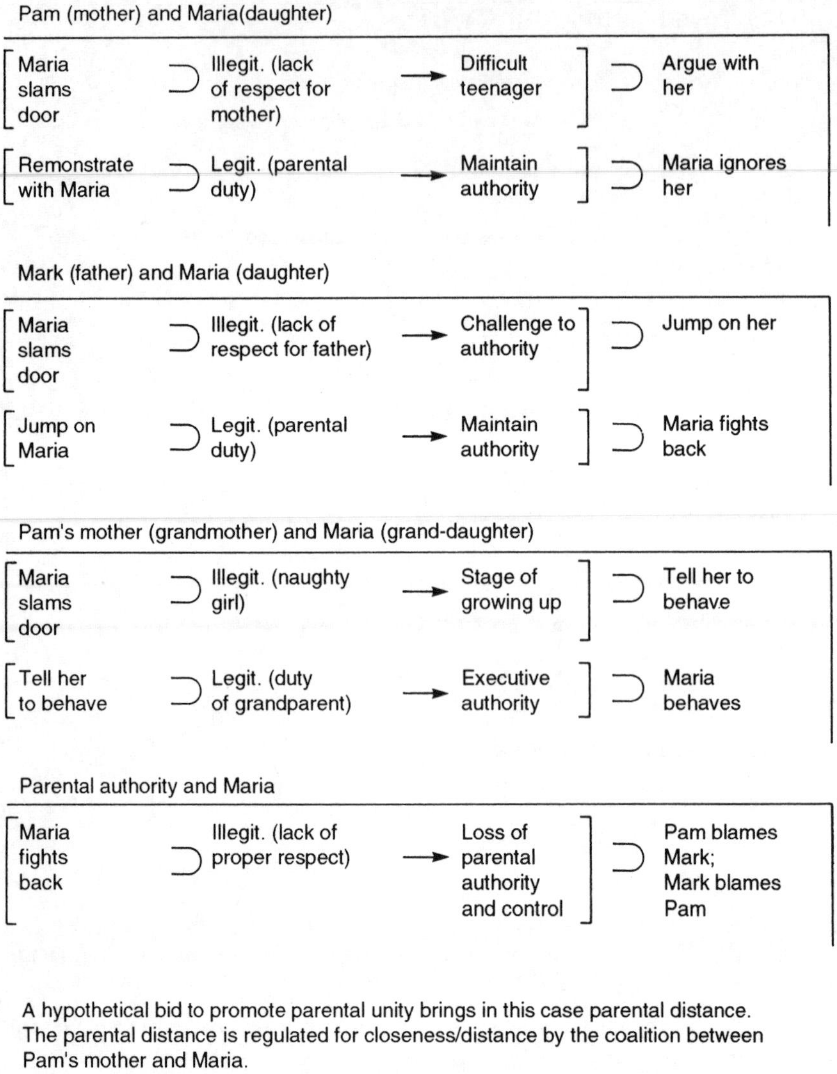

A hypothetical bid to promote parental unity brings in this case parental distance. The parental distance is regulated for closeness/distance by the coalition between Pam's mother and Maria.

Fig. 17.8a Regulative rules and parental authority: differing perspectives on the same behaviour.

(see Figure 17.9). These categories refined the earlier hypotheses. All families exhibited escalating distress which was to be expected in the context of a psychiatric clinic.

The characteristics distinguishing families exhibiting suicidal behaviour were:

    1 a threat of imminent systemic dissolution (the family was about to break up);

    2 a context of mutual negative connotation of all behaviours; and

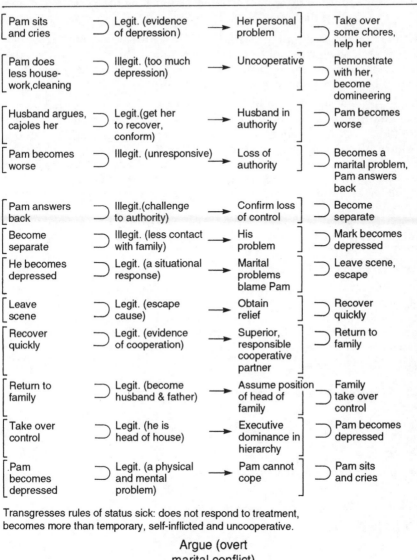

Mark's construing of Pam's problem

Pam sits and cries	Legit. (evidence of depression)	Her personal problem	Take over some chores, help her
Pam does less housework, cleaning	Illegit. (too much depression)	Uncooperative	Remonstrate with her, become domineering
Husband argues, cajoles her	Legit. (get her to recover, conform)	Husband in authority	Pam becomes worse
Pam becomes worse	Illegit. (unresponsive)	Loss of authority	Becomes a marital problem, Pam answers back
Pam answers back	Illegit. (challenge to authority)	Confirm loss of control	Become separate
Become separate	Illegit. (less contact with family)	His problem	Mark becomes depressed
He becomes depressed	Legit. (a situational response)	Marital problems blame Pam	Leave scene, escape
Leave scene	Legit. (escape cause)	Obtain relief	Recover quickly
Recover quickly	Legit. (evidence of cooperation)	Superior, responsible cooperative partner	Return to family
Return to family	Legit. (become husband & father)	Assume position of head of family	Family take over control
Take over control	Legit. (he is head of house)	Executive dominance in hierarchy	Pam becomes depressed
Pam becomes depressed	Legit. (a physical and mental problem)	Pam cannot cope	Pam sits and cries

Transgresses rules of status sick: does not respond to treatment, becomes more than temporary, self-inflicted and uncooperative.

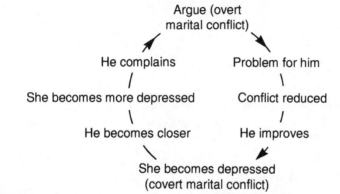

Argue (overt marital conflict)

He complains — Problem for him

She becomes more depressed — Conflict reduced

He becomes closer — He improves

She becomes depressed (covert marital conflict)

Fig. 17.8b Regulative rules in a cycle of family depression.

3 a family tradition of conflict management by one member adopting the sick role.

All the families seen in the context of a family therapy clinic for the first assessment session exhibited relational conflict. This is not surprising in that a condition for referral to the clinic by the referring psychiatrist would have been the presence of relational conflict.

Similarly, for all the families interviewed, there was a pattern of escalation of that relational conflict. In a context of failing attempted solutions and the development of a crisis it appeared that more of one behaviour, 'A', was leading to more of another behviour, 'B', which in turn led to more of 'A'. This is the process Bateson referred to as 'schizmogenesis', i.e. a pattern of behaviour, attempting to promote stability, leads to 'runaway'. The more one person does to convince, cajole, influence, directly bargain or demand, the more the other demurs, rejects, withdraws or refuses. The conflict is present in the organized interaction, not in the person.

Total negative connotation

An important factor distinguishing the suicidal families from the non-suicidal was that of total negative connotation. In the process of escalation the person who became suicidal was perceived as totally deviant as a person, rather than a person exhibiting deviant behaviours. No matter how they acted, whatever they did was perceived as wrong

a) The threat of imminent dissolution

	Threat of imminent dissolution	No threat
Suicidal	14	—
Non-suicidal	—	6

$\chi < .001$ after Yates correction   N = 20

b) The presence of negative connotation

	Total deviance: a negative connotation of all behaviour	Partial deviance
Suicidal	14	—
Non-suicidal	1	5

$\chi < .02$ after Yates correction   N = 20

c) A family tradition of conflict management by the 'sick role'

	Tradition of sickness	No tradition
Suicidal	13	1
Non-suicidal	2	4

$\chi < .001$ after Yates correction   N = 20

Fig. 17.9 Categories distinguishing 'suicidal' from 'non-suicidal' families.

by their family. This was reflected in the psychiatric ward situation described earlier. Furthermore, the family were perceived negatively by the identified patient. The context then was of mutual negation.

The case which refined this factor of total negative connotation was a family where a teenage daughter was construed as deviant and not able to do anything correctly (see Figure 17.9b). In this family there was no threat of the daughter leaving, nor did she have a history of symptomatic behaviour to resolve conflict. The parents were the complainants, and the mother the identified patient.

The threat of imminent dissolution

The factor which clearly demarcated the suicidal from the non-suicidal families was the threat of a complete breakdown of the family, or relational, system. One member had left or was about to leave. Suicidal behaviour at such a time is an attempt to maintain systemic coherence. Rather than being seen as a destructive negative act, it is possible to see it as part of a pattern of interactions to negotiate change. Instead of suicidal behaviour being an 'end process', the punctuation of a process of escalation, it can be construed as a strategy for recalibrating thresholds of distress in a process of continuing negotiation.

A tradition of distress management

In the suicidal families there appeared to be a family repertoire of distress management by the expression of physical or psychological problems. These problems regulated conflict or distress, albeit temporarily, and in some ways contributed to further distress in a context of developmental change.

In the negative cases where there was a tradition of the symptomatic management of conflict but no presence of suicidal behaviour, the symptoms (depression) kept the partners separate rather than together. It could be proposed, then, that when symptoms keep a family together and also resolve conflict, then suicidal behaviour may occur at a time of separation. When symptoms keep partners separate then separation is not a critical issue; it is togetherness that becomes problematical.

For suicidal behaviour to occur then there need to be three factors present. When someone is about to leave, everyone involved sees the rest of the family negatively and there is a tradition of episodes of illness keeping the family together at times of conflict. These factors can be expressed as distinguishing categories (see Figure 17.9) or as family rules (see Figure 17.10).

Discussion

This study attempted to describe suicidal behaviour at different levels of understanding and entailed an elaborate set of descriptions. Although such a 'thick' detailed description takes time, it is rich in understandings which can be woven together to represent the dynamic interplay of ideas.

(a) *Threat of imminent dissolution*

Escalation of conflict

Systemic viability		
Any act	Independent act ᐳᐳᐳ	System about to cease

(b) *The presence of total illegitimacy*

Escalation of conflict

Mutual negative connotation		
Any act	Deviant act ᐳᐳᐳ	Illegitimate: example of a totally deviant person

(c) *A family tradition of conflict management by the 'sick role'*

History of the system (a family tradition)

Relational conflict		
Any act	Escalation of symptoms ᐳᐳᐳ	Legitimate: maintain unity

Fig. 17.10   Rules distinguishing 'suicidal' from 'non-suicidal' families.

Personal meaning was seen as resident within relational contexts which were informed by cultural conditions. It is possible to propose that there was an ecology of ideas which emerged from this constellation of descriptions. The use of constellation, rather than stratified hierarchy, is deliberate. This places an emphasis on perspectives of a universe where the configuration of the constellation appears different according to where the observer is standing. The problem of a stratified hierarchy metaphor is that it can appear that a higher level determines what goes on at a lower level. A consideration of different perspectives proposes a greater understanding of the formal relationship between realms of a constellation. As Bloch[88] says, quoting Gertrude Stein, 'There is no there, over there'.

The different levels of observation generated differing sets of data and further levels of enquiry for each level. The newspaper data generated further questions about the construing and reporting of deviancy, and particularly about causal trains in chronic mental illness. The psychiatric ward research promoted a strategy for the management of suicidal behaviour by the research act itself. The letters from women generated an interest in the personal construing of biography of the realm of mental illness in women. The hospital interview data stimulated an assessment strategy for suicidal behaviour and a coordinated interdisciplinary crisis policy for mental health in the local area.[4] The third stage generated three distinguishing categories of suicidal behaviour which could be investigated in a more rigorous trial. These categories could be used clinically for the recognition of warning signs of escalating behaviour and, therefore, for prevention strategies.

Although this methodological approach does not control conditions as in a formal clinical trial, it does propose hypotheses which could be tested in such a way. It is useful as a preliminary conceptual tool which stays close to the natural setting of the behaviour, and close to the accounts of those involved in that behaviour. As a methodology it has, therefore, propositional, clinical and conceptual validity. The results of this research can be presented either as categories (see Figure 17.9) for further research validation using quantitative studies, or as processual rules (see Figure 17.10) for validation using qualitative studies. It is hoped that both views complement each other.

The aim of this work was not to formally prove a point but to develop an ecosystemic research paradigm. Although this methodology was crude, it represented an attempt to base research on clinical consultations where the researcher was required to act as a clinical anthropologist.[89] The same approach could be made towards any of the chronic problems besetting modern Western civilization where understandings are found to be wanting.

The main principles of this approach were to:

- (a) see what happens in practice;
- (b) develop propositional hypotheses;
- (c) organize 'fields' in which to study the phenomenon;
- (d) test hypotheses within these contextual 'fields';
- (e) adopt methodology appropriate for each contextual 'field'; and
- (f) refine hypotheses including negative cases.

References

1 Wells, N. *Suicide and Deliberate Self-harm*. London: Office of Health Economics, no. 69, 1981.

2 Riskin, J., Faunce, E. An evaluation of family interaction research. *Fam Proc* 1972; **11**: 365–455.

3 Lask, B. Family therapy outcomes research. *J Fam Ther* 1979; **1**: 87–91.

4 Aldridge, D., Rossiter, J. A strategic assessment of deliberate self harm. *J Fam Ther* 1984; **6**: 113–25.

5 Aldridge, D. Family interaction and suicidal behaviour: A brief review. *J Fam Ther* 1984; **6**: 309–22.

6 Aldridge, D., Dallos, R. Distinguishing families where suicidal behaviour is present from families where suicidal behaviour is absent. *J Fam Ther* 1986; **8**: 243–52.

7 Aldridge, D. Treating self mutilatory behaviour: a social strategy. *Fam Sys Med* 1988; **6**: 5–19.

8 Aldridge, D. Goal setting, the patient's assessment of outcome and recognition of therapeutic change. *Comp Med Res* 1988; **3**: 89–97.

9 Bynner, J., Stribley, K. M. *Social Research: Principles and Objectives.* Harlow: Longman, 1978.

10 Smith, H. W. *Strategies of Social Research: The Methodological Imagination.* London: Prentice-Hall, 1975.

11 Parker, A. The meaning of attempted suicide to young parasuicides: a repertory grid study. *Br J Psychol* 1981; **139**: 306–12.

12 Reiss, D., Oloveri, M. E. Family stress as community frame. *Mar Fam Rev* 1983; **6**: 61–83.

13 Dallos, R., Aldridge, D. Handing it on: family constructs, symptoms and choice. *J Fam Ther* 1987; **9**: 39–58.

14 Douglas, J. *The Social Meanings of Suicide.* Princeton, New Jersey: Princeton University Press, 1967.

15 Geertz, C. *The Interpretation of Cultures.* New York: Basic Books, 1973.

16 Siegal, L., Friedman, J. The threat of suicide. *Dis Nerv Sys* 1955; **16**: 45–51.

17 Hunter, R., McAlpine, I. *Three Hundred Years of Psychiatry.* Oxford: OUP, 1963.

18 Miner, J. R. Suicide in relation to climatic and other factors. *Am J Hyg* 1922; **2**: 111.

19 Durkheim, E. *Suicide.* New York: Macmillan, 1951.

20 Henry, A. F., Short, J. L. *Suicide and Homicide.* Glencoe, Illinois: The Free Press, 1954.

21 Holinger, P. C., Offer, D. Prediction of adolescent suicide: a population model. *Am J Psychiat* 1981; **139**: 302–6.

22 Shepherd, D. M., Barraclough, B. M. Work and suicide: an empirical investigation. *Br J Psychiat* 1980; **136**: 469–78.

23 Fabrega, H. An ethnomedical perspective of medical ethics. *J Med Phil* 1990; **15**: 593–625.

24 Aldridge, D. Making and taking health care decisions. *J Roy Soc Med* 1990; **83**: 720–23.

25 Leach, E. *Culture and Communication: The Logic by which Symbols are Connected.* London: Cambridge University Press, 1976.

26 Bateson, G. *Steps to an Ecology of Mind.* London: Granada, 1973.

27 Fernandez, J. The mission of metaphor in expressive culture. *Curr Anthropol* 1974; **15**: 119–45.

28 Evans, G. Deliberate self-poisoning in the Oxford area. *Br J Prev Med* 1967; **21**: 97–107.

29 Bostock, F. T., Williams, C. L. Attempted suicide as an operant behaviour. *Arch Gen Psychiat* 1974; **31**: 482–6.

30 Sifneos, P. E., Manipulative suicide. *Psychiat Quart* 1966; **40**: 525–37.

31 Ginsburg, G. P. Public conceptions about attitudes about suicide. *J Health Soc Behav* 1971; **12**: 201–7.

32 Sale, I., Williams, C. L., Clark, J., Mills, J. Suicide behavior: community attitudes and beliefs. *Suicide* 1975; **5**: 158–68.

33 Jeffrey, R. Deviant patients in casualty departments. *Sociol Health Illness* 1979; **1**: 90–108.

34 Burvill, E. Suicide in Western Australia, 1967. Analysis of coroners' records. *Aust NZ J Psychiat* 1981; **5**: 37–44.

35 Hawton, K., Catalan, J. *Attempted Suicide: A Practical Guide to its Nature and Management.* Oxford: OUP, 1982.

36 Freud, S. *Mourning and Melancholia. Collected Papers, Vol. 4.* London: Hogarth Press, 1925.

37 Jung, C. *Psychiatric Studies.* New York: Pantheon, 1957.

38 Rank, O. *The Myth of the Birth of the Hero.* New York: Vintage Books, 1969.

39 Adler, A. F. Suicide. *J Ind Psychol* 1958; **14**: 57–62.

40 Stengel, E. *Attempted Suicide: Its Social Significance and Effects.* Oxford: OUP, 1958.

41 Kreitman, N. *Parasuicide.* Chichester: Wiley, 1977.

42 Brenman, M. On teasing and being teased: the problem of moral masochism. *Psychoanal Study Child* 1952; **7**: 264–85.

43 Johnson, F. G., Frankel, B. G., Harvis, G. K., Whitehead, P. C. Self injury in London, Canada: a prospective study. *Can J Pub Health* 1975; **66**: 307–16.

44 Morgan, H. G. *Death Wishes? The Understanding and Management of Deliberate Self-harm.* Chichester: Wiley, 1979.

45 Bach, Y., Rita, G. Habitual violence and self-mutilation. *Am J Psychiat* 1974; **131**: 1018–20.

46 Ballinger, B. R. Minor self-injury. *Br J Psychiat* 1971; **118**: 535–8.

47 Lukianowicz, N. Suicidal behaviour: an attempt to modify the environment. *Br J Psychiat* 1972; **121**: 387–90.

48 Kelly, G. Suicide: the personal construct point of view. In: Shneidman, E., Farebrow, N. L. (eds.) *The Cry for Help.* New York: McGraw Hill, 1955.

49 Kelly, G. *The Psychology of Personal Constructs.* New York: McGraw Hill, 1955.

50 Haley, J. *Leaving Home.* New York: McGraw Hill, 1980.

51 Richman, J., Rosenbaum, M. A clinical study of the role of hostility and death wishes by the family and society in suicidal attempts. *Isr Ann Psychiat Rel Disc* 1970; **8**: 213–31.

52 Watzlawick, P., Weakland, J. *The Interactional View*. New York: W. W. Norton, 1977.

53 Murthy, V. Personality and the nature of suicide attempts. *Br J Psychiat* 1969; **115**: 791–5.

54 Schrut, A. Some typical patterns in the behavior and background of adolescent girls who attempt suicide. *Am J Psychiat* 1968; **125**: 69–74.

55 Watzlawick, P., Beavin, J., Jackson, D. *Pragmatics of Human Communication*. New York: W. W. Norton, 1967.

56 Bowlby, J. *Attachment and Loss. Vol. 2 Separation, Anxiety and Anger*. London: Hogarth Press, 1973.

57 Byng-Hall, J. Symptom bearer as marital distance regulator: clinical implications. *Fam Proc* 1980; **19**: 355–65.

58 Tabachnick, N. D. Interpersonal relations in suicide attempts. *Arch Gen Psychiat* 1961; **4**: 42–7.

59 Rosenbaum, M., Richman, J. Family dynamics and drug overdoses. *Life Threat Behav* 1972; **2**: 19–25.

60 Tuckman, J., Connor, H. E. Attempted suicide in adolescents. *Am J Psychiat* 1962; **119**: 228–32.

61 Reiss, D. Varieties of consensual experience. I A theory of relating family interaction to individual thinking. II Dimensions of a family's experience of its environment. *Fam Proc* 1971; **10**: 1–35.

62 Reiss, D. *The Family's Construction of Reality*. Cambridge, Mass.: Harvard University Press, 1981.

63 Pearce, W. B., Cronen, V. E. *Communication, Action and Meaning*. New York: Praeger Scientific, 1980.

64 Bancroft, J., Skrimshire, A., Casson, J., Harvard-Watts, D., Reynolds, F. People who deliberately poison or injure themselves: their problems and their contacts with helping agencies. *Psychol Med* 1977; **7**: 289–303.

65 Bateson, G. *Mind and Nature*. Glasgow: Fontana, 1979.

66 Beer, S. *Platform for Change*. London: Wiley, 1975.

67 Maturana, U., Varela, F. *Autopoiesis and Cognition: The Realization of the Living*. Dordrecht, Holland: Reidel, 1980.

68 Zborowski, M. Cultural components in responses to pain. *J Soc Iss* 1952; **4**: 16–30.

69 Zola, I. L. Medicine as an institution of social control. *Sociol Rev* 1972; **20**: 487–504.

70 Mechanic, D. Perception of parental responses to illness: a research note. *J Health Hum Behav* 1966; **6**: 253–7.

71 Atkinson, J. M. *Discovering Suicide: Studies in the Social Organization of Sudden Death*. London: Macmillan, 1978.

72 Blumer, H. Society as symbolic interaction. In: Manis, J. G., Metyler, B. N. (eds.) *Symbolic Interaction: A Reader in Social Psychology*. Boston: Allyn and Bacon, 1972.

73 Denzin, N. K. *The Research Act: A Theoretical Introduction to Sociological Methods*. Chicago: Aldine, 1970.

74 Cohen, S., Young, J. *The Manufacture of News. Deviance, Social Problems and the Media*. London: Constable, 1973.

75 Bateson, G. The position of humour in human communication. *Macy Foundation Conference IX*: 1953; 1–47.

76 Harré, R., Secord, P. F. *The Explanation of Social Behavior*. Totowa, New Jersey: Littlefield Adams, 1973.

77 Jackson, D. Family rules: marital quid pro quo. *Arch of Gen Psychiat* 1965; **12**: 589–94.

78 Aldridge, D. *Suicidal Behaviour: An Ecosystemic Approach*. Milton Keynes: The Open University, 1985.

79 Laing, R. *The Politics of the Family*. London: Tavistock, 1969.

80 Palazzoli, M. S., Boscolo, L., Cecchin, G., Prata, G. *Paradox and Counterparadox*. New York: Jason Aronson, 1973.

81 Tuchman, J., Youngman, W. F. A scale for assessing suicide risk of attempted suicides. *J Clin Psychol* 1968; **24**: 17–19.

82 Bancroft, J., Skrimshire, A., Simkin, S. The reasons people give for taking overdoses. *Br J Psychiat* 1976; **128**: 538–48.

83 Bancroft, J., Hawton, K., Simkin, S., Kingston, B., Cumming, C., Whitewell, D. The reasons people give for taking overdoses: a further enquiry. *Br J Med Psychol* 1979; **52**: 353–65.

84 Heather, N. The structure of delinquent values: a repertory grid investigation. *Br J Clin Psychol* 1979; **18**: 263–75.

85 McCall, G., Simmons, J. L. *Issues in Participant Observation: A Text and a Reader*. London: Addison-Wesley, 1969.

86 Sluzki, C. Process of symptom production and patterns of symptom maintenance. *J Marital Ther* 1981; **7**: 273–80.

87 Wassenaar, D. Brief strategic therapy and the management of adolescent Indian parasuicide patients in the general hospital setting. *S Afr J Psychol* 1987; **17**: 93–8.

88 Bloch, D. Mode or modality. *Fam Sys Med* 1987; **5**: 3–4.

89 Aldridge, D., Pietroni, P. Research trials in general practice: towards a focus on clinical practice. *Fam Pract* 1987; **4**: 311–15.

18 Research strategies in a hospital setting: the development of appropriate methods

David Aldridge

Summary

Designing appropriate research methods is seen as a developmental process. Three related areas of clinical research are proposed; physiological experimentation, theoretical development and clinical outcomes. The dialogue between clinicians in a hospital setting, where the criteria for the assessment of clinical criteria for research are negotiated, is seen as beneficial in promoting understanding between practitioners. Research also stimulates the academic life of the department.

Introduction

This chapter is a report of preliminary research in the medical faculty at the University of Witten/Herdecke from January 1987 until September 1987. The aim of the initial project is to establish specific research strategies for music therapists in a hospital setting and to develop a range of methodological approaches appropriate for unconventional medicine.

The intention of the researcher in the project is to devise a way of researching into the phenomena of a particular therapeutic approach (music therapy), in a way which generates exciting ideas pertinent to the practitioners (in this case, music therapists), and which is applicable to the institutional context (the hospital). This way of working while meeting specific needs also considers the ecological niche in which those needs reside; i.e. the particular research interventions are designed to fit into the broader setting in which they are applied. This 'fit' is made not only on the practical grounds of clinical practice and patient access, but also in terms of philosophy, as will be demonstrated later.[1]

Orthodox and complementary medical practitioners are currently seeking ways of carrying out research which addresses the needs of clinicians and considers the whole person. This project keeps such clinical and holistic perspectives in mind. This work is also happening at a time when other research commentators[2,3] are advocating broad research perspectives which include qualitative and quantitative data.

The setting

The university hospital at Witten/Herdecke is a large general hospital which serves the immediate community. It has inpatient and outpatient facilities. The underlying philosophy of the hospital is anthroposophical after the teachings of Rudolf Steiner.

Anthroposophical medicine is an extension of orthodox medical practice. Its basic tenets are:

1 Each person is a unique individual and treatment decisions must recognize this individuality.

2 Scientific, artistic and spiritual insights, which recognize the whole person, need to be applied together in our therapeutic endeavours.

3 Life has meaning and purpose. If these qualities are lost then there is a deterioration of health.

4 Illness may provide opportunities for positive change and new balance in a person's life.

Creative music therapy has been an important part of the therapeutic approaches since the hospital first began.[4] As a discipline it has always been part of the medical faculty and enjoyed the cooperation of medical practitioners. For a researcher it is an ideal virgin environment to formulate research strategies. There is no established way of researching. The only stipulation is that the methodology maintains the integrity of music therapy and does not attempt to impose a restrictive methodology on the practice.

Method

The general methodological approach is that of ethology or clinical anthropology[5] where initial careful observations are used as a platform on which to build further endeavours.

The researcher met the five hospital music therapy staff collectively, and then singly each month for six months. He also went out into the hospital and interviewed those senior medical practitioners who were known to be interested in music therapy either because they were regular referrers to the music therapists or because they professed an interest in music therapy. These interviews were then written up as an internal paper and submitted departmentally and to those previously interviewed for comment. All practitioners involved were then invited to a common meeting and asked for their comments about the work so far. This meant that the work stayed close to the comments of the practitioners directly or peripherally involved.

From these early discussions it was possible to see what common areas of interest were available to build on. This chapter is a report of the results of those discussions.

Three areas of research

Three areas are recommended for the research in the music therapy department (see Figure 18.1). These areas of interest emerged from the discussions with the doctors in the hospital who were asked directly what they wanted to see from the music therapy department and how

Figure 18.1 Proposed research structure

	Physiological work	*Clinical studies*	*Theoretical work*	*Publications*
Year one	Establish physiological criteria of change in therapist–patient interaction	Single case studies, develop methods and working relationships	Literature reviews, theory development Symposium	Case studies, and position papers
Years two and three	Continue work on identified clinical problems, refine hypotheses	Continue work on refining hypotheses, look for long-term changes	Collect case examples from recorded work	
	Prepare research report and further proposals		Develop theory and define techniques	Prepare clinical outcomes papers

None of these areas of work is exclusive, but each part will inform the other. For the sake of practicality and to avoid confusion, it may help to think of these three areas: physiological work, teaching/theory work and the clinical case studies. Not all therapists will want to concentrate on all three areas. The clinical case study work and the physiological work will provide a framework for more refined and formal research studies. These studies will inform, and be informed by, the developing theory. This approach gives the work both conceptual and practical coherence. Knowledge gained in this way has meaning for the practitioners and retains the integrity of therapeutic practice which is enlivened by the rigour of a naturalistic science.

much they were willing to cooperate, and from extensive talks with the music therapists.

A significant feature in developing research ideas was to get music therapists to present their taped work to the researcher, and to say what questions were raised by that work. All the discussions focused on clinical practice, not idealized abstractions about research.

The three areas for future research are as follows:

1 Physiological

The aim of this part of the research is to discover the physiological implications of improvising music with a therapist. As the music therapy department shares its accommodation with the department of physiology there are opportunities for continuing dialogues.

The questions to be asked are:

What changes occur during the process of playing music together

    (a) in the individuals concerned, and

    (b) in the interaction between patient and therapist?

What are the implications of those changes

    (a) for the patient, and

    (b) for the course of the therapy?

There has been a limited amount of work on the influence of receptive music on physiological parameters. However, there has been little work on the interaction between therapist and patient playing music together. This investigation of mutual influence in therapy is potentially of great benefit in understanding therapist/patient interaction in contexts other than music therapy.

The initial part of this programme will monitor the heart rate of the patient and the heart rate of the therapist, and the playing of the therapist on the piano and the playing of the patient on a drum. These will be recorded in real time onto a videotape recording of the session. It will be possible to see observed changes in the therapeutic interaction on the videotape and correlated changes in the other parameters. Each interaction will occur in a variety of contexts: rest, playing a composed work and creative improvised playing. In some ways this is an attempt to monitor the physiology of creative dialogues, a feature which many of us try to include in our clinical practice.

2   Theoretical

This work will focus on the taped work of the therapy sessions. Nordoff Robbins music therapists always audiotape their work, and have a system for indexing their tapes. This careful observation, which is accessible to another clinician/researcher, is a significant feature of any research approach and emphasizes the rigour of the therapists.

The questions to be asked are:

How do music therapists talk about their work?

What are the questions they ask of their own therapeutic endeavour?

How can the adult work be documented in an acceptable way?

Can some terms be defined in a way which can form a common vocabulary for talking about music therapy with our peers and colleagues?

How does the therapy work?

What happens during the course of therapy?

What is the relationship between the music and the patient as a whole person?

Can a patient's state of health or illness be heard in the way in which they improvise music; and if so, how can this be demonstrated?

These questions are concerned with internal validity.

3 Clinical

This clinical work will concentrate on understanding clinical outcomes and questions of therapeutic changes. It will be carried out within the context of the hospital wards and in cooperation with interested doctors and therapists.

The questions to be asked are:

What changes during the process of therapy in terms of the patient's problem?

How is this change recognized by the music therapist?

How can this change be communicated to other professional practitioners?

What is evidence of therapeutic change for the patient?

What are the clinical criteria of the referring practitioners in terms of patient referral, therapeutic change and clinical prognosis?

How can observed changes be documented and correlated with those of other practitioners and family members?

These questions are concerned with external validity.

It is important to note that in this approach the process of therapy and outcome are *not* separate activities. It is convenient to consider them as separate but this does not happen in clinical practice. Similarly, clinician and researcher work together, not separately.[5,6,7,8]

Implications for practice

The implications for the music therapy department, and the university hospital, are set out below.

We have developed a way of working which satisfies the members of the music therapy department and their various needs. Research solutions have not been imposed upon the therapists, they have been developed with the therapists. The three areas of research, clinical, experimental and theoretical, are all inter-related, yet separate. While maintaining a picture of the whole research endeavour it is possible to implement particular strategies appropriate to the level of investigation. A holistic strategy does not mean that everything must be all lumped together in an infinite series of multiple variables, rather that each part is understood in relationship to other parts and to the whole.

By following a programme which is flexible, different clinicians are allowed to follow their own interests. Some therapists, for instance, are more interested in the physiological experiments while others are more concerned with theoretical issues about health indices and wellbeing.

Methodological development

Each of the previous areas has its own detailed protocol, which again is being refined in another round of investigation.[9]

Although the development of an appropriate methodology takes time initially, it is satisfying in the long run. A benefit of working in this way is that the clinicians are intimately involved with the research. Research is seen as applicable in practice, and as belonging to the clinicians. The traditional split between research and clinical practice is avoided. In this context the researcher is a facilitator and guide, and the clinician actively engages in the research process. When methodology meets the needs of the clinicians, and is based upon their epistemology, then research endeavours are likely to be completed.

The development of research methodology is not pursued as an activity separate from the epistemology which underlies the therapeutic activity. Rather than impose an alien methodology upon music therapy it has been a policy within the department to develop rigorous methods which are isomorphic with the underlying premises of music therapy. Many of the published research studies about music and music therapy from the United States so far have been from a standpoint of music psychology. In general they have been reductionist and, in particular, cerebral.[3] While concentrating on the mechanics of perception they have neglected the questions of music as an artistic activity, the relationship between music and healing processes within the body, the implications of music for health, and the inter-relationship between body, mind and spirit. Similarly, there has been no investigation of the relationship between therapist and patient.

By applying rigid methodologies without due regard for the nature of the therapy itself and the persons involved, those studies have been unscientific. They have lacked internal validity. Methodology is intended to serve science. Science is not the servant of methodology.[8] By restricting our questions to those which can only be answered by orthodox methodologies we ignore the possibility of finding the very answers for which we seek.

Clinical dialogues

By pursuing a research policy which involves a variety of clinicians the work of the department is linked to other practitioners within the hospital. This has meant that a number of bridges have been built between different practitioners. The advantage for research and clinical practice is that a many-sided picture of the patient is composed. Furthermore, continuing clinical dialogues are encouraged between practitioners.

Academic life

In reviewing the literature, writing papers, and talking about theoretical issues, the academic life of the department is enlivened. The staff are encouraged to read articles outside their usual range of reading, and new material is introduced. There are also benefits for the students in the music therapy department and the medical school in that by concentrating on clinical case studies and individual tuition it is possible to add an extra dimension to their teaching.

Single case study designs[10] are a particularly effective way of teaching students. It allows them to follow their own interests under expert supervision. They are responsible for their own learning but this is guided by a tutor. By following case study designs it is possible to prepare material for the production of case studies and theses for examination.

For the staff it means that they can prepare papers for publication based upon their own clinical practice but with the added overlay of a formal research instrument. In time this builds a repertoire of case studies all based upon a similar format.

Research in context

There are several reasons why the research project within the department of music therapy developed so well and these are related to the hospital setting.

1 Own interest

The idea of carrying out a research programme was not imposed; it came out of an interest shown by the music therapists themselves and their desire to grow as a department. The fact that all the music therapists in the department are trained in the Nordoff Robbins approach[4] has enabled a consistency of approach.

2 Timing and validity

The time was right for the development of research. As a department the music therapists were aware that there was a need to develop academically. Similarly, the music therapy staff were looking to formulate research methods which could be validated internally on their own terms as clinicians, yet would satisfy external criteria of validity. In our early discussions we considered the audiences for our work: the broader audience of the professional culture; the smaller audience of our music therapy peers; and finally, ourselves. In addition the hospital and medical faculty were actively seeking new research endeavours.

3 Reflexive

The music therapists were already questioning their own work in terms of theory building, clinical efficacy and therapeutic process. The research has always attempted to stay close to those questions and to relate each part of the work to the whole.

Having an overview has maintained a necessary cohesion between differing ideas and interests. Each person does not have to know what every other person is doing in detail. This allows for academic independence. However, all the parts relate to a commonality of interest which promotes cohesion and gives meaning and structure to all the research endeavours. To work in this way means that staff members can be both independent and interdependent. By maintaining a commonality of purpose different members can follow their own interests without feeling that they are disloyal to their colleagues.

4 Hospital ethos

The whole ethos of the hospital community is one of a cooperative culture of like-minded people. The art therapies, eurhythmy and music therapy are recognized by the medical staff as having a legitimate place within the whole therapeutic approach. This integration, clinically, theoretically and methodologically, is worthy of its own research study. When art and medicine meet in such a setting it is possible to begin dialogues between practitioners from differing clinical backgrounds where beauty, inspiration and the deepest longings of the human spirit are seen as essential for health.

5 Holistic approach

The commonality of background at the hospital, which is founded in anthroposophy, maintains a cohesive framework at times of dissent. When superficial disagreement occurs there is recourse to a deeper unity both at an epistemological level and in the tradition of working. In a health setting where the author has worked recently, where the talk was of 'holistic' medicine and multidisciplinary practice, superficial disagreement led to the exposure of deep fundamentally opposed medical epistemologies and professional differences. The academic tradition at Herdecke, which remains true to its holistic approach yet is responsive to change, encourages a true scientific endeavour where both imagination and rigour work together.

Perhaps the most important feature of working at Herdecke is the acceptance of differing levels of understanding of particular phenomena. Orthodox medicine, while making many advances, still has severe limitations in understanding the human being as a whole person. By refusing to accept simplistic and reductionist solutions Herdecke is preparing a way for the future of medical science understandings. It is only in the field of applied clinical research methodologies which grapple with complexity that the difficult area of chronic illness will be tackled in the later part of the twentieth century. However, as Lynch[11] says in his book about the medical consequences of loneliness:

> Examining the nature of living together, understanding the nature of human dialogue, and blending a scientific understanding of human companionship within a philosophical framework that will allow us to appreciate its complexity will not be an easy matter (p. 231).

It is my contention that music is this dialogue.

6 External influence

A tradition of anthroposophy and the secure underpinning of practice with epistemology was further enhanced by the ready acceptance of people from outside the hospital to bring in new ideas. Academic tolerance is surely the mark of an intellectual climate in which ideas can grow. At Herdecke there was this readiness to consider a broad spectrum of ideas as Steiner himself advocated.[12] This did not mean an uncritical acceptance, but it did mean a willingness to listen in good faith.

Conclusion

There is no one paradigm for scientific research. When we consider music therapy we must consider both art and science. This dichotomy is of our own making. No such split exists either in the music or in our own health for that matter. When we enforce the split we run the risk of losing the music and the essential properties of healing.

It is my intention to develop methods which sensitively articulate what is pertinent to the experience of playing music together and the implications for the health of a person. By listening to various colleagues it is possible to begin to attempt to answer their questions using their criteria. Our over-riding emphasis is to return constantly to the music as it is used creatively in clinical practice to test out our emerging hypotheses.

Our methodological approach of commitment to mutual dialogue in research reflects the approach of creative music therapists to their work and anthroposophists of medicine. I hope that as a community of scientists and artists, linked by our common fraternity as practitioners, we can extend these dialogues to other practitioners whatever their disciplines and training.

References

1 Aldridge, D. Treating self-mutilating behaviour; a social strategy. *Fam Sys Med* 1988; **6**: 5–19.

2 Bunt, L. G., Hoskyns, S. L. A perspective on music therapy research in Great Britain. *J Br Music Ther* 1987; **1**: 3–6.

3 Clarke, E., Hoskyns, S. L. Starting research in music therapy. In: *Proc 3rd Music Therapy Day Conference*, City University, London, February 1987.

4 Nordoff, P., Robbins, C. *Creative Music Therapy.* New York: John Day, 1977.

5 Aldridge, D., Pietroni, P. Research trials in general practice: towards a focus on clinical practice. *Fam Pract* 1987; **4**: 311–15.

6 Aldridge, D., Pietroni, P. The clinical assessment of acupuncture for asthma therapy. *J Roy Soc Med* 1987; **80**: 222–4.

[7] Lincoln, S. Y., Guba, E. G. *Naturalistic Inquiry.* Beverly Hills: Sage, 1985.

[8] Pietroni, P., Aldridge, D. Summary of discussion on BMA Report. *Hol Med* 1987; **2**: 95–102.

[9] Aldridge, D., Verney, R. Forschungsbericht Musiktherapie Januar 1987 bis September 1987. Research report to the Medical Faculty, University of Witten-Herdecke, W. Germany (unpublished).

[10] Barlow, H., Hersen, M., Jackson, M. Single case experimental designs. *Arch Gen Psychiat* 1973; **29**: 319–25.

[11] Lynch, J. J. *The Broken Heart: The Medical Consequences of Loneliness.* New York: Basic Books, 1977.

[12] Steiner, R. *Theosophy.* New York: Anthroposophic Press, 1971.

Section 3

19 Acupuncture as a treatment for chronic pain

C. A. Vincent

Introduction

Traditional Chinese medicine has developed over a period of at least 3000 years,[1] and there is a large and rather daunting literature. The most important early written record is the *Yellow Emperor's Classic of Internal Medicine*[2] probably written about 300 BC. The origins of acupuncture, its place in the systems of medicine and philosophy of ancient China, and the application of these traditional ideas to diagnosis and treatment of disease have been discussed in several important books.[1,3,4] Scientific research into acupuncture has a number of different aspects. Experimental studies have sought to demonstrate short-term analgesic effects and examine the biochemical and physiological mechanisms that underlie such effects.[5,6] In this chapter, however, I will be primarily concerned with the evaluation of acupuncture as a treatment for chronic pain and other disorders. Even when the scope of the review is narrowed to the clinical evaluation of acupuncture there is still a large literature; certainly many hundreds of papers have been published in English. Many of these, however, are primarily descriptive, of poor quality and little value.

The main criticisms revealed against acupuncture are firstly that the theories underlying traditional acupuncture are implausible and irrelevant to modern medicine, and secondly that any effects acupuncture has are simply those of an appealing placebo.[7] I shall only briefly discuss the traditional ideas in any detail; the reader is referred to the books cited above. The approach I shall take is that the traditional ideas need to be understood in outline, but that questions about efficacy can be asked without considering them in detail. The treatment may be effective whether or not the theory is valid.

The most important questions, in my view, are:

1 Does acupuncture have a beneficial effect on any individual disease or disorder?

2 Is this effect primarily, or even partly, due to the action of the needles (and associated treatments), or is it due to psychological processes? To put it another way, is acupuncture just a placebo, or is there some specific treatment effect?

This book describes a number of approaches to the evaluation and understanding of the treatment process, pointing out the value of observational studies, single case designs and controlled trials. There are a large number of descriptive studies of acupuncture,[8] and some single case designs.[9] I do not want to dispute the value of such approaches. I will assume, though, that controlled trials are the final arbiter of the efficacy of a therapy,[10] and concentrate on their methodology and results.

I begin by sketching the ideas underlying traditional acupuncture, briefly considering their validity and relevance to the evaluation of acupuncture treatment. I then discuss some methodological issues, particularly the definition of an appropriate placebo control for acupuncture. The most urgent task for researchers of acupuncture treatment is to establish an agreed and satisfactory methodology for its evaluation. I will then briefly review controlled trials of acupuncture for chronic pain and a variety of other disorders. A chapter of this length cannot possibly attempt a comprehensive account and the reader is advised to consult the various review papers that are cited, and from there the individual studies.

Finally, I will comment on the small group of studies which do appear to have used a satisfactory placebo control and offer some suggestions for the conduct of future trials.

Traditional acupuncture

A thorough understanding of the concepts and theory underlying the practice of traditional acupuncture is not essential to assess individual studies, but certain aspects (such as point location) need to be considered. The reader also needs to appreciate that the diagnosis made by traditional acupuncturists can be quite independent, and quite foreign, to more orthodox medical approaches.

The core ideas of traditional acupuncture are as follows. Energy flows within the body along lines known as channels or meridians. There are 14 main channels, some associated with an organ of the body, and a number of subsidiary channels. The state of a person's health is dependent on the balance of energy in the system and the overall level of energy. In the treatment of disease, needles are inserted in the classical acupuncture points located on the channels and are manipulated with the aim of restoring the energy flow to a state of balance, and so restoring the patient to a state of health. Any disease or disorder should be reflected in an imbalance of this system and should, in principle, be amenable to treatment. Traditionally oriented acupuncturists are often prepared to treat a wide range of conditions.

Diagnosis for a traditional acupuncturist will encompass the medical history, the patient's psychological state and the impact of the patient's lifestyle on their complaint. The patient's state of health, and hence the state of the energy system, will also be inferred from subtler signs such as the quality of the pulse, the colour of the tongue, the complexion and the patient's smell. The pulse diagnosis is especially complex as twelve pulses are discerned, each with different qualities, corresponding to the twelve main meridians. The resulting diagnosis is usually couched in terms that are entirely different from orthodox medical diagnosis.[3]

Types of acupuncture

The traditional acupuncturist may treat patients with similar conditions (in orthodox medical terms) in very different ways, according to the (traditional) diagnosis they have made. For instance, ten different patients with migraine might be treated in ten different ways. In contrast, many practitioners use orthodox diagnoses and a corresponding prescription or 'formula' of points for each dysfunction or disease. Where this approach is taken, the formula has usually been derived from traditional Chinese ideas, even though the practitioners may no longer subscribe to them. Most clinical trials employ this approach. Only a very few allow the individual approach of traditional acupuncture.[7,11]

In some modern forms of acupuncture classical point locations play no part. The locations can be trigger points, tender areas, points in the same dermatome as the pain, etc.,[12] and electrical stimulation is often employed. There are also hybrid techniques such as electro-acupuncture according to Voll[13] and Ryodoraku therapy[14] which are derived from traditional acupuncture but refined and systematized using electrical methods of diagnosis and treatment. As yet, however, they have not been systematically evaluated. With so many methods available it is obviously crucial that each study specifies its particular methods as closely as possible, as differences in technique may explain apparently discrepant findings.

Practitioners of traditional acupuncture may criticize the formula approach on the grounds that it gives inferior results and is not in keeping with the spirit of traditional acupuncture. The attention paid to the individual patient during a traditionally based diagnostic session is no doubt valuable, regardless of the validity of the traditional ideas. Whether traditional acupuncture gives superior results is an empirical matter, and to my knowledge no study has yet addressed this question.

Validity of traditional ideas

Numerous books have been published about traditional approaches to diagnosis and treatment,[1,3] but there have been very few attempts to evaluate these methods of diagnosis. Cole[15] carried out a series of small studies examining the reliability and validity of the pulse diagnosis. She concluded that the pulse diagnosis 'is not apparently a means of objective analysis, but offers subjective meaning to the practitioner and is a vehicle for a meaningful and helpful interaction with the patient'. Further studies on the process of diagnosis and treatment would be extremely useful. Whether or not the traditional ideas were substantiated, such research would help to rid acupuncture of its reputation for irrationality.[16]

A considerable amount of work has been carried out, especially in China, on the possible anatomical basis of meridians and points. 'Propagated Channel Sensation' refers to the sensations experienced by a small proportion of people when acupuncture points are needled; these sensations tend to run along the acupuncture meridians – though it is not clear whether the subjects, who are presumably Chinese, know in advance where the meridian pathways are supposed to be. Changes in skin resistance and temperature have also been suggested as providing evidence for the existence of meridians.[17] Reviewing this work, Macdonald[18] acknowledges that sensations may follow meridian lines but suggests that such phenomena can be explained without postulating the existence of a meridian system. Meridians have also been detected by the injection of radio-tracers into acupuncture points, but more recent work suggests that the pattern of spread of the radio-tracer corresponds to vascular drainage of the tracer.[19] In China, work on research on meridian phenomena continues, but most Western researchers would probably dismiss the idea of a meridian system. At the very least, we must conclude that the existence of meridians remains unproven.

Research on acupuncture points has been more fruitful, and there are definite links between the observations made by acupuncturists and phenomena observed by other clinicians and scientists. As we shall see, a discussion of the existence and location of acupuncture points is crucial for a proper evaluation of the clinical studies. Macdonald[18] makes a number of comments. Firstly, it is difficult to be precise about the location of acupuncture points. Their position is usually assessed according to the size and shape of the patient, and while there is reasonable agreement about the locations of the fundamental points,[7] the number of points continues to grow.[18] Secondly, there is evidence that they become tender when a patient is sick, and there is certainly considerable overlap with the independently developed concept of trigger points.[20,21] Thirdly, it is possible that acupuncture locations have some kind of neurophysiological basis, perhaps corresponding to the termination of peripheral nerve endings. For our purposes, it is important to realize that while acupuncture locations may provide useful therapeutic guidelines, it is unlikely they have a precise and constant location. The effect of acupuncture may be stronger at some points than others, but this is unlikely to be an all-or-nothing phenomenon.

Methodology of acupuncture trials

Many studies of acupuncture treatment are seriously flawed by methodological problems.[7] Poor design, inadequate measures and statistical analysis, lack of follow-up data and substandard treatment are all too common. The most important problems are the measurement of outcome, design and choice of control group. Outcome measures are discussed elsewhere in this volume, and by Vincent and Chapman.[22] The main issues addressed here are the question of whether trials of acupuncture should be single blind or double blind, the definition of an appropriate control group, and methods of testing the adequacy of the control. Controlled trials may encompass comparisons of acupuncture with a waiting list group, an alternative treatment or a placebo. The main methodological problems arise with the placebo control.[23]

Single blind or double blind trials?

The expectations of both patients and clinicians (as well as a variety of other factors) may affect the outcome of a trial. There is therefore a need to 'blind' both patients and clinicians to the allocation of the treatments under test. In a single blind trial, patients do not know whether they are receiving a true or a control treatment, and in a double blind trial the clinicians do not know either.[7]

It is questionable whether double blind trial methodology can be applied to acupuncture. Reports have appeared of so-called double blind trials in which patient progress has been assessed by an independent clinician, who was unaware of treatment allocation.[24,25] This independent assessment is a valuable addition to any trial, but does not make it double blind. In both these trials, the clinician giving the treatment inevitably knew whether he was giving true acupuncture or a sham, control treatment. Such trials are therefore single blind, with independent assessment.

It is difficult to see how a trial of acupuncture could be double blind. It would mean that the person giving the treatment would not know whether he was giving true or sham treatment, and he would therefore have to have little or no experience as an acupuncturist! It is possible that the sites to be needled could be marked on the patient by an experienced acupuncturist and then treated by a technician who had been merely trained in needling technique,[26] but it is questionable whether a technician would produce the same quality of treatment as an experienced acupuncturist.

Most discussions of the methodology of acupuncture trials have now recognized that they need to be single blind. It is important to emphasize, though, that this is not because complementary medicine is allowed, or demands, different standards of proof. It would, for instance, be possible to carry out a single blind trial comparing two surgical techniques: the patient would be unaware of which technique was being used. A double blind trial, however, would mean that the surgeon would also have to be unaware of the choice of technique – hardly feasible, when the surgeon is providing the treatment. The same logic applies to trials of acupuncture or any other skilled treatment.

Placebo control conditions used in acupuncture trials

A bewildering variety of control procedures have been used in acupuncture trials. In some, all acupuncture procedures are matched with those in the true treatment group except that needles are not inserted into the patient; instead they are rubbed against the skin[27] or glued to it.[28] It seems unlikely that patients would accept these procedures as credible forms of treatment, as even those with no experience of acupuncture treatment are likely to know that needle insertion is involved. This type of placebo cannot therefore be recommended, as if the control is not perceived as a bona fide treatment then the trial will not be valid.

In the most commonly used control treatment, needles are actually inserted but at incorrect, theoretically irrelevant sites. Usually this has simply meant carrying out a procedure similar to the true treatment at nearby, non-classical locations. Depth of insertion and stimulation are the same; only location differs. This procedure, which is termed 'sham' or 'mock' acupuncture, has been used as a placebo in a great many studies.[24,25,26,29] The reasons for sham acupuncture being used as a placebo treatment derive from traditional theory. For acupuncture to be effective, according to the theory, needles must be inserted at designated classical points.[1] Acupuncture at non-classical sites (sham acupuncture) was consequently assumed by most investigators to be ineffective, and therefore ideal as a placebo. This assumption needs to be questioned.

To begin with, there is some doubt as to whether acupuncture points and non-points can be reliably distinguished.[18] Even if they can, there is evidence that acupuncture at non-classical locations may have analgesic effects.[12,23] Stimulation at classical point locations may produce superior analgesia,[30] but there is no reason to suppose that the non-classical locations are completely inert. Controlled trials have also shown significant therapeutic benefits from both classical and non-classical locations.[8,24] These are sometimes interpreted to mean that acupuncture is no more than a placebo, but an equally plausible interpretation is that both forms of acupuncture have some effect but that exact point locations are not very important.[12] Studies of the acupuncture treatment of back pain, for instance, show no difference between sham (non-classical site) acupuncture and true acupuncture[26,29,31,32,33] but acupuncture has shown an advantage over a true placebo control.[34] To demonstrate a significant difference between acupuncture at different sites would in fact be quite difficult. As Lewith and Machin[35] point out, if true and sham acupuncture both have specific effects, then a trial with very large subject numbers would be needed to show a difference between them.

Finally, we should note that it is by no means necessary to think in terms of classical/non-classical point locations. Melzack *et al.*[20] have pointed out the correspondence between acupuncture points and trigger points, and Liu[36] between acupuncture points and motor points. Some practitioners[37] only needle trigger points for the relief of pain, and thereby avoid the associations with traditional Chinese theory. It seems that stimulation at many different sites, whether or not they be classical point locations, may produce analgesic effects in a particular area of the body.[12,35,38,39] The sham acupuncture control condition relies on the quite opposite assumption that some (non-classical) locations are therapeutically inert.

Acupuncture at non-classical sites (sham acupuncture) cannot be assumed to be a placebo. A sham acupuncture control condition really only offers information about the most effective sites of needling, not about the specific effects of acupuncture. This fundamental error has bedevilled the majority of controlled trials of acupuncture. It is therefore vital to find a control condition that does not suffer from these defects, which in practice means one with small or non-existent specific physiological effects.

Solutions to the problem of the acupuncture control

Mock TENS

The first plausible solution to the problem outlined above was the introduction of mock transcutaneous electrical nerve stimulation (TENS) as a control condition in acupuncture trials. In this procedure, transcutaneous electrical nerve stimulators are used in the usual way, except that no current actually passes between the electrodes. Patients are sometimes told that they are receiving subliminal pulse therapy and they will therefore not feel the current. This control was first used in a trial of acupuncture in the treatment of back pain,[34] in which acupuncture was found to be superior to mock TENS. Mock TENS has also been used in trials of acupuncture for post-herpetic neuralgia[40] and migraine[41]; acupuncture was of no value for post-herpetic pain, and of doubtful benefit in the treatment of migraine. While these results are disappointing in terms of acupuncture's efficacy, they suggest that mock TENS is an acceptable control.

Minimal acupuncture

Vincent and Richardson[7] suggested that it would be possible to use a form of sham acupuncture that involves only minimal surface stimulation. In minimal acupuncture, needles are placed away from classical or trigger points, inserted only 1–2 mm and stimulated extremely lightly. Vincent[23] suggests that this procedure minimizes the specific effects of the needling while maintaining its psychological impact. The fact that the minimal acupuncture may have some physiological effect would make this control condition a somewhat sterner test of true acupuncture than a completely inert placebo. It might therefore be unsuitable as a control for a form of acupuncture where surface needling is used.[34] However, this disadvantage is perhaps outweighed by the fact that the treatment and control are almost identical in the eyes of the patient.

Minimal acupuncture has been used as a control condition in several studies, though not always described in this way. True acupuncture was, for instance, found to be superior to minimal in a trial of the acupuncture treatment of migraine.[42]

Another interesting way of ensuring an inert acupuncture placebo was that of Jobst *et al.*[75] who, for the control condition in a trial of acupuncture for disabling breathlessness, deliberately chose a place (the knee) where needling was expected to have no effect. A difficulty with this might be that patients would not see this as being a credible treatment for breathlessness.

My own preference in the choice of placebo is minimal acupuncture, as it can be matched almost exactly to the true treatment. It may have a slight therapeutic effect, but this can be minimized by very shallow insertion of the needles. Even if there is a small effect, the trial is not invalidated; it is just slightly harder to demonstrate a difference between treatment and control.

Assessing the adequacy of control conditions

A difficulty with any control condition, and especially one of a different form from the true treatment, is that it may have a different psychological impact. If mock TENS, say, has a lesser psychological impact than acupuncture, then a significant difference might simply mean that acupuncture was the more powerful placebo. Mock TENS has, however, been shown to have considerable therapeutic power,[43] though it can vary depending on how it is presented to the patient.[44] From this point of view an acupuncture control condition might be preferable as different forms of acupuncture are likely to have a similar psychological impact.

Whatever the choice of control group, it is valuable to check the adequacy of the control. It is not feasible to assess every psychological variable that may be of importance, but it is possible to make some assessment of the adequacy of whichever control procedure one is using. For instance, Vincent[42] chose to assess the credibility of the acupuncture treatment and the control, as the credibility of a treatment appears to be an important aspect of its therapeutic power.[45,46,47] Petrie and Hazelman[48] found that acupuncture and mock TENS had equal credibility as treatments when demonstrated to patients but no study has yet assessed the relative credibility of acupuncture and mock TENS with patients having a course of treatment. It is clearly important that this is done, as the results may differ from those where the techniques are simply demonstrated.

The circumstances of every trial are different. The fact that minimal acupuncture and mock TENS are equally credible to acupuncture in one study does not necessarily mean that they will be in all. An assessment of credibility of treatment is therefore a valuable addition to any controlled study. If the treatment and control turn out not to be equally credible then the results of the study must be interpreted in the light of this information.

The evaluation of acupuncture treatment

An enormous number of reports of the therapeutic efficacy of acupuncture have been published but many are little more than rough descriptions of the immediate effects of acupuncture. For instance, Zang[49] treated 192 patients with bronchial asthma, reporting immediate improvement in 98.9% and clinical remission in 76.5%. These results appear impressive, but have not been matched in more careful studies (see below). As Prance *et al.* point out,[50] such studies appear to be conducted by people who accept *a priori* the effectiveness of acupuncture and are only seeking to describe the results achieved. The acupuncture literature is over-run with descriptive studies, most of which are of such poor quality that nothing can be concluded from them. This is not to say that descriptive, or uncontrolled, studies do not have their place. If acupuncture has not been tried for a particular disorder, then it is perfectly reasonable to begin with an exploratory study. For instance, Filshie[51] assessed the use of acupuncture for pain associated with malignancy by reviewing case notes. The study is by no means a controlled trial, but is certainly a useful preliminary report. Single case studies may also provide valuable information about the treatment process, but will not provide evidence of the efficacy of a treatment across a range of patients,[9,52] which can really only be achieved with randomized clinical trials.[10]

Several types of controlled trial can be distinguished:

1 No-treatment or waiting list control. Acupuncture has, for instance, been shown to be superior to waiting list control in the treatment of neck and back pain.[11,53] These studies at least suggest that any changes observed are not simply due to the passage of time, but cannot tell us whether acupuncture has any advantages over other treatment options.[8]

2 Acupuncture as an addition to an existing treatment. For instance, Gunn *et al.*[54] found that the addition of acupuncture to standard therapy produced a significant improvement in low back pain patients.

3 Acupuncture compared to another treatment. There are, for instance, a number of studies comparing acupuncture with TENS.[55,56]

4 Acupuncture compared with placebo control. These studies assess the crucial question of whether the effects of acupuncture are simply due to psychological factors. Although other types of controlled trials are considered, I shall place most emphasis on those with a placebo control.

Acupuncture for chronic pain

Several reviews of the use of acupuncture in the treatment of chronic pain have now appeared.[8,35,57,58,59] All have commented on the poor quality of most of the studies, and all have stated that this severely limits the conclusions that can be drawn from the review. Richardson and Vincent[8] reviewed all English language controlled trials of acupuncture published before 1986. They concluded that there was good evidence for the short-term effectiveness of acupuncture for low back pain, mixed results for headache, and some encouraging preliminary results for cervical pain and arthritis. The proportion of patients helped varied from study to study but commonly fell in the region of 50–80%. Follow-up periods, however, were disappointingly short and evidence for longer term benefits was weak. They suggested that the response rate and degree of benefit obtained were higher than might be expected from a placebo response, but cautioned that very few studies used a satisfactory placebo control. The extent to which acupuncture was producing benefit by psychological mechanisms had not really been established.

In addition to the basic reviews, two meta analyses of the literature on chronic pain have been reported. Meta analysis is a discipline that critically reviews and statistically combines the results of previous research. The purposes of such a procedure include increasing overall statistical power, resolving uncertainty between conflicting reports and improving estimates of the size of the effect being investigated.[60] However, it should be emphasized that although these techniques have the potential for resolving questions about the efficacy of acupuncture, they cannot compensate for the poor quality of studies they set out to combine. For instance, if the placebo control is unsatisfactory in the original studies, then biased estimates will be produced in the final meta analysis.

Patel and colleagues[58] reviewed all randomized controlled trials of acupuncture for chronic pain that measured outcome in terms of the numbers of patients improved. They attempted a statistical pooling of the results and concluded that the results favoured acupuncture, though various methodological problems precluded a definite conclusion. Combining the results of these studies, however, does not seem very sensible. There are only 14 trials, of very variable standard. They address the treatment of various chronic pain problems, and they appear to use eight different control groups. It is not clear what any statement about the superiority of acupuncture over a control can mean in these circumstances.

A more comprehensive meta analysis, and the most recent review available, was produced by Ter Riet and his colleagues.[59] They decided not to attempt a statistical pooling of results, arguing that the studies were on the whole too poor and too disparate to allow their results to be combined. Their report is therefore perhaps best considered a critical review. They identified 51 reports of acupuncture for chronic pain involving some kind of control or group comparison, which had not been previously reported. Each study was scored on 18 methodological criteria, some weighted more heavily than others, with a maximum possible score of 100.

Only eleven studies scored 50 or more points, with the best study obtaining 62% of the maximum score. Positive and negative results were approximately equally divided in the higher quality studies, whether a cut-off score of 40 or 50 points was taken. Studies were also separated into four categories of pain: headache, musculoskeletal (spine), musculoskeletal (other) and miscellaneous. The pattern of results did not change, however. Results are equivocal for all four groups, though the treatment for musculoskeletal problems of the spine (mostly low back pain) show slightly more positive results.

The overall conclusions of all reviewers are similar. Studies are generally methodologically poor. Acupuncture appears to produce some benefits for patients with chronic pain, but it is not clear how long they last or whether they are psychologically mediated. When acupuncture is compared with alternative treatments (such as TENS), the results are equivocal.[8] When acupuncture is compared with a placebo control, the results are also equivocal. Flaws in the placebo control may bias the results of some of these studies against acupuncture. Studies with acceptable placebos are considered below.

Acupuncture for other disorders

Studies of acupuncture for chronic pain are poor. Studies of acupuncture for other disorders are, with some exceptions, generally worse.[61] Vincent and Richardson[61] reviewed the use of acupuncture for asthma, deafness, hypertension, psychiatric disorders, smoking and obesity. They concluded that the studies on hypertension, obesity and psychiatric disorders were so poor that nothing could be concluded from them. Studies on asthma and deafness were of a higher standard and are considered below. Studies on the treatment of smoking and drug addiction are also considered in a separate section. It should be noted that treatments for obesity, smoking and addictions generally are a rather special case as they tend to use auricular acupuncture. The mechanisms that may operate for musculoskeletal pain may not have much in common with those mediating any effect of ear acupuncture.

Deafness

The treatment of sensorineural deafness by acupuncture is interesting. It reads like a cautionary tale for researchers.[61] Early studies from China claimed 80–90% success rates.[62] However later, more careful studies involving audiometric evaluation failed to find any effect.[61] Finally, in 1982 a report appeared from the Beijing Research Institute of 1000 cases treated over 20 years, concluding that in the vast majority of cases acupuncture does not have any beneficial effect on deafness. Thus the earlier enthusiasm generated by reports based on subjective impressions of improvement has not been sustained when more careful studies have been carried out. Two controlled studies of acupuncture for tinnitus have also been carried out, but neither found it to be of any value.[61]

Asthma

Several experimental studies have reported short-term effects of acupuncture on asthma,[61] though not all have used a placebo control. For instance, Tashkin and colleagues[63] demonstrated the superiority of acupuncture over placebo in the treatment of metacholine induced asthma. It has proven more difficult, though, to demonstrate the effects of acupuncture as a therapy for asthma. Tashkin[64] failed to demonstrate any effects of classical acupuncture on chronic asthma. Christensen[76] showed a modest effect on both subjective and objective measures, with true acupuncture proving superior to sham. Jobst[75] showed an improvement in patient ratings of breathlessness and exercise tests, true acupuncture being superior to sham. All three of these studies are small – 24 patients at most. The results are equivocal, perhaps because of the low power of the studies. Nevertheless the results are sufficiently encouraging to warrant a larger scale trial.

Acupuncture in the treatment of addictions

Vincent and Richardson[61] reviewed seven studies of acupuncture in the treatment of smoking. They concluded that acupuncture seemed to be as successful as many other techniques, but there was nothing to

Table 19.1 Acupuncture for chronic pain: studies with acceptable placebo controls

Authors	Population	N	Design	Control	Type of acupuncture	Dependent measures	Follow-up	Results
Hansen & Hansen 1983	Facial pain	16	Cross-over	Minimal acupuncture	Classical; 10 daily sessions	Daily pain ratings	4 week	66% patients improved. True acupuncture. sig. > control
Macdonald *et al.* 1983.	Low back pain	17	Group comparison	Mock TENS	Tender areas & trigger points. Some EA. Up to 10 sessions	Various pain VASs, mood, independent clinician's assessment	None	Acupuncture sig. > placebo for pain relief, activity, physical signs in pain area
Petrie & Langley 1983	Cervical pain	13	Group comparison	Mock TENS	Classical; 8 sessions, twice weekly	Self-ratings	None	84% acupuncture group reported good pain relief. Acupuncture sig. > placebo
Lewith *et al.* 1983	Post-herpetic neuralgia	62	Group comparison	Mock TENS	Classical & auricular; 6–8 sessions	Daily records, sleep moderation, sleep disturbance	2 month	Sig. improvement in only 7 patients in each group. No sig. difference between groups
Dowson *et al.* 1984	Migraine headache	48	Group comparison	Mock TENS	Classical: 6 sessions	Frequency, duration, intensity, medication	24 week	56% acup. and 30% placebo showed 33% pain relief. 44% acup. and 57% placebo less frequent headaches. No sig. difference between groups
Petrie & Hazelman 1986	Chronic neck pain	25	Group comparison	Mock TENS	8 sessions, twice weekly	Daily diary: pain intensity,	1 month	45% of acup. group & 30% of

Lehmann et al. 1986	Chronic low back pain	53	Group comparison	Mock TENS	EA group and TENS group (all groups had additional treatment)	Physician assessment. VRS measures of pain & disability, medication	6 month	placebo group show sig. response. No sig. difference between groups EA sig. >TENS and mock TENS
Ballegaard et al. 1986	Severe angina	26	Group comparison	Minimal acupuncture	Classical; 7 sessions over 3 weeks	Exercise tests, pain diaries, medication	3 week	Acup. sig. > control for cardiac work capacity only
Vincent 1989	Migraine	30	Group comparison	Minimal acupuncture	Classical; 6 weekly sessions	4 × daily ratings of pain and medication	1 year	43% reduction in weekly pain score for acup. group, 14% for control. Acup. sig. > control for pain levels, but not for medication reduction
Dickens & Lewith 1989	Osteoarthritis	13	Group comparison	Mock TENS	Classical; 6 sessions over 2 weeks	Daily. VAS pain scores medication sleep, grip, tenderness	3 week	76% reduction in pain in acup. group. 10% in control, but no sig. difference between groups
Ballegaard et al. 1990	Moderate angina	49	Group comparison	Minimal acupuncture	Classical; 10 sessions over 3 weeks	Exercise tests, pain diaries, medication, wellbeing	6 month	Reduction of 50% in attacks & medication. No sig. difference between groups

suggest it was of any special benefit. Ter Riet and colleagues evaluated studies of acupuncture in the treatment of smoking, heroin addiction and alcohol addiction using very similar criteria to those in their previous reviews.[59,65] As before, studies were of generally low quality, with the difference that low quality studies were more likely to show that acupuncture was beneficial than high quality ones. Only one of eight positive studies[66] scored over 50 points out of 100. Only three of 15 studies on smoking showed positive results.

Striking features in these studies were the inadequate numbers of patients, and lack of biochemical validation. Three out of five studies on heroin addiction claimed a positive result, but these studies are of very poor quality. A pilot study and a later controlled trial[66] showed that acupuncture could help prevent relapse for alcoholics. These studies appeared to be carefully designed and implemented, but have been subject to a number of criticisms,[67] in particular that drop-out rates were very high from the control group.

Studies with an acceptable placebo control

This brief account of reviewers' conclusions makes depressing reading. Very few controlled trials of acupuncture meet acceptable methodological requirements. In my view, and that of other authors,[35,59] an inappropriate placebo control is the most serious problem and completely invalidates many of the studies. It seems important, therefore, to separate out those studies with an acceptable placebo, to see if different conclusions can be drawn. I have suggested that minimal acupuncture (in some form) and mock TENS are both plausible as control groups, though some reviewers have directed criticism at the mock TENS control.[59] Table 19.1 shows all the studies that I am aware of that use either of these control groups,[18,34,40,41,42,68,69,70,71,72,73,74] in the treatment of chronic pain.

There are only twelve studies, and they concern the treatment of a variety of disorders. Only five of the studies show a significant advantage of acupuncture over placebo, though several others show a non-significant advantage. However, the trials are very small, with four involving less than 20 subjects. It is doubtful if many of them have sufficient power to conclude that a non-significant result definitely shows acupuncture to be equivalent to placebo. The probability of a Type II error – failing to detect an actual difference – is high.

The standard of the studies is also very variable, with methodology scores ranging from 28 to 57 on Ter Riet's ratings. A cautious interpretation of these studies is that the results for post-herpetic neuralgia and angina suggest that acupuncture is ineffective. Acupuncture may well be helpful for low back pain but its efficacy for migraine remains to be resolved.

The conclusions from a selective review of placebo controlled studies are similar, then, to those of other reviews. Acupuncture may be effective for some types of chronic pain, but the results are equivocal in many cases. The principal conclusion must be, though, that there are still, after

20 years of research, too few adequate studies to permit firm conclusions to be drawn.

Conclusions

Disappointingly little has been achieved by literally hundreds of attempts to evaluate acupuncture. Major methodological flaws are apparent in the vast majority of studies. Some tentative conclusions can be drawn, however. Acupuncture does not appear to be helpful for deafness and drug addiction and further investigations are probably unnecessary. Controlled studies have shown positive findings for low back pain, and equivocal results for migraine and asthma. Nevertheless, larger scale studies are warranted for all these disorders, though other types of musculoskeletal pain, tension headache and arthritis are also possible candidates.

Controlled trials of any treatment have become an immensely difficult and technical undertaking. They are expensive, time-consuming and ideally require collaboration between practitioners and researchers and consultation with a statistician. It is not really possible for complementary practitioners in private practice to mount such trials, and it is very difficult for a professional association or college. However, it is clear that there is no longer any point in conducting small, preliminary studies of acupuncture treatment. There are dozens of such studies, with some encouraging findings. The only way that acupuncture can gain full acceptance as a valid form of treatment is through good controlled trials that are large enough to answer the questions they pose.

Recommendations for the conduct of clinical trials are made throughout this book, and Ter Riet's[59] list of criteria is a good starting point for anyone designing a trial of acupuncture. Specific points I would emphasize, after reviewing the existing research on acupuncture, are:

1 Trials should be single blind; it is not feasible to conduct double blind trials. Some trials are nevertheless incorrectly described as double blind.

2 A range of outcome measures should be used, preferably with some independent assessment. An adequate follow-up is essential.

3 Considerable care needs to be taken in the choice of control group, especially with placebo controls. For a placebo, I suggest a form of acupuncture treatment that is designed to have minimal effects. It will be the option that is the closest match to the true treatment and avoids the difficulties inherent in randomizing patients to a non-acupuncture treatment.

4 It is very useful to check the adequacy of any control treatment with a measure of credibility, or similar assessment, as the choice of control is frequently a matter for criticism.

5 Trials have generally been too small to permit firm conclusions. Ter Riet[59] implies that 50 patients per group are needed. This may not be necessary. However, preliminary calculations of the necessary size for a reasonable power need to be carried out (see Pocock, Chapter 3).

References

[1] O'Connor, J., Bensky, D. *Acupuncture: A Comprehensive Text.* Shanghai College of Traditional Chinese Medicine. Chicago: Eastland Press, 1981.

[2] Veith, I. *The Yellow Emperor's Classic of Internal Medicine.* Berkeley, California: University of California Press, 1972.

[3] Kaptchuk, T. *The Web That Has No Weaver: Understanding Chinese Medicine.* New York: Congdon Weed, 1983.

[4] Lu, G.-D., Needham, J. *Celestial Lances: A History and Rationale of Acupuncture and Moxa.* Cambridge: Cambridge University Press, 1980.

[5] Chung, S.-H., Dickenson, A. Pain, enkephalin and acupuncture. *Nature* 1980; **283**: 243–4.

[6] Price, D. D., Rafii, A., Watkins, L. R., Buckingham, B. A psychophysical analysis of acupuncture analgesia. *Pain* 1984; **19**: 27–42.

[7] Vincent, C. A., Richardson, P. H. The evaluation of therapeutic acupuncture: concepts and methods. *Pain* 1986; **24**: 1–13.

[8] Richardson, P. H., Vincent, C. A. Acupuncture for the treatment of pain: a review of evaluative research. *Pain* 1986; **24**: 15–40.

[9] Vincent, C. A. The treatment of tension headache by acupuncture: a controlled single case design with time series analysis. *J Psychosom Res* 1990; **34**(5): 553–61.

[10] Pocock, S. J. Current issues in the design and interpretation of clinical trials. *Br Med J* 1985; **290**: 39–42.

[11] Coan, R. M., Wang, G., Ku, S. L., Chan, Y. C., Ozer, F. T., Coan, P. L. The acupuncture treatment of low back pain: a randomized controlled study. *Am J Chin Med* 1980; **8**: 181–9.

[12] Melzack, R. Acupuncture and related forms of folk medicine. In: Melzack, R., Wall, P. D. (eds.) *Textbook of Pain.* London: Churchill Livingstone, 1984.

[13] Voll, R. Twenty years of electroacupuncture therapy using low-frequency current pulses. *Am J Acup* 1975; **3**: 291–314.

[14] Okazaki, K. Ryodoraku for migraine headache. *Am J Chin Med* 1975; **3**: 61–70.

[15] Cole, P. Acupuncture and pulse diagnosis in Great Britain. Unpublished PhD thesis, University of Sussex, 1975.

[16] Skrabanek, P. Acupuncture and the age of unreason. *Lancet* 1984; **ii**: 1169–71.

[17] Zhaowei, M., Zongxiang, Z., Xianglong, H. Progress in the research of meridian phenomena in China during the last five years. *J Trad Chin Med* 1985; **5**(2): 145–52.

[18] Macdonald, A. J. R. Acupuncture analgesia and therapy. In: Wall, P. D., Melzack, R. (eds.) *Textbook of Pain.* 2nd ed. London: Churchill Livingstone, 1989.

[19] Lazorthes, Y., Esquerre, J.-P., Simon, J., Guiraud, G., Guiraud, R. Acupuncture meridians and radiotracers. *Pain* 1990; **40**: 109–12.

[20] Melzack, R., Stillwell, D. M., Fox, E. J. Trigger points and acupuncture points for pain: correlations and implications. *Pain* 1977; **3**: 3–23.

[21] Travell, J. G., Simons, D. G. *Myofascial Pain and Dysfunction. The Trigger Point Manual.* Baltimore: Williams and Wilkins, 1983.

[22] Vincent, C. A., Chapman, C. R. Pain measurement in trials of acupuncture. *Acup Med* 1989; **6**: 14–19.

[23] Vincent, C. A. The methodology of controlled trials of acupuncture. *Acup Med* 1989; **6**: 9–13.

[24] Gaw, A. C., Chang, L. W., Shaw, L. C. Efficacy of acupuncture on osteoarthritic pain: a double blind controlled trial. *New Eng J Med* 1975; **293**: 375–8.

[25] Henry, P., Baille, H., Dartigues, J. F., Jogeix, M. Headache and acupuncture. In: Pfaffenrath, V., Lundberg, P. O., Sjaastad, O. (eds.) *Updating in Headache.* Berlin: Springer Verlag, 1985.

[26] Godfrey, C. M., Morgan, P. A controlled trial of the theory of acupuncture in musculoskeletal pain. *J Rheumatol* 1978; **5**: 121–4.

[27] Borglum-Jensen, L., Melsen, B., Borglum-Jensen, S. Effect of acupuncture on headache measured by reduction in number of attacks and use of drugs. *Scand J Dent Res* 1979; **87**: 373–80.

[28] Gallachi, G. Acupuncture for cervical and lumbar syndrome. *Scheiz Med Wschr* 1981; **111**: 1360–66.

[29] Mendelson, G., Selwood, T. S., Kranz, H., Kidson, M. A., Scott, D. S. Acupuncture treatment of chronic back pain: a double blind placebo controlled trial. *Am J Med* 1983; **74**: 49–55.

[30] Reichmanais, M., Becker, R. O. Relief of experimentally induced pain by stimulation at acupuncture loci: a review. *Comp Med East West* 1977; **5**: 281–8.

[31] Lee, P. K., Andersen, P. W., Modell, J. H., Saga, S. A. Treatment of chronic pain with acupuncture. *JAMA* 1975; **232**: 1133–5.

[32] Edelist, G., Gross, A. E., Langer, F. Treatment of low back pain with acupuncture. *Can Anaesth Soc J* 1976; **23**: 303–6.

[33] Yue, R. W. M. Acupuncture for chronic back and neck pain. *Acup Electro-Ther Res* 1978; **3**: 323–4.

34 Macdonald, A. J. R., Macrae, K. D., Master, B. R., Rubin, A. P. Superficial acupuncture in the relief of chronic low back pain. *Ann Roy Coll Surg Eng* 1983; **65**: 44–6.

35 Lewith, G. T., Machin, D. On the evaluation of the clinical effects of acupuncture. *Pain* 1983; **16**: 111–27.

36 Liu, Y. K., Varela, M., Oswald, R. The correspondence between some motor points and acupuncture loci. *Am J Chin Med* 1977; **3**: 347–58.

37 Baldry, P. E. *Acupuncture, Trigger Points and Musculoskeletal Pain.* London: Churchill Livingstone, 1989.

38 Chapman, C. R., Wilson, M. E., Gehrig, J. D. Comparative effects of acupuncture and transcutaneous stimulation on the perception of painful dental stimuli. *Pain* 1976; **2**: 265–83.

39 Stewart, D., Thompson, J., Oswald, I. Acupuncture analgesia: an experimental investigation. *Br Med J* 1977; **275**: 67–70.

40 Lewith, G. T., Field, J., Machin, D. Acupuncture compared with placebo in post-herpetic pain. *Pain* 1983; **16**: 361–8.

41 Dowson, D., Lewith, G. T., Machin, D. The effects of acupuncture versus placebo in the treatment of headache. *Pain* 1985; **21**: 35–42.

42 Vincent, C. A. A controlled trial of the treatment of migraine by acupuncture. *Clin J Pain* 1989; **5**: 305–12.

43 Thornsteinsson, G., Stonnington, H. H., Stillwell, G. K., Elveback, L. R. The placebo effect of transcutaneous nerve stimulation. *Pain* 1978; **5**: 31–41.

44 Langley, G. B., Sheppard, H., Johnson, M., Wigley, R. D. The analgesic effects of transcutaneous nerve stimulation and placebo in chronic patients. *Rheumatol* 1984; **2**: 1–5.

45 Borkovec, T. D., Nau, S. D. A. Credibility of analogue therapy rationales. *J Behav Ther Exp Psychiat* 1972; **3**: 257–60.

46 McGlynn, F. D., McDonnel, R. M. Subjective ratings of credibility following brief exposure to desensitization and pseudotherapy. *Behav Res Ther* 1974; **12**: 141–6.

47 Shapiro, D. A. Comparative credibility of treatment rationales: three tests of expectancy theory. *Br J Clin Psychol* 1981; **20**: 111–22.

48 Petrie, J., Hazelman, B. Credibility of placebo transcutaneous nerve stimulation and acupuncture. *Clin Exp Rheumatol* 1985; **3**: 151–3.

49 Zang, J. Immediate anti-asthmatic effect of acupuncture in 192 cases of bronchial asthma. *J Trad Chin Med* 1990; **10**: 89–93.

50 Prance, S. E., Dresser, A., Wood, C., Fleming, J., Aldridge, D., Pietroni, P. Research on traditional Chinese acupuncture – science or myth: a review. *J Roy Soc Med* 1988; **81**: 588–90.

51 Filshie, J., Redman, D. Acupuncture and malignant pain problems. *Eur Soc Surg Oncol* 1985; **11**(4): 389–94.

[52] Barlow, D. H., Hersen, M. *Single Case Experimental Designs.* 2nd ed. New York: Pergamon, 1984.

[53] Coan, R. M., Wong, G., Coan, P. L. The acupuncture treatment of neck pain: a randomized controlled study. *Am J Chin Med* 1982; **9**: 326–32.

[54] Gunn, C. C., Milbrandt, W. E., Little, A. S., Mason, K. E. Dry needling of muscle motor points for chronic low back pain. *Spine* 1980; **5**: 279–91.

[55] Laitinen, J. Acupuncture and transcutaneous nerve stimulation in the treatment of chronic sacro-lumbalgia and ischialgia. *Am J Chin Med* 1976; **4**: 169–75.

[56] Fox, E. J., Melzack, R. Transcutaneous nerve stimulation and acupuncture: comparison of treatment for low back pain. *Pain* 1976; **2**: 141–8.

[57] Bhatt-Sanders, D. Acupuncture for rheumatoid arthritis: an analysis of the literature. *Sem Arth Rheu* 1985; **14**(4): 225–31.

[58] Patel, M., Gutzwiller, F., Paccaud, F., Marazzi, A. A meta-analysis of acupuncture for chronic pain. *Int J Epidemiol* 1989; **18**(4): 900–6.

[59] Ter Riet, G., Kleijnen, J., Knipschild, P. Acupuncture and chronic pain: a criteria based meta-analysis. *J Clin Epidemiol* 1990; **11**: 1191–9.

[60] Sacks, H. S., Berrier, J., Reitman, D., Ancona-Berk, V. A., Chalmers, T. C. Meta-analysis of randomized controlled trials. *New Eng J Med* 1987; **316**: 450–5.

[61] Vincent, C. A., Richardson, P. H. Acupuncture for some common disorders: a review of evaluative research. *J Roy Coll Gen Pract* 1987; **37**: 77–81.

[62] Rosen, L. Acupuncture and Chinese medical practices. *Volta Rev* 1974; **76**: 340–50.

[63] Tashkin, D. P., Bresler, D. P., Kroening, R. J. Comparison of real and simulated acupuncture and isoproterenol in metacholine induced asthma. *Ann Allergy* 1977; **39**: 379–87.

[64] Tashkin, D. P., Kroening, R. J., Bresler, D. P. A controlled trial of real and simulated acupuncture in the management of chronic asthma. *J Allergy Clin Immunol* 1985; **76**: 855–64.

[65] Ter Riet, G., Kleijnen, J., Knipschild, P. A meta-analysis of studies into the effect of acupuncture on addiction. *Br J Gen Pract* 1990; **40**: 379–82.

[66] Bullock, M. L., Culliton, P. D., Olander, R. T. Controlled trial of acupuncture for severe recidivist alcoholism. *Lancet* 1989; **i**: 1435–9.

[67] Anon. Many points to needle. *Lancet* 1990; **i**: 20–21.

[68] Hansen, P. E., Hansen, J. H. Acupuncture treatment of chronic facial pain – a controlled crossover trial. *Headache* 1983; **23**: 66–9.

[69] Petrie, J. P., Langley, G. B. Acupuncture in the treatment of chronic cervical pain: a pilot study. *Clin Exp Rheumatol* 1983; **1**: 333–5.

[70] Petrie, J. P., Hazelman, B. L. A controlled trial of acupuncture in neck pain. *Br J Rheumatol* 1986; **25**: 271–5.

[71] Lehmann, T. R., Russell, D. W., Spratt, K. F. Efficacy of electroacupuncture and TENS in the rehabilitation of chronic low back pain. *Pain* 1986; **26**: 277–90.

[72] Ballegaard, S., Jensen, G., Pedersen, F., Nissen, V. H. Acupuncture in severe, stable angina pectoris. *Acta Med Scand* 1986; **220**: 307–13.

[73] Dickens, W., Lewith, G. T. Single-blind, controlled and randomized clinical trial to evaluate the effect of acupuncture in the treatment of trapezio-metacarpal osteoarthritis. *Comp Med Res* 1989; **3**(ii): 5–8.

[74] Ballegaard, S., Pedersen, F., Pietersen, A., Nissen, V. H. Effects of acupuncture in moderate, stable angina pectoris. *J Int Med* 1990; **227**: 25–30.

20 Biofeedback

Sandra Horn

Introduction

When an organism engages in purposive (goal-directed) behaviour, rapid and accurate knowledge of the results of its actions (feedback) is crucial. Without it, behaviour could not be adjusted so as to keep the organism moving toward the goal.

In physiological systems, too, feedback enables constant modulation of the processes to take place, so that the system stays within defined limits. These systems are self-governing, and do not usually impinge on consciousness.

Biofeedback is the use of instrumentation to enhance and transform biological information, which is normally imperceptible, into signals which can be perceived by the senses and modified by learning. That is, it is a means by which learned self-control of physiological activity may be effected.

What kind of learning?

In the 1960s, Neal Miller and his associates demonstrated that autonomic functions such as heart rate, blood pressure, and the rate of formation of urine could be modified by operant conditioning in laboratory rats.[1] The theoretical basis for this kind of learning is that any behaviour which is rewarded, or which results in satisfaction, tends to be reinforced. They went on to show that modifications in blood pressure could also be achieved by human subjects, albeit that the changes were smaller and less consistent.[2] Miller wrote that in animal experiments, rewards are a kind of feedback; in human learning, information that success is being achieved serves as a reward. Instrumentation can provide the feedback and thus the reward. In Miller's view, the relatively poorer results achieved by humans suggests that humans are as smart as rats, but we may not yet be as clever at training them (humans). He pointed out the capacity of humans to influence visceral responses by voluntary or involuntary changes in the rate or depth of breathing, or changes in tension in skeletal muscles, and he felt that these things should be controlled for in further experiments, so that the specific effects of biofeedback could be evaluated.

He might also have considered the use of contemplation as a mediational mechanism; human beings are possibly the only animals able to attain visceral changes by thinking about calming or arousing situations. From Miller's behaviourist point of view, these influences get in the way of pure operant conditioning of physiological activity. The implication is that better visceral responses could be obtained in their absence. However, if biofeedback is to be an effective clinical tool rather than a laboratory procedure, it may be that these very influences need to be incorporated into treatment. Perhaps human learning proceeds more effectively if the cerebral cortex plays its part.

Miller described studies on human subjects which demonstrated that different types of feedback produced different magnitudes of response; studies in which individual subjects produced very different rates and magnitudes of response under the same conditions of treatment; and those which appeared to show that 'many hours of arduous practice' might be necessary in order to achieve a therapeutic response. Nevertheless, in spite of these problems, he felt that the principle of learned visceral changes had been established, and the way had been opened for what was potentially a powerful new technique in the maintenance or restoration of healthy functioning in body systems.

The early work on biofeedback was followed by a wave of enthusiasm for the technique, which led to attempts to demonstrate its usefulness in a variety of disorders. In particular, it has been used in disorders:

1 which are 'silent' (asymptomatic) such as hypertension;

2 in which early warning signals are disrupted or attenuated, such as in faecal incontinence secondary to lesions of the spinal cord or nerves;

3 in which the information about disturbed functioning tends to be received late in its development, as in pain associated with muscle tension, for example. The early build-up of tension often goes undetected until a critical point is reached at which pain will be experienced.

In such cases, biofeedback offers the hope of alleviation without the use of drugs or other invasive techniques. As Marcer has pointed out,[3] this may be a crucial factor where the condition is silent but pharmacological treatments tend to produce unpleasant side effects, thus leading to problems in compliance with drug regimes. Hypertension is a case in point.

Biofeedback has also been used in conditioning of the musculoskeletal system: for example, in neuromuscular re-education after stroke; in muscle tension control in headache and other types of pain; and in the treatment of focal dystonias, notably spasmodic torticollis. In these cases, the most common form of feedback is that from electromyographic recordings (EMG) transformed into visual or auditory signals. More recent developments have included electronic devices designed to feed back information about movement, position or pressure. Basmajian[4] has described the use of head position monitors, foot placement and foot position monitors in cerebral palsy. In other studies, recordings have been taken of variables such as skin temperature, galvanic skin response, electrical activity in the brain (EEG) and cardiac rhythm (ECG). Skin temperature and changes in the electrical activity of the skin are related to the arousal/relaxation response, and so may be used as general indicators of a range of associated phenomena, such as blood pressure, cardiac output, and tone in skeletal muscles. Data from

EMG and ECG, on the other hand, gives more direct and specific information, such as the state of tension in a group of muscles or the presence of cardiac arrhythmias. There are four basic ways in which this information is transformed and fed back to the subject.

Types of biofeedback

Binary auditory feedback

There are two states of the feedback signal, and they change from one to the other when a predetermined criterion is reached. An example of this type of feedback is a high-pitched tone sounding when the signal is above criterion, and changing to a low pitch when criterion is reached. Olton and Noonberg[5] give the example of a criterion of 30°C skin temperature as the target. The change in pitch tells the operator if skin temperature is above or below criterion, but not by how much. More detailed feedback is possible with an analogue signal.

Analogue auditory feedback

In this condition, there is a continuous relationship between the character of the signal and the magnitude of the response. This gives more information to the subject, as knowledge about the closeness of the response to the target is available.

In Eufemia and Wesolowski's[6] study on tension headache, for example, EMG activity in the frontalis muscles was fed back in the form of a series of clicks. The frequency of the clicks increased with increasing muscle tension.

Binary visual feedback

This type of feedback usually incorporates a light or array of lights, which come on when the target level of the response is reached.

Analogue visual feedback

The level of activity is translated into a continuous read-out, which may be in the form of a needle moving across a dial, a series of numbers, bands of colour, and so on. Any number of imaginative possibilities exist, but as in all forms of feedback, the clarity of the signal and the target, and the speed, reliability and accuracy of the feedback, are crucial. Large[7] used a visual analogue scale with a needle on a dial in his study of chronic musculoskeletal pain.

Combined feedback

Some researchers have also used a combination of auditory and visual displays. For example, Cozean, Pease and Hubbell[8] used both visual analogue (oscilloscope) and auditory analogue signals in their study of the treatment of gait dysfunction after stroke. It is not clear whether this increase in information enhances learning, or inhibits it by splitting the attention of the subject. There is no firm evidence for the superiority of this technique, nor has there been a definitive study on the type of feedback most likely to facilitate learning.

Rugh[9] has argued that biofeedback users tend to prefer instruments which deliver slow auditory clicks with long time constants, which carry relatively little information and therefore permit relatively low levels of arousal. Instruments which demand high levels of information-processing produce higher levels of cognitive arousal, which might inhibit muscular relaxation and other important components of learned self-control. These are interesting ideas, as yet unsubstantiated.

Does biofeedback work?

If biofeedback is to be an effective clinical tool, its specific effects must be demonstrated and it must be shown to produce results which are longlasting, which generalize to situations outside the treatment room, and which can be maintained eventually in the absence of feedback.

Since the early days of biofeedback research, the results of numerous studies have confirmed the finding that such things as heart rate, blood pressure, skin temperature, electrodermal activity, salivation, alpha activity in EEG, and tension in single motor units and selected muscles can be brought under voluntary control. In spite of its widespread clinical and research usage over the years since the 1960s, however, biofeedback has failed to live up to the promise of those early studies. It has not always been possible to replicate promising-looking research, and much of the work has been poorly controlled or ill-devised.

Establishing the specific effects of biofeedback has been a major diffi-culty. Many of the techniques used have also involved muscular relaxation, with or without mental imagery. (Anecdotal evidence also suggests that some subjects use relaxing imagery of their own accord.) Those undergoing biofeedback are usually sitting or lying down and engaged in the quiet contemplation of a visual or auditory signal, and so it is important that biofeedback itself is shown to produce faster or greater gains than these simpler techniques alone, particularly as the physiological variables undergoing conditioning are likely to be in-fluenced by the level of arousal.

Hume[10] has highlighted the absence of adequate baselines and appropriate control procedures in much of the literature. He underlines the argument that many of the clinical uses of biofeedback are directed towards decreasing activity in such variables as heart rate, blood pressure and muscle tension, and therefore the appropriate control is a standard relaxation procedure, which is intended to lower physiological arousal in general.

Another area of difficulty is the relationship between the disorder under treatment and the physiological process undergoing conditioning.

Relationship between the learned response and the disorder

A particular difficulty in evaluating the efficacy of biofeedback has arisen when it has been used to treat conditions in which the link between the physiological process undergoing modification and the disorder is indirect, or not well established.

An example of the use of biofeedback training in a condition in which the disorder and the physiological response are not closely related is the treatment of migraine by voluntary raising of the temperature of the fingers. Thermal biofeedback has also been used in effecting voluntary vasodilation in the fingers in conditions such as Raynaud's phenomenon. In the case of Raynaud's, the link between the control of temperature in the hand and the syndrome is clear. Even when they are between attacks, patients with the primary disease and with Raynaud's phenomenon secondary to other disorders exhibit lower baseline digital temperatures than controls. Studies such as those carried out by Surwit and Fenton[11] and Freedman, Lynn, Ianni and Hale[12] have demonstrated that temperature feedback enhances voluntary vasodilation in the fingers of those with the disorder. Yocum, Hodes, Sundstrom and Cleeland[13] carried out a retrospective review of 23 patients' records. Twelve had Raynaud's phenomenon and eleven had the primary disease. After biofeedback training, all patients could elevate their baseline digital temperatures.

Improvement, both by subjective report and decreased incidence of ulcers, was maintained in about half the patients after a year. At 18-month follow-up, four out of seven patients could still elevate their digital temperatures. The reasons for the success of these four patients and the attenuation of the response in the others is not clear and merits further investigation, but the initial effect of the feedback was well demonstrated.

In the case of migraine, on the other hand, the link between digital vasodilation, leading to raised digital temperature, and the activity of the extracranial arteries is not at all clear. Indeed, there are good reasons why the blood supply to the cranium should not be affected by the temperature of the fingers! Nevertheless, voluntary vasodilation in the fingers has been used as a potential treatment for migraine. Two arguments have been put forward for this approach:

1 Increased peripheral blood flow is associated with increased relaxation. Relaxation might be an effective treatment for migraine.

2 Increased blood flow to the periphery might cause a corresponding decrease in flow in the extracranial vessels, and this in turn might reduce vasodilation, and so reduce pain.

Neither of these arguments is supported by scientific evidence. While it is true that relaxation is often accompanied by increased peripheral blood flow, the converse is not true. Neither is there any evidence that increased blood supply to the fingers results in blood being diverted from the extracranial vessels.

In a review of the literature, Holmes and Burish[14] concluded that there is no evidence that finger temperature biofeedback training is an effective technique for treating migraine. Many of the studies in the review confound biofeedback effects with those from psychotherapy or various forms of relaxation training. Where an effect has been demonstrated, it is usually related to the relaxation response.

Holmes and Burish also considered the case of tension headache. There is a widespread assumption that this type of headache is related to an increase in muscle tension, and so biofeedback training aimed at decreasing the tension by conditioning the EMG output of the frontalis muscles has been undertaken in a number of studies. Most researchers have assumed the tension/pain relationship and some, such as Budzynski *et al.*[15] and van Boxtel and van der Ven,[16] have demonstrated it, while others have failed to find any such relationship in headache sufferers, or have found a degree of vasoconstriction in some subjects as well – as in Tunis and Wolff.[17] In the study by Borgeat, Elie and Larouche,[18] 33 tension headache sufferers underwent pretreatment training, during which they were taught to increase frontal muscle tension. Subjective pain responses showed that 14 of them demonstrated a positive correlation between increased tension and head pain, and the remaining 19 did not. Subsequent biofeedback training resulted in different patterns of learned response between the two groups, but there was no difference in clinical improvement. Neither group was convincingly helped by the training.

Studies by Harper and Steger[19] and Epstein and Abel[20] have shown no relationship between frontalis muscle tension and headache in most of their cases. It may be that other craniofacial muscles show an increase in tension associated with headache; this has not been established. Whether or not this is true, there would seem to be little value in conditioning the response in muscles where there is little or no evidence of increased tension. Just as questions of placebo, individual differences, baseline measures, adequate controls or the effects of relaxation must be considered, future researchers must address the question of the relationship between the disorder and the response to be conditioned.

The technique of biofeedback is not well served by attempts to condition responses with little or no established relationship to the disorder under treatment.

Individual differences

Hume also reiterated the need for attention to the feedback parameters and to individual characteristics of the subjects (patients). This is a move away from simple operant conditioning as demonstrated in laboratory animals, but it may be an important missing link between the promising-looking laboratory data and the relatively disappointing clinical applications of the technique.

When Miller said that humans are as smart as rats but we are not yet as good at training them, he was ignoring the part played in the learning process by those very human subjects; they are not only smarter but much more complex and variable. Some individuals demonstrate start-ling abilities in visceral control, but it may be that these are not dependent on biofeedback. They may be analogous to inherent differences, such as those seen in hypnotic susceptibility, for example. Differences in learning ability and learning style may also be important. These may be related to personality type, as suggested by Eysenck,[21] who argued that introverts and extraverts will respond to different learning regimes. Rotter[22] has also put forward the concept of 'locus of control' as an individual characteristic which may be important in determining treatment outcome. Craig, Franklin and Andrews[23] have developed a locus of control scale to measure the extent to which an individual perceives events as being a consequence of his own behaviour (internal locus of control) or the result of luck or the influence of powerful others (external locus of control). In a retrospective study of headache treated by biofeedback, Hudzinski and Levenson[24] measured locus of control and found that patients under 40 years old and with an internal locus had benefited most from treatment. Hart[25] has suggested that differences in preference for cognitive structure will predict success in biofeedback versus relaxation training. While these studies do not amount to conclusive evidence of the influence of individual differences in personality on treatment outcome, they suggest it is an area meriting further study.

Subgroup differences

Middaugh[26] has also argued that within groups of individuals under-going biofeedback, certain subgroups may benefit more than others, but that this differential effect may be lost in the statistical analysis. She quotes four studies in which pretreatment characteristics had a strong effect on outcome:

1 Four groups of ten normal subjects were compared on the ability to contract the abductor hallucis muscle in the foot. One group had EMG feedback; one had sensory stimulation; one was an unassisted control group; and one received no training but was a test-retest control group. Overall, only the feedback group improved significantly, but the unassisted controls did almost as well. A more detailed look at the results showed that the subjects who did well in the control group had good initial control of the muscle, while those who did well in the feedback group had poor initial ability and only made significant gains when pro-vided with feedback.

2 Twenty four women with stress urinary incontinence were treated either with manometric biofeedback (n = 13) or with Kegel exercises and verbal feedback (n = 11). Both groups im-proved, but the biofeedback group showed greater improve-ment. Again, a detailed look at the pretraining characteristics of the groups revealed that those who did well in the Kegel group started with better control over the pelvic floor muscles than did the failures, while in the biofeedback group, those patients who had poor initial control showed improvement.

3 Thirty three children with spina bifida and associated faecal incontinence were treated with either behaviour modification alone, or with behaviour modification coupled with biofeedback. Overall, 64% of the children achieved a 50% reduction in incontinence, and 33% became completely continent. There appeared to be no difference between the groups statistically. However, in a subgroup of children (27%) with low lesions, good rectal sensation and high rates of incontinence, biofeedback was statistically superior.

4 Two groups of stroke patients received treatment for upper limb function. One (n = 18) had biofeedback and the other (n = 17) standard physiotherapy. Both groups improved significantly and maintained their gains, but dividing them up into early and late entry into treatment and mild or severe stroke suggested that the severe group responded best to early biofeedback intervention.

Middaugh's detailed analyses of outcome data suggest that there is a need to consider not only individual differences in patients, but also different subsets of patients based on relevant pretreatment parameters, if a true assessment of the effect of biofeedback is to be made.

Other intervening variables

The role of such variables as attitude to treatment, motivation, family support, and other factors which are hard to measure has been ignored by behaviourists in the field of biofeedback research. These things may have little or nothing to do with operant conditioning of physiological responses, but everything to do with the development of biofeedback as an effective clinical tool. Johnston and Steptoe[27] have commented that 'There is no convincing evidence that biofeedback leads to greater blood pressure reductions than those which are produced with simpler relaxation techniques ... Nevertheless it is wise to be pragmatic about the use of biofeedback. Many clients like it, and consider that it assists them to relax successfully. Biofeedback can also provide a vivid demonstration of the way in which physiological processes affect physical responses, and can thereby reinforce the therapeutic rationale.' Those engaged in therapeutic learning cannot afford to ignore factors such as whether the client likes the technique, or that it provides a vivid demonstration of the principle, as these may be powerful positive influences on the learning process.

In contrast, the study by Little *et al.*[28] of the treatment of hypertension in pregnancy by biofeedback and relaxation demonstrates the strong negative effect of some background factors. All of the very young (19 and under) working-class women who were in the group required admission to hospital. That is, they were treatment failures. The authors comment that these women appeared to be in a high state of anxiety and to have few resources. Learning, whether it is biofeedback based or not, is not likely to be facilitated if these background factors are left unattended.

Wittrock, Blanchard and McCoy[29] found that three things were related to outcome in their studies on the treatment of essential hypertension by thermal biofeedback:

1 Initial level of expectation of benefit (higher expectation = more success);

2 Whether the patient practised at home between sessions;

3 The amount of in-session increase in hand temperature; responders made progressively greater gains, while non-responders failed to show gains at all.

These appear to be a combination of motivation and another factor – conditionability? – which is possibly an inherent difference.

The studies of Patel and her co-workers[30,31] on hypertension are among the most impressive in terms of good experimental design and long-term results. Their behavioural programme includes educational films and slides about blood pressure, how emotions affect the body, concepts of relaxation and biofeedback, and opportunities for the patients to ask questions and discuss problems. Treatment combines relaxation and meditation, biofeedback and stress management training. Patients are also encouraged verbally, shown their blood pressure records, instructed to practise relaxation and meditation at home and to incorporate the habits into daily routines. This is a long way from operant conditioning, but it is effective learning of self-control of visceral responses, and it incorporates biofeedback. It appears to be a way forward, and demonstrates the power of a combined approach in treating a condition which is subject to many influences; for example, stress, diet, smoking and heredity.

In hypertension, as in some of the other conditions treated more or less successfully by biofeedback, the active participation of a well-informed subject might be the key to a positive outcome.

The future

Middaugh[26] has made a plea for a shift in emphasis in biofeedback research, away from piling up study on study, and toward a more thoughtful interpretation of clinical and experimental findings and the development of a clearer conceptual framework. She highlights the need for a match between what the patient needs and what the biofeedback can contribute; for attention to be paid to the characteristics of those patients who do well and those who do not; and for further studies on different types of procedures and their effects on different types of patient. With regard to Middaugh's first point, mention has already been made of the good match between hand temperature conditioning and Raynaud's syndrome, and the necessity of establishing the role of increased muscle tension in so-called tension headache before attempting treatment with EMG biofeedback. Middaugh also points out that in neuromuscular re-education, training may need to take place on three different levels:

1 The establishment of control of a disordered muscle or muscle group;

2 The control of combinations of muscle groups in order to effect the desired change in movement or posture;

3 The production of multiple movements and adjustments with appropriate coordination, timing and balance, in order to carry out the required task.

Success at level 1 of training does not guarantee success at level 3. The treatment goal needs to be broken down into discrete tasks, each one of which is an essential precursor to the next. Each task may need a somewhat different approach or different instrumentation. Unless this task analysis is undertaken before treatment commences, results are bound to be disappointing. It is not that the technique fails, but that it is applied without sufficient rigour. To date, too few studies have been carried out under rigorous conditions, and it seems likely that some of the poor results reported can be attributed to methodologies based more on hope than precision.

Middaugh's second plea is for attention to be paid to those who do well and those who do not. Many studies contain some subjects who simply do not respond to the treatment. There are a number of possible reasons for this:

1 Some people cannot alter their visceral responses during biofeedback. They are, perhaps, comparable to those who cannot be hypnotized. If this is the case, it may be that a pretreatment trial will identify them and they should be excluded from biofeedback training and offered alternative methods of treatment.

2 People may respond differentially to different training regimes. Some may need short frequent sessions, others may need longer sessions but at less frequent intervals. It may be that these differences are related to personality type, as suggested by Eysenck, who argues that extraverts learn best with short bursts of input and introverts learn best with longer. Learning may be enhanced if these groups are identified before treatment, and given different regimes.

3 Locus of control may be another factor in learned self-control. It is not yet clear whether it is an abiding characteristic, or a trait that can change as learning proceeds. If it is proved to be a relatively strong and stable personality trait, it is likely that those with an external locus of control will do badly under biofeedback. If, on the other hand, it is shown to change as learning takes place, so that those who start off with an external locus become more internal, then the conditions under which the change is likely to occur must be identified. Some studies have suggested that change does take place and that it predicts success.[23] It may be that biofeedback assists that change, as it demonstrates to the subject that self-control is taking place.

Future researchers might well add locus of control measures to others at pretreatment screening.

4 Patel and others have shown the importance of giving information to subjects and increasing motivational factors. These additions do not detract from the effects of biofeedback; rather, they enhance them. By and large, treating people like laboratory rats undergoing operant conditioning produces positive but small changes during biofeedback. In order to magnify those changes into therapeutically useful responses, human factors in learning need to be taken into account. These could include the use of educational sessions, the encouragement of intertreatment practice, the keeping of logbooks to record progress and setbacks for discussion with therapy staff, and so on.

5 In addition to the need for attention to interpersonal and intrapersonal characteristics and other human factors, there is a need for the characteristics of the conditions under treatment to be considered. In neuromuscular re-education, for example, biofeedback can enhance weak or intermittent sensory feedback, but it cannot restore function where the naturally occurring feedback is completely absent. Where the underlying problem has been precisely identified and the treatment matched to the need, as in some forms of neuromuscular re-education using biofeedback, results have tended to be impressive. However, there is another whole area of biofeedback in which the training is aimed at reducing the level of tension in skeletal muscles and autonomic arousal in general. The treatment of various types of pain and some disorders of the cardiovascular system come under this area. The evidence for biofeedback being superior to other simpler techniques such as relaxation training is not clear here. However, it can be said that studies have shown that for some people, including those who 'like' biofeedback, it may be the method of choice. Again, pretreatment screening should identify those for whom biofeedback will enhance and sustain the relaxation response.

It is a relatively simple matter to measure a variable such as pulse rate under conditions of relaxation instruction with and without feedback, and to discover the subject's preferred mode.

6 Finally, the mode of feedback may be an important factor. Is the response to auditory input better than to visual? Are clicks better than tones? Do coloured lights produce a stronger response than white light? Is the onset of a favourite piece of music when the target response is reached a good piece of feedback? Do direct read-outs of EMG and blood pressure produce more efficient learning than read-outs transformed into either lights or noises? We do not yet know the answers to these questions. It may be that the difference between one mode and the next is insignificant, or it may be that it holds the key to greatly improved results. Perhaps giving subjects a choice of mode enhances learning. Further studies on different types of feedback and their

effects on different subjects are overdue.

It is now more than 20 years since biofeedback began to be used as a therapeutic technique. While results have been mixed, it has been possible to tease out the most promising trends. They have, without exception, come from studies in which biofeedback has been used with precision, with close attention being paid to the characteristics of the subjects and their conditions, and a good match between the subject's needs and what biofeedback could offer. More work remains to be done to tease out all the factors contributing to its successful use.

References

1   Miller, N. E. Biofeedback: evaluation of a new technique. *New Eng J Med* 1974; **290**: 684–5.

2   Miller, N. E., DiCara, L. V., Solomon, H., Weiss, J. M., Dworkin, B. Learned modifications of autonomic functions: a review and some new data. *Circ Res Suppl 1* 1970; **27**: 3–11.

3   Marcer, D. *Biofeedback and Related Therapies in Clinical Practice*. London: Croom Helm, 1986.

4   Basmajian, J. Biofeedback in rehabilitation: a review of principles and practices. *Arch Phys Med Rehabil* 1981; **62**: 469–75.

5   Olton, D. S., Noonberg, A. R. *Biofeedback: Clinical Applications in Behavioural Medicine*. New Jersey: Prentice-Hall, 1980.

6   Eufemia, R. L., Wesolowski, M. D. The use of a new relaxation method in a case of tension headache. *J Behav Ther Exp Psychiat* 1983; **14**(4): 355–8.

7   Large, R. G. Prediction of treatment response in pain patients: the illness self-concept repertory grid and EMG feedback. *Pain* 1985; **21**: 279–87.

8   Cozean, C. D., Pease, W. S., Hubbell, S. L. Biofeedback and functional electric stimulation in stroke rehabilitation. *Arch Phys Med Rehabil* 1988; **69**: 401–5.

9   Rugh, J. D. Instrumentation in biofeedback. In: Gatchel, R. J., Price, K. P. (eds.) *Clinical Applications of Biofeedback: Appraisal and Status*. New York: Pergamon, 1979.

10   Hume, W. I. *Biofeedback: Research and Therapy*. New York: Eden Press, 1976.

11   Surwit, R. S., Fenton, C. H. Feedback and instructions in the control of digital temperature. *Psychophysiology* 1980; **17**(2): 129–32.

12   Freedman, R. R., Lynn, S. J., Ianni, P., Hale, P. A. Biofeedback treatment of Raynaud's disease and phenomenon. *Biofeedback Self-regul* 1981; **6**: 355–65.

13   Yocum, D. E., Hodes, R., Sundstrom, W. R., Cleeland, C. S. Use of biofeedback training in treatment of Raynaud's disease and phenomenon. *J Rheumatol* 1985; **12**(1): 90–93.

14 Holmes, D. S., Burish, T. G. Effectiveness of biofeedback for treating migraine and tension headaches: a review of the evidence. *J Psychosom Res* 1983; **27**: 515–32.

15 Budzynski, T. H., Stoyva, J., Adler, C. S., Mullaney, D. J. EMG biofeedback and tension headache: a controlled outcome study. *Psychosom Med* 1973; **35**(6): 484–96.

16 Van Boxtel, A., van der Ven, J. R. Differential EMG activity in subjects with muscle contraction headaches related to mental effort. *Headache* 1978; **17**: 233–7.

17 Tunis, M. M., Wolff, H. G. Studies on headache: cranial artery vasoconstriction and muscle contraction headache. *Arch Neurol Psychiat* 1954; **71**: 425–34.

18 Borgeat, F., Elie, R., Larouche, L. M. Pain response to voluntary muscle tension increases and biofeedback efficacy in tension headache. *Headache* 1985; **25**: 387–91.

19 Harper, R. G., Steger, J. C. Psychological correlates of frontalis EMG and pain in tension headache. *Headache* 1978; **18**: 215–18.

20 Epstein, L. H., Abel, G. G. An analysis of biofeedback training effects for tension headache patients. *Behav Ther* 1977; **8**: 37–47.

21 Eysenck, H. J. *The Structure of Human Personality*. London: Methuen, 1970.

22 Rotter, J. B. Generalised expectancies for internal vs. external control of reinforcement. *Psychol Monographs* 1986; **80**: 1–28.

23 Craig, A. R., Franklin, J. A., Andrews, G. A scale to measure locus of control of behaviour. *Br J Med Psychol* 1984; **57**: 173–80.

24 Hudzinski, L. G., Levenson, H. Biofeedback behavioural treatment of headache with locus of control pain analysis: a 20-month retrospective study. *Headache* 1985; **25**: 380–6.

25 Hart, J. D. Predicting differential response to EMG biofeedback and relaxation training: the role of cognitive structure. *J Clin Psychol* 1984; **40**(2): 453–7.

26 Middaugh, S. J. On clinical efficacy: why biofeedback does – and does not – work. *Biofeedback Self-Regul* 1990; **15**(3): 191–208.

27 Johnston, D., Steptoe, A. Hypertension. In: Peace, S., Wardle, J. (eds.) *The Practice of Behavioural Medicine*. Oxford: OUP, 1989.

28 Little, B. C. *et al.* Treatment of hypertension in pregnancy by relaxation and biofeedback. *Lancet* 1984; **8382**: 865–7.

29 Wittrock, D. A., Blanchard, E. B., McCoy, G. C. Three studies on the relation of process to outcome in the treatment of essential hypertension with relaxation and thermal biofeedback. *Behav Res Ther* 1988; **2**(1): 53–66.

30 Patel, C. H., North, W. R. S. Randomised controlled trial of yoga and biofeedback in the management of hypertension. *Lancet* 1975; **2**: 93–5.

[31] Patel, C. H., Marmot, M. G., Terry, D. J. Controlled trial of biofeedback-aided behavioural methods in reducing mild hypertension. *Br Med J* 1981; **282**: 2005–8.

21 Environmental medicine: principles and practice of evaluation

George T. Lewith

Summary

This chapter reviews the clinical trial methodology that has been suggested to evaluate the use of food exclusion and challenge as a treatment for a variety of different chronic conditions. Environmental medicine encompasses the individual's reaction to foods, chemicals and other environmental factors. This chapter concentrates primarily on the clinical trial methods employed to evaluate food intolerance alone, and suggests the approaches that may be employed within clinical trials to assess the validity and significance of food exclusion diets in a number of chronic conditions.

Introduction

Environmental medicine covers a broad range of problems. For some people it is known simply as 'food allergy', while in other instances the term 'clinical ecology' has been used. Environmental medicine encompasses a huge area and includes illnesses that may be attributable to foods, chemicals, other inhaled substances such as dust or mould spores, and even, in some instances, electromagnetic radiation. However, for the purposes of this chapter I shall be concentrating specifically on the assessment and evaluation of dietary factors as possible triggers for illness.

The report on food intolerance and food aversion published by the Royal College of Physicians in 1984[1] sets out an excellent framework for evaluating food reactions.

Food allergy is defined as a form of food intolerance in which there is also evidence of an abnormal immunological reaction to food.

Food aversion comprises both psychological avoidance and physiological intolerance. The individual avoids food for psychological reasons and experiences unpleasant bodily reactions caused by the emotions associated with food ingestion.

In those who have reproducible adverse reactions to foods, a number of factors can be isolated. These include:

1 A lack of particular enzymes, for instance lactase deficiency.

2 A pharmacological effect, perhaps due to large amounts of caffeine in coffee or tea.

3 An unexplained histamine releasing effect in unsensitized individuals. Such reaction which can result from the consumption of shellfish, strawberries, or other foods.

4 An irritant effect on the mucous membranes of the mouth or bowels, such as that caused by highly spiced curry.

5 An indirect effect caused by the fermentation of unabsorbed food residues in the lower bowel.

Food intolerance is defined as a reproducible, unpleasant and adverse reaction to specific foods. It is not psychologically based. This must occur even when the food is eaten blind – for instance, disguised in a puree or soup. It is such food intolerance, or food sensitivity, which forms the basis of environmental medicine's approach to dietary management. There is, as yet, no complete immunological or biochemical explanation for such reactions, but they can nevertheless be validated clinically.

The cycle of food sensitivity

Food sensitivity or food intolerance is frequently responsible for low grade, chronic symptomatology. It does not appear to cause the abrupt and obvious urticarial or allergic reaction that may result from ingestion of strawberries. It is essential for those wishing to investigate environmental medicine to understand the fundamental difference between food allergy and food intolerance or food sensitivity.[2] The cycle of the food reactions that may occur with food intolerance has been described elsewhere.[3] However, it is important to outline these general principles yet again as they form such an important basis for deciding on the exact clinical trial methodology that can be used to evaluate this area.

Food intolerance appears to be based on the concept of *masked sensitivity*. This means that, if an individual develops migraine in response to a particular group of foods, it is very difficult, if not impossible, clearly to associate the ingestion of a particular food with migraine. It is usually because the food is eaten very frequently, often many times during any day. Foods which appear to fall under the category of masked sensitivity are often those to which the patient is addicted.

The most straightforward way to unmask food sensitivity is to ask the individual either to fast or to avoid foods which you suspect may be triggering a masked sensitivity. After a short period of time the food sensitive individual will become *hyper-reactive*. This means that further food challenge will result in a clear food reaction, triggering symptoms that have cleared on food avoidance. Unmasking a food sensitivity can take anything between one to six weeks. Hyper-reaction also occurs on a variable time base. Sometimes the hyper-reactive phase just lasts for a week and sometimes it may be present for many months or years. An individual may hyper-react to many foods. Sometimes the ingestion of a small amount of one food may be enough, while in other instances all foods which may trigger a masked sensitivity need to be ingested before a hyper-reaction occurs. The quantity of food or foods required to trigger a hyper-reaction is also very variable.

Subsequent to the phase of hyper-reaction an individual will become food *tolerant*. This in effect means that they can tolerate a small amount of the food to which they have a masked sensitivity without developing symptoms. Food tolerance may occur in one month, or may never occur at all. An individual may be tolerant to one of the foods which triggers a masked sensitivity, but not to another. In general, however, if the level of tolerance is abused then *active sensitization* will occur. This leads directly to masked sensitivity, food addiction, and further chronic symptoms. The area of food tolerance is again very variable, as a group of individuals with the same diagnosis may at one extreme require just a minor modification to their diet because they are very food tolerant, while those at another end of the spectrum may require a very rigorous diet for the rest of their lives. These concepts are summarized in Figure 21.1.

Food intolerance does not follow a specific dietary pattern. While it is possible to demonstrate that illnesses such as migraine, irritable bowel syndrome, and rheumatoid arthritis may respond to appropriate food avoidance, the exact foods in question will vary from individual to individual. Food intolerance almost invariably involves several foods and usually there are one or two 'major' foods. These are foods which are frequently used in the manufacture of other foodstuffs, for instance

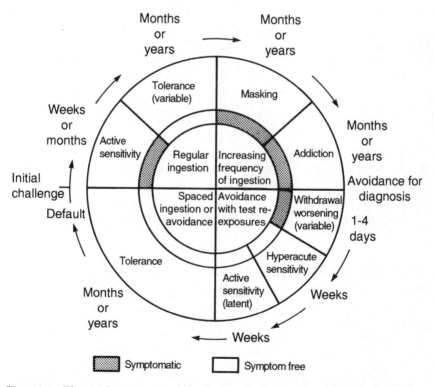

Fig. 21.1 The cyclic concept of food allergy. The upper part represents the natural history prior to diagnosis, the lower part the sequence which follows specific diagnosis. (After Radcliffe[3])

wheat, milk or yeast. There are also a number of 'minor' foods involved, such as chocolate, tomatoes, potatoes and onions, and these are usually much easier to avoid than yeast or wheat.

The cycle of masked sensitivity, hyper-reaction and food tolerance has been described clinically on numerous occasions. We do not, however, have an immunological, physiological or biochemical basis through which we can understand its complete mechanism, although we understand some aspects of this phenomenon.[4]

The clinical evaluation of food sensitivity must therefore be prefaced by these empirical but consistent clinical observations. When designing clinical trials, the following items must therefore be taken into account.

1 Food sensitivities are almost invariably multiple. While an individual may tolerate one food, by introducing a second apparently chemically unrelated food their tolerance to the first food may alter.

2 The time base of the cycle of masked sensitivity, hyper-reaction and tolerance can vary enormously from individual to individual.

3 A single conventional diagnosis can have as its root cause a very wide range of potential food sensitivities.

4 As we do not understand the exact mechanism of food sensitivity, certain types of feeding methods may be questionable ways of evaluating food sensitivity. For instance, if there is an oral component to food sensitivity, then nasogastric feeding could be both an inappropriate and inexact method of 'blinding' the patient. Placing food into capsules is open to similar criticisms, as well as the fact that food capsules may simply not contain enough food volume to elicit a reaction.

In spite of these problems, the central hypothesis within environmental medicine with respect to food sensitivities can be tested in a proper and coherent manner. The fundamental question which must be asked is:

> Does this disease improve on food avoidance and can it be aggravated by food reintroduction, preferably on a blind basis?

Endpoint measurement

Environmental medicine is frequently utilized to manage chronic illness such as migraine, irritable bowel, arthritis, skin diseases such as eczema, and generalized undifferentiated illness.[5,6,7,8,9,10,11,12,13] However the vast majority of these illnesses are based on clinical diagnoses rather than detailed laboratory investigations. As a consequence, endpoint measurement designed to assess the success or failure of a particular therapeutic intervention is often difficult.

Those attempting to evaluate environmental medicine must therefore of necessity rely on general assessments that can be obtained from observing the patient clinically, patient symptom diaries, as in the case of migraine or irritable bowel, and general scoring systems particularizing the evaluation of ill health or wellbeing. There are a number of well-established methods for evaluating such 'soft' endpoints, but all such techniques are open to the criticism that they lack the objectivity and clarity of an abnormal laboratory test that becomes normal after some specific treatment.

Outcome measurements and the definition of endpoints in the evaluation of clinical trials are dealt with thoroughly elsewhere within this book. It is, however, vital that the investigator considers endpoint measurement in some detail and attempts to draw together acceptable and well-validated techniques for outcome measurement, relevant to the specific clinical situation requiring assessment. It is quite inappropriate to pilot new measurement techniques at the same time as attempting to evaluate a new phenomenon. If it is not possible to find an appropriate method of measuring outcome and a new one must be designed, then this must be evaluated prior to embarking on the clinical trial.

The diagnosis of food sensitivity

A wide range of investigations has been suggested to aid the diagnosis of food sensitivity. In many instances there has been confusion in the investigator's mind between food sensitivity and food allergy. In some instances reputable doctors have deliberately and knowingly muddied the waters, claiming that food allergy tests were ineffective when in fact food sensitivity or intolerance, rather than food allergy, was being assessed.

An excellent review of the diagnostic tests available is to be found elsewhere.[14] Its conclusions are currently valid and quite clear: there is no reliable test available with which to evaluate food intolerance accurately.

While many tests, both conventional and unconventional, can help guide the clinician, none is definitive. Conventional testing methods based on scratch tests and a variety of blood tests such as RAST are simply not reliable indicators of food intolerance. Unconventional testing methods, such as those based on acupuncture techniques, cytotoxic testing or applied kinesiology, tend to be very operator- or laboratory-dependent and therefore are not consistently reliable in the context of a clinical trial. As a consequence, as far as food intolerance is concerned, the only reliable technique is symptom clearance based on food avoidance with subsequent symptom provocation on repeated, and ideally blind, reintroduction of the offending foods.

Case studies

Basing our assessment of environmental medicine solely on food exclusion diets makes assumptions which do not hold water in a clinical setting. For instance, a patient with migraine may have environmental triggers based primarily on foods, but secondarily on other inhaled environmental factors; for example, high levels of mould spores during warm, damp weather in the autumn and spring may trigger eczema. The assumption of a clinical investigator might be that if a patient fails to respond to dietary exclusion then they do not have an environmental problem. This assumption would be incorrect. It would be more appropriate to state that an individual with migraine who fails to respond to a food exclusion diet *does not have an environmental problem based on food intolerance*. Other environmental problems cannot, however, be excluded on the basis of investigations which have simply made no attempt to measure what might be complex environmental factors.

If we are to institute clinical trials within environmental medicine, we must be aware of such difficulties. We must also accept, however, that it is impossible for us to evaluate such complexity within the context of conventional clinical trial methodology. It is in this area that we must begin to analyse individual case studies with some care. The clinical situations that occur in day-to-day medical practice do represent a valid experience and, as such, carefully recorded individual case studies are of vital importance in this complex area.

Case studies can provide consistent and reproducible data within any particular individual. This data is, however, not blind. Information obtained in this manner allows us to understand complex clinical problems and furthermore may spearhead the design of more incisive, detailed and broader clinical evaluation.

Beginning a clinical trial: the variability of responses to food sensitivities

It has been suggested that many illnesses may respond to appropriate food exclusion diets providing the correct food intolerances can be isolated. Migraine, rheumatoid arthritis and eczema[5,6,7,8,9,10] are all illnesses in which food intolerance has been demonstrated to play an established part. However food intolerance alone, while it may be of major importance, may not represent the only initiating factor and contact sensitivity or underlying psychological problems may also be implicated. Consequently the expected resolution rate based on food exclusion alone will vary from about 75% to 95%, depending on chance and the population studied. Therefore, before embarking on a clinical trial the researcher should be aware that food exclusion alone is most unlikely to produce 100% response in any population with chronic illness.

The diagnosis of specific food intolerances represents a very major difficulty when initiating a clinical trial. Some researchers have attempted to use conventional scratch tests,[15,16] RAST[17,18] and, in some instances, cytotoxic tests[19,20] as the basis for defining food intolerance prior to entry into a clinical trial. As suggested earlier, none of these investigations is completely reliable and therefore they form a poor, or at best limited, diagnostic basis for entry. The most logical and watertight basis for diagnosing food sensitivity is the use of highly restrictive diets.

Two major techniques have been used: the use of elemental diets[21,22] and the use of oligo antigenic diets.[10,23,24]

Elemental diets involve providing those entering a clinical trial with a good supplement based on a small range of essential nutrients. Oligo antigenic diets involve using very restricted dietary regimes or simple restriction to lamb, pears, carrots, and one or two other vegetables, all of which are most unlikely to be responsible for any food-based reactions.

Many investigators have ascertained the foods most likely to trigger food intolerance in any specific illness.[25] These rank orders of foods are usually based on carefully monitored open studies of patients with specific diagnoses. The foods that are least likely to trigger reactions can then be used as the bases around which an oligo antigenic diet can be designed.

It is possible to use the standard fast and food reintroduction techniques in order to isolate food intolerance. These techniques are described in detail elsewhere.[26,27] They are, however, cumbersome and require an individual to follow a very restricted and carefully monitored period of fasting and food reintroduction. It usually takes at least three to four weeks to establish a diet involving, say, ten foods, and is simply too time-consuming, demanding and complex to be an acceptable method upon which to base a clinical trial.

Total parenteral nutrition is another possible alternative. Improvement in Crohn's disease has also been noted when parenteral nutrition has been provided during an acute relapse.[28,29] While these approaches may be acceptable in life-threatening situations, such as an acute exacerbation of inflammatory bowel disease, it is neither ethical nor reasonable to place migraine patients on intravenous drip for ten days in order to ascertain whether they are food allergic.

Having selected a population with a consistent diagnosis, such as migraine or rheumatoid arthritis, it will then be necessary to monitor their illness carefully over a period appropriate to the illness while receiving whatever dietary regime is deemed appropriate. In a periodic disease such as migraine this may be over a period of one or two months prior to entry. The investigator should begin to see the illness responding during this period, providing, of course, that it is food based.

Time based response to food intolerance

Clinicians within the field of environmental medicine are well used to the fact that individuals with the same illness have a different time scale for response to food avoidance. Some patients with very severe migraine may respond completely to the appropriate food avoidance within a week, while others may take four to six weeks. Patients with rheumatoid arthritis and eczema have a tendency to respond more slowly to food avoidance than those with urticaria, migraine or irritable bowel. Any study involving food exclusion must therefore be allowed to continue for a period of at least three months in order to ascertain in detail the exact response that an individual may have to any particular food exclusion regime. In some instances, depending on the illness, the period of food exclusion may be substantially extended. For instance, some studies on inflammatory bowel disease have used survival curve analysis to look at 'time to the next relapse' as the most important endpoint for assessing treatment outcome.[30] In these situations a study period of 18 months or two years may be needed, during which the patient will continue with the recommended dietary regime.

Patient compliance and nutritional status

Dietary investigations are usually carried out on an outpatient basis. They frequently require the patient to sustain restrictive diets for prolonged periods and this necessarily will raise difficulties in relation to patient compliance and the general nutritional adequacy of any particular diet. In order to aid compliance, the help of a dietician, nutritionalist or nurse is essential. Patients must have free access to and continuing support from the clinical team responsible for the investigation. Furthermore, a nutritional analysis of the proposed dietary regime is essential. If basic nutrients are missing from the diet, then these must be provided by the use of a safe supplement.

Open or descriptive studies

Many of the initial studies on food intolerance were open, descriptive studies of how a population with a specific diagnosis responds to a particular food exclusion regime. In the majority of early studies, a spring water fast followed by detailed food reintroduction, along with careful monitoring of the subsequent clinical response, has been used as the basis for diagnosing food intolerance. An enormous number of such studies exists and provide the basic reference point from which further, more detailed and rigorous clinical investigation may flow. Such studies have allowed us to define the foods to which patients are most likely to become intolerant. They have also allowed us to define the illnesses which are most likely to respond to food exclusion. Open studies are, however, uncontrolled and by and large do not involve the use of subsequent food challenge. While they form an essential framework around which further investigation may be built, they do not in themselves provide definitive evidence for the value of food exclusion in specific illnesses. It is essential that some kind of control or blind challenge be introduced in order to validate the observations of the open studies available.

Sodium cromoglycate

A number of studies have used oral sodium cromoglycate to 'block' allergic responses happening within the gut. While the exact mechanism of food intolerance remains unclear, we are aware that a number of histamine-related phenomena occur directly within the gastrointestinal tract and appear to play an important part in mediating food intolerance. As sodium cromoglycate acts as a membrane stabilizer, thereby diminishing histamine-mediated responses, it is logical to presume that this conventional medication may modify the normal masked sensitivity reactions experienced by those suffering from food intolerance. The use of sodium cromoglycate in capsule form can be explored by the use of conventional, double blind, cross-over studies in a very coherent scientific manner. The drug appears to work in patients with food intolerance only while it is being taken and for a very short period afterwards. Consequently it is both reasonable and clinically applicable to suggest blind, placebo controlled, cross-over studies. Such studies do indeed demonstrate clear improvement in those patients receiving oral sodium cromoglycate as compared to controls in illnesses such as eczema, as well as its well-accepted place in the management of asthma.[32,33,34]

Challenge

Having ascertained whether a patient improves on an appropriate exclusion, it is then appropriate to challenge that patient with foods, hoping that symptoms will then be provoked. Ideally food challenge should be on a blind basis. A number of points are of central importance when considering challenge, as masked sensitivity clearly behaves in a very different way to the kind of immediate allergic reaction which may occur in allergic individuals after the ingestion of shellfish, fish or strawberries.

Having obtained symptom clearance in individual patients or groups of patients, it should be expected that some of the individuals will be in a state of tolerance and consequently single challenges may not produce symptom recurrence. If an individual is to have symptoms provoked by food challenge, then challenges must be repeated, ideally two or three times a day for a period of at least two weeks. If symptoms are provoked very swiftly in any particular individual, then the case for symptom clearance and provocation on food challenge is clearly proven and it is not necessary to go on continually challenging the patient and therefore making them ill. If, however, no symptom recurrence occurs at first, then challenges should be repeated over at least two weeks before suggesting that the challenge experiment has failed.

Challenges may be open or blind. In open challenges the patient will eat a food they either suspect or know will provoke symptoms. In many ways open food challenge is the simplest technique to employ, as it involves least thought and food preparation. It is, however, unblinded and consequently much more likely to evoke a placebo response or a psychologically based allergic response.

Blind challenge can involve a number of different techniques:

1 *Challenge with food capsules.* This involves placing the potential offending food into food capsules and giving them to the patient on a placebo or controlled blind basis. In other words, in some instances the patient will receive a provoking food, while in other instances a placebo or non-provoking food. This represents a problem, as it is almost impossible to get enough food into capsules. Furthermore, patients will frequently be aware of which food they are taking, as foods are rarely colourless,

odourless and tasteless. Absorption through the oral mucosa may well play a part in food intolerance. If this is the case, then food capsules do not represent a real food challenge, as only part of the mechanism of food intolerance will be triggered. Capsules are unlikely to disgorge their contents until the small intestine, so it may well be that mechanisms involving the stomach mucosa are also excluded.[35,36]

2 *Nasogastric feeding*. Feeding the food by nasogastric tubes directly into the stomach overcomes the objections of volume, taste, colour and texture. However, it is impossible to repeat nasogastric food challenge over a prolonged period of, say, two weeks. Furthermore, any oral absorption mechanisms that may be involved will be bypassed. While nasogastric challenge is better than challenge by capsules, it is not ideal. Challenge through nasogastric tubes and by capsules can easily be carried out on a blind basis, but because they may be poor challenge methods they may fail to illicit the proper response that occurs within food intolerance and, as a consequence, they must be considered second best.[37]

3 *Pureed or disguised foods*. A number of studies have challenged with soups or pureed foods or food disguised in some way, so that the placebo challenge exactly matches the real thing.[23,38] For instance, a soup could be made either with wheat flour or with soya flour. One may be safe, while the other likely to cause food reaction. The patient can then be challenged on a blind basis and on a number of occasions during any one day. One such study involved the use of specially prepared foods courtesy of Heinz Ltd.[38] This is probably the ideal method of blind food challenge, although it is both complex and difficult to match real and placebo foods for texture, taste and consistency.

There are obviously no ideal methods of challenging. Each method of food challenge brings with it its own problems. The methods outlined above are those that have been most frequently used, and involve tried and tested techniques. None is perfect, but nevertheless symptom provocation, based on blind food challenge, is an essential part of the rigorous investigation of food sensitivities and must necessarily be one of the aspects involved in any clinical trial designed to evaluate food intolerance.

Special patients

In any study group there will be patients who are slow to react to food challenges because of their intrinsic tolerance, and those who will react very promptly, swiftly and reproducibly to single food challenges. It is quite reasonable to select this 'highly reactive' group and use them as a model for food challenge by doing repeated and controlled experiments on a small number of known and reliable reactors. This may well provide the methodology through which new serological investigations for food intolerance can be validated.

Study method

From the morass of data and problems presented it may now seem almost impossible to design a clinical study to evaluate food intolerance. This is not the case, but it is necessary to understand the complexity and variability of the issues involved prior to embarking on a study. The methodological problems should be considered under the following broad headings:

1 *Define the disease*. As a general rule illnesses tend to disappear or become far less common when you wish to study them. Pick a common disease which has a clearly defined diagnosis.

2 *Search the literature*. Make sure that there are at least some very open or descriptive studies suggesting that food sensitivity may be important in the particular illness you wish to study.

3 *Decide the nature of the study*. Studies within environmental medicine, with respect to food sensitivity can take many forms.

   a) **Open studies**   These involve simply taking a group with a known diagnosis, placing them on a food exclusion diet and monitoring their progress.

   b) **Case studies**   This is appropriate for very complex problems in which it may be necessary to explore an individual and complicated environmental problem in depth.

   c) **Controlled studies**   This involves placing one group of randomly allocated patients on a diet and comparing them with a matched control group who are not receiving a diet. A variety of different statistical methods can be applied in these studies, one of which may be to monitor the patients over a prolonged period to look for the relapse rates in the control versus the treatment group.

   d) **Controlled studies with food challenge**   This is the most complex, but also the most scientifically watertight method of evaluating food intolerance. The first phase involves a controlled trial, comparing those excluding particular foods with those on a normal diet. The second phase involves taking the treatment group, who have hopefully improved, and challenging them using one of the methods of food challenge outlined, in order to provoke symptoms.

4 *Assess the illness and the treatment*. Having decided on the disease and the type of study that is appropriate and for which resources are available, a method of assessing the illness should be clearly defined, along with the endpoints which will define the success or failure of the proposed treatment. Ideally the investigator should employ a well-used and clearly validated method for evaluating the particular illness to be studied.

5 *Statistical aspects*. Prior to entry into a study an assessment should be made of what the likely treatment success might be. Based on this 'guestimate', appropriate statistical tables can be

consulted and an evaluation of how many patients should ideally be entered into the study in order for it to be of statistical significance. The study should be discussed with a statistician prior to entry, as this is the best way to get both good advice and statistical cooperation.

6 *Baseline measurement.* A period of baseline measurement prior to entry into the trial is ideal. This should be appropriate to the illness being studied. If, for instance, you are studying migraine then patients should complete daily diaries for a period of one month prior to entry into the study, in order to evaluate the frequency, severity and type of headaches that they experience while being monitored. This monitoring should then continue during the phase of food exclusion for all groups of patients entering the study. A time period of at least three months should then be used to evaluate the effects of diet. This may well be extended, depending on the illness being studied.

7 *Food challenges.* Ideally, blind food challenges should then be part of the third phase of the study, in order to confirm the value of the original food exclusion.

A number of different methods of food exclusion have been suggested. The one that has been most widely used and is probably most acceptable to patients and researchers alike is that of a restricted or oligo antigenic diet.

Conclusion

Environmental medicine has been subjected to more clinical trials than most other areas of complementary medicine. Many of these have used conventional trial methodology with great success. Food intolerance as a cause for illness is possible to evaluate cogently and coherently using a combination of the techniques mentioned. In this chapter I have attempted to outline some of the approaches that have been used to evaluate environmental medicine and this certainly represents a formidable body of work from which any investigator should obtain substantial benefit.

References

1 Royal College of Physicians and British Nutritional Foundation. Food intolerance and food aversion. *J Roy Coll Phys* 1984; **19**(2): 4–5.

2 Lewith, G. T., Kenyon, J. N. *Clinical Ecology*. Wellingborough: Thorsons, 1985; 9–13.

3 Radcliffe, M. J. Diagnostic use of dietary regimes. In: Brostoff, J., Challacombe, S. J. (eds.) *Food Allergy and Food Intolerance*. London: Bailliere Tindall, 1987; 806–22.

4 Stokes, C. R., Miller, B. G., Bourne, F. J. Animal models for food sensitivity. In: Brostoff, J., Challacombe, S. J. (eds.) *Food Allergy and Food Intolerance*. London: Bailliere Tindall, 1987; 286–300.

5 Monro, J., Cavini, C., Brostoff, J. Migraine is a food allergic disease. *Lancet* 1984; **2**: 719–21.

6 Mansfield, L. E. The role of food allergy in migraine: a review. *Ann Allergy* 1987; **58**(S): 313–17.

7 Atherton, D. J., Sewell, M., Soothill, J. F., Wells, R. S., Chilvers, C. E. D. A double blind crossover trial of antigen avoidance diet in atopic eczema. *Lancet* 1987; **1**: 401–3.

8 Atherton, D. J. Breast feeding and atopic eczema. *Br Med J* 1983; **287**: 775–6.

9 Darlington, G., Jump, A., Ramsey, N. Dietary treatment of rheumatoid arthritis. *Practitioner* 1990; **234**: 456–60.

10 Darlington, L. G., Mansfield, J. R., Ramsey, N. Placebo-controlled blind study of dietary manipulation therapy in rheumatoid arthritis. *Lancet* 1986; **2**: 236–8.

11 Brown, M., Gibney, M., Husband, P. R., Radcliffe, M. Food allergy in polysymptomatic patients. *Practitioner* 1981; **225**: 1651–4.

12 Alun Jones, V., Shorthouse, M., McLaughlan, P. Food intolerance: a major factor in the pathogenesis of irritable bowel syndrome. *Lancet* 1982; **2**: 1115–17.

13 Hunter, J. O., Alun Jones, V. Studies in the pathogenesis of irritable bowel syndrome produced by food intolerance. In: Read, N. W. (ed.) *The Irritable Bowel Syndrome*. New York: Grune and Stratton, 1985; 221–37.

14 Royal College of Physicians and British Nutritional Foundation. Food intolerance and food aversion. *J Roy Coll Phys* 1984; **18**(2): 9–11.

15 Shapiro, R. S., Eisenberg, B. C. Allergic headache. *Ann Allergy* 1965; **23**: 123–6.

16 Lessoff, M. H., Buisseret, P. O., Merrett, T. G., Merrett, J., Wraith, D. G. Assessing the value of skin prick tests. *Clin Allergy* 1980; **10**: 115–20.

17 Monro, J. A., Brostoff, J., Carini, C., Zilkha, K. J. Food allergy in migraine. *Lancet* 1980; **2**: 1–4.

18 Freed, D. L. J. Laboratory diagnosis of food intolerance. *Practitioner* 1981; **225**: 873–91.

19 Black, A. P. A new diagnostic method in allergic disease. *Pediatrics* 1956; **17**: 716–24.

20 Lehman, C. W. The leucocytic food allergy test: a study of reliability and reproducibility. Effect of diet and sublingual drops on this test. *Ann Allergy* 1980; **45**: 150–8.

21 Hill, D. J., Lynch, B. C. Elemental diet in the management of severe eczema in childhood. *Clin Allergy* 1982; **12**: 313–15.

22 O'Morain, C., Segal, A. W., Levi, A. J. Elemental diets in the treatment of acute Crohn's disease. *Br Med J* 1980; **281**: 1173–5.

23 Egger, J., Carter, C. M., Wilson, J. W. Is migraine food allergy? A double blind trial of oligo antigenic diet treatment. *Lancet* 1983; **2**: 865.

24 Grant, E. C. Food allergies and migraine. *Lancet* 1979; **1**: 966–9.

25 Radcliffe, M. J. Clinical methods for diagnosis. *Clin Immunol Allergy* 1982; **2**: 205–20.

26 Rowe, A. H. Food allergy: its manifestations, diagnosis and treatment. *JAMA* 1928; **91**: 1623.

27 Rowe, A. H., Rowe, M. D. *Food Allergy: Its Manifestations and Control and The Elimination Diet*. Springfield, Illinois: Charles C. Thomas, 1972.

28 Dickinson, R. J., Ashton, M. G., Axon, A. J. Controlled trial of intravenous hyperalimentation and total bowel rest as an adjunct to the routine therapy of acute colitis. *Gastroenterology* 1980; **79**: 1199–1204.

29 Driscoll, R. M., Rosenberg, J. H. Total parenteral nutrition in inflammatory bowel disease. *Med Clin N Am* 1978; **62**: 185–201.

30 Alun Jones, V., Dickinson, R. J., Workman, E. Crohn's disease: maintenance of remission by diet. *Lancet* 1985; **2**: 177–80.

31 Pagnelli, R., Levinsky, R. J., Brostoff, J., Wraith, D. G. Immune complexes containing food proteins in normal and atopic subjects after oral challenge and the effect of sodium cromoglycate on autogen absorption. *Lancet* 1979; **1**: 1270–2.

32 Ortolani, C., Postovello, E., Zanussi, C. Prophylaxis of adverse reactions to foods. A double blind study of oral sodium cromoglycate for the prophylaxis of adverse reactions to foods and additives. *Ann Allergy* 1983; **50**: 105–9.

33 Atherton, D. J., Soothill, J. F., Edridge, J. A controlled trial of oral sodium cromoglycate in atopic eczema. *Br J Dermatol* 1982; **106**: 681–5.

34 Wraith, D. G., Young, G. V. W., Lee, T. H. The management of food allergy with diet. In: Nalcrom, M., Pepys, J., Edwards, A. M. (eds.) *The Mast Cell*. Geneva: Ciba-Geigy, 1979; 443.

35 May, C. D., Bock, S. A. A modern clinic approach to food hypersensitivity allergy. *Ann Allergy* 1979; **33**: 166–88.

36 Bahna, S. C., Ghandi, M. D. Milk hypersensitivity – practical aspects of diagnosis, treatment and prevention. *Ann Allergy* 1983; **50**: 295–301.

37 Finn, R., Cohan, M. N. Food allergy: fact or fiction. *Lancet* 1978; **1**: 426–8.

38 Pike, M., Atherton, D. J. Atopic eczema. In: Brostoff, J., Challacombe, S. J. (eds.) *Food Allergy and Food Intolerance*. London: Bailliere Tindall, 1987; 589.

22 Research into homoeopathic treatment of rheumatological disease: why and how?

Peter Fisher

Summary

Rheumatology is the most developed area of clinical research into homoeopathy. Several double blind trials investigating the efficacy of homoeopathy have been published; their methods, results and criticisms are described. Development research to improve homoeopathic treatment is also required. A new method of development research, based on a computerized database, is described. Future priorities are discussed.

Introduction

More clinical research has been done into the homoeopathic treatment of rheumatological conditions than any other group of diseases, and several clinical trials of rigorous design have been published in major, peer-reviewed conventional medical journals. It is too early to speak of a tradition, but we now have considerable experience of research in this area and its pitfalls. An evolution of methodology is perceptible. The particular problems of homoeopathy are driving the development of new and innovative methods, methods which may be of value to other complementary therapies, and in mainstream medicine.

Sceptics sometimes say that research in the complementary therapies is a waste of time: prejudice within the medical and scientific establishment is too deep-seated, and the established practices of complementary therapists will not be changed by research findings. Yet it is only just over a decade since the first double blind study of homoeopathic treatment was published in a conventional journal. There is no question that this publication and its successors have influenced conventional medical opinion in favour of homoeopathic treatment, and have led to shifts of opinion within the homoeopathic community. This is not to say that prejudice no longer exists, or that there is any room for complacency.

What is the question?

But before even thinking about methodology we need to address a more fundamental issue: what are the objectives of research. The question is: 'What is the question?'! There is a danger that a preoccupation with methodology will lead complementary medical researchers to neglect this vital initial consideration. As all experienced clinical researchers know, the most common cause of failed research is that the question which the research was intended to answer was never clearly defined, or if it was, was subsequently modified. Obviously a vague question will generate a vague answer, a complex question, a complex answer – which in practice often means no clear result. Contrariwise, once the question is clearly defined, the method required to find the answer is only a short step away.

Obviously there is an enormous range of questions which might be posed, but they can usefully be divided into four classes:

Efficacy

Does this treatment give benefit compared to another treatment, usually placebo?

The double blind study, despite its drawbacks, is the method of choice for answering questions of this type. It is the most rigorous method, and the most familiar to medical sceptics and the regulatory authorities, who are important targets of such research.

Development research

Which homoeopathic medicine or prescribing strategy is most effective in which situation?

The complexity and very large number of variables involved in homoeopathic prescribing make problems of this class particularly interesting and difficult to answer. It could be argued that development research should precede efficacy research, so that it is the efficacy of the optimal treatment that is being assessed. In fact, for pragmatic reasons, research aimed at showing efficacy has so far taken priority.

There are no ready-made solutions to the problems of development research. But once the question is clearly framed, the outlines of the methodology required quickly become evident. At the Royal London Homoeopathic Hospital (RLHH) we are currently implementing an innovative method to determine the optimal treatment in different situations. Some of our early findings are summarized below.

Basic research

How does this treatment work?

This is a central question for homoeopathy, revolving around the high 'ultra-molecular' dilutions, in which no molecule of the starting substance persists. It is the claims made for these dilutions which make homoeopathy an *a priori* absurdity for its opponents.

There is no lack of theories[1,2,3] concerning the nature of the information contained in the ultra-molecular dilutions. Some of these theories propose important developments in physics.[4] But even the best of these are, at present, little more than informed speculation. In my opinion the time is not yet ripe to tackle questions of this class; we have still to prove beyond doubt that there is indeed a question here to be answered!

Epistemology

What is the nature of the question?

The rationale of conventional drug treatment of rheumatic disease is based on blocking or in some other way interfering with the inflammatory and pain mediating mechanisms. Homoeopathy has always opposed, and defined itself in contradistinction to, such allopathic therapeutics.

Although the mode of action of homoeopathy is unknown, it is clear that it acts in a different way. Further, it seems very unlikely that a comprehensive understanding of homoeopathy will be possible within the mechanistic framework of contemporary bioscience. Like most complementary therapies, homoeopathy is, traditionally at least, vitalistic.

Traditional homoeopathic theory involves a 'spirit-like vital force', the *vis mediatrix naturae*. Although it is possible to practise homoeopathy very successfully without reference to this theoretical conception, a deeper understanding of its basis will require a 'new vitalism'. This will demand an entirely new medical paradigm comparable in its scale and implications to Darwin's theory of evolution.

For pragmatic reasons, I will here confine myself to dealing with the first two classes of question.

Published research: a review

Rheumatoid arthritis

It was the seminal work of Drs Robin and Sheila Gibson of the Glasgow Homoeopathic Hospital which proved the practicality of rigorous trials of homoeopathy. Their studies of rheumatoid arthritis, carried out in collaboration with the Glasgow Centre for Rheumatic Diseases, were the first studies of homoeopathy to achieve publication in a peer-reviewed conventional medical journal.

Their first study[5] was published in the *British Journal of Clinical Pharmacology* in 1978. The trial was of large scale: 195 patients with rheumatoid arthritis (RA) inadequately controlled on non-steroidal anti-inflammatory drugs (NSAIDs: the standard first-line treatment for RA) alone. Patients who had previously been treated with slow-acting anti-rheumatic drugs (SAARDs: gold, d-penicillamine, etc.) were excluded from the trial.

Patients were allocated to active or placebo treatment. The active treatment group were assigned alternately to high-dose enteric-coated aspirin or homoeopathy as indicated. 'As indicated' means that the homoeopathic doctors could prescribe any homoeopathic medicine, in whichever potency they considered indicated. Those patients receiving aspirin stopped their previous NSAIDs on trial entry, while those in the homoeopathy group were permitted to continue. The patients were treated for twelve months and assessed at the beginning and end of the period by a standard battery of tests for RA disease activity.

The results were quite impressive for homoeopathy: at the end of the year 42.6% of the homoeopathic treatment group had stopped all other treatment and were better than they had been at the beginning; a further 24% of the homoeopathy group were better at the end of the trial but remained on conventional medication. In contrast, only 14.6% of the aspirin group were maintained and improved on this treatment. One hundred percent of the placebo group dropped out of the trial within six weeks (Figure 22.1).

However, this study attracted fierce criticism[6] from a conventional rheumatologist, principally on the grounds that while the homoeopathic prescribers were free to prescribe any homoeopathic medicine, only aspirin was available to the conventional doctors. Also that the placebo used (sucrose – sugar!) was easily recognizable, so that the study was not truly double blind, and that the homoeopaths were more committed to their therapy than the other doctors involved.

The nature of the question being posed played a central role in the ensuing debate. The critic assumed that the question was 'How does homoeopathy compare with conventional therapy or placebo in the treatment of rheumatoid arthritis?', concluding that the study design

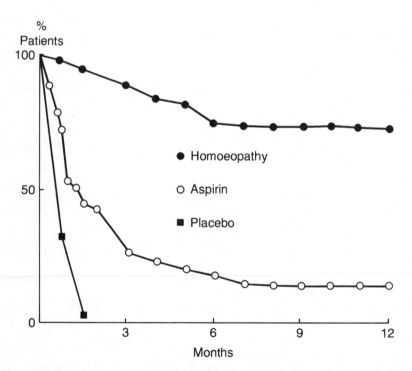

Fig. 22.1 Drop-out over 12 months in rheumatoid arthritis patients treated with homoeopathy, high dose aspirin, and placebo.[5,9] (Reproduced by permission of the *British Homoeopathic Journal*)

was inadequate to address this question. In replying, the authors stated that their null hypothesis had in fact been 'That homoeopathy is ineffective and detrimental to the patient' and that they had refuted this hypothesis.[7] They did, however, concede that the trial design was not ideal, and proceeded to a better design.

Double blind trial

Gibson *et al.*'s second clinical trial[8] was of improved design, being truly double blind. It involved 46 RA patients, again inadequately controlled on conventional first-line treatment. The subjects remained on their previous therapy but received, in addition, homoeopathy as indicated or matching placebo for three months, double blind.

The patients were classified according to whether they had good or poor homoeopathic prescribing symptoms (R and U patients respectively), and equal numbers of R and U patients were assigned to the treatment groups. Assessment was in terms of a standard battery of indices of RA activity: visual analogue score (VAS) of pain, articular index of joint tenderness, grip strength, finger joint circumference, duration of morning stiffness and functional index. Blood tests were also done.

The results were again favourable to homoeopathy with statistically significant changes ($p < 0.01$ or 0.005) for all indices except joint circumference (subsequent work has revealed that joint circumference is a poor criterion in RA, and it is now rarely used). The two homoeopathic prescribing physicians also judged whether the patients had received active or placebo treatment – and were correct in 37 of the 46 cases. There were no significant changes in blood tests (haemoglobin, ESR, rheumatoid serology). R patients responded better than U patients. But the study was criticized on the grounds that the attempt to match the groups for R and U patients and other variables meant that it was not truly randomized.

In a follow-up study[9] the patients in the placebo group changed to active treatment, and showed an improvement similar to that experienced by the active treatment group in the first part of the study. No patient reported side effects from homoeopathy in any of these studies.

Osteoarthritis

Gibson *et al.*'s clinical trials were all of one disease/any medicine type (box 1), in which any homoeopathic medicine could be prescribed to patients within a defined group. In 1983, the first attempt at a different kind of study, assessing the effect of a single homoeopathic medicine, was published[10] (box 2). This was a three-way cross-over, double dummy, double blind clinical trial comparing the homoeopathic medicine Rhus toxicodendron 6x (Nelson) with the NSAID Fenoprofen and placebo.

The method is less complex than it sounds; because the homoeopathic and conventional medicines cannot be made to look alike and are taken in a different way, it was necessary to have two placebos for the study to be truly blind. Thus each patients took three different combinations:

```
┌─────────────────────────────────────────┐
│                                         │
│          Efficacy research              │
│           methodology                   │
│                                         │
│       One disease/any medicine          │
│                                         │
│   Question: Is homoeopathy, taken as a  │
│   whole, more effective than another    │
│   treatment or placebo in this          │
│   condition?                            │
│                                         │
│   Method: Double blind controlled       │
│   clinical trial.                       │
│                                         │
│   Investigates the efficacy of          │
│   homoeopathy as a system. May          │
│   obscure the fact that some remedies   │
│   are effective, others not.            │
│                                         │
│   Reference[8]                          │
│                                         │
└─────────────────────────────────────────┘
```

Box 1

```
┌─────────────────────────────────────────┐
│                                         │
│          Efficacy research              │
│           methodology                   │
│                                         │
│       One disease/one medicine          │
│                                         │
│   Question: Is this homoeopathic        │
│   medicine more effective than another  │
│   treatment and/or placebo?             │
│                                         │
│   Method: Double blind controlled       │
│   clinical trial.                       │
│                                         │
│   Investigates the efficacy of a        │
│   particular homoeopathic medicine.     │
│   The most rigorous method. Strict      │
│   prospective selection of suitable     │
│   patients essential, recruitment       │
│   may be slow.                          │
│                                         │
│   References[10,12,13]                  │
│                                         │
└─────────────────────────────────────────┘
```

Box 2

active Rhus toxicodendron + placebo Fenoprofen, placebo Rhus toxicodendron + active Fenoprofen, and double placebo. The sequence in which they received the treatments was random. Thirty three patients with osteoarthritis of hips and knees on X-ray were recruited and received each of the three treatments for two weeks each, in random sequence. Patients were recruited at the RLHH and in the rheumatology outpatient clinics of two conventional hospitals. Assessment was in terms of VASs of pain at rest, on movement and at night.

The results were negative with respect to the homoeopathic medicine; there were no significant differences between the VAS scores of patients receiving active Rhus tox and placebo, whereas Fenoprofen caused highly significant improvement in symptoms. However, active Rhus tox was clearly different from placebo, in that five patients experienced exacerbation of their symptoms while taking it, in two cases severe enough to require withdrawal from the trial. This trial was methodologically rigorous but open to criticism from the homoeopathic viewpoint.[11] A number of points were raised, including the short (two week) treatment period and the relatively low potency. However, the most telling criticism was that the prescribing criteria for Rhus tox had not been fully applied. Although mention was made of some of the features considered essential for a successful prescription of Rhus tox, it is clear that these were not applied as strictly as normal in homoeopathic practice.

Fibrositis

Two competing interpretations of the result of this study emerged: either it was a 'true negative' reflecting the fact that Rhus tox is ineffective, or it was a 'false negative' due to flaws in the trial design. To resolve the divergence between these two interpretations, our group at St Bartholomew's Hospital embarked on a series of clinical trials.

Our first, pilot, study explored the use of a limited range of homoeopathic medicines in the treatment of fibrositis (also known as primary fibromyalgia).[12] Twenty four patients were recruited in outpatients, and each was prescribed one of three homoeopathic medicines: Arnica montana, Bryonia alba, Rhus toxicodendron, in 6c potency. Since these three medicines would not be expected to cover all cases of fibrositis, each prescription was given a 'goodness-of-fit' score, indicating how well indicated it was. Thus score 2 = three or more typical prescribing features, score 1 = one or two typical features, score 0 = no definite indication.

This study showed Rhus tox to be the most frequently indicated homoeopathic medicine for fibrositis, prescribed in 42% of cases, and well-indicated (i.e. score 2) in 25%. The main finding of this study was that improvement is correlated with strong prescribing indications, irrespective of which medicine was prescribed (Figure 22.2).

We were encouraged by this result to proceed to a definitive study. This was similar in conception to the osteoarthritis study of Shipley *et al.*,[10] being double blind with cross-over. Again the patients had fibrositis, but only those in whom Rhus tox was unequivocally indicated were admitted to the trial.

Patients received Rhus tox 6c (Boiron) and matching placebo, in random sequences, for one month each. Assessment was in terms of VASs of pain and sleep and tender point count. I judged the patients' eligibility for trial entry but, as an additional precaution, I had no further contact with the patients until after they had completed the trial. The medication was dispensed and assessments performed by a clinical metrologist

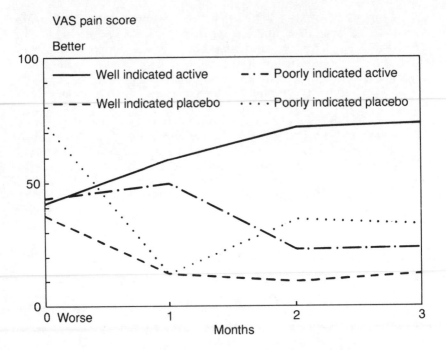

Fig. 22.2   The effect of indication score on visual analogue pain score over three months in patients with fibrositis treated with Arnica, Bryonia and Rhus tox 6c.[12]

(research nurse), who was also blind. The results were positive, showing highly significant improvement of objective and subjective parameters. There was a reduction of about 25% in tender point count (this is the most reliable measure of fibromyalgia). This trial was published in the *British Medical Journal* in 1989.[13]

A further trial is currently underway; the entry criteria are the same (fibrositis with Rhus tox definitely indicated). But we are using Rhus tox 30c (an 'ultra-molecular' dilution) and a longer (three month) treatment period. The study is of uncrossed, parallel group design. It has been designed to yield results which will be directly comparable (at one month) to those of the previous study described above.

Rigour versus realism

Some critics have complained that the clinical improvements in this and other trials were relatively modest. Here again, the question of objective is crucial. The intention of these studies was to demonstrate the efficacy or otherwise of homoeopathic treatment as rigorously as possible, and this placed restraints on the homoeopathic doctors. A longer treatment period and the freedom to prescribe other potencies and medicines would probably have yielded a more impressive response. But it would also have introduced a larger number of variables and increased patient drop-out, which would have reduced its scientific rigour.

There is always a 'trade-off' between scientific rigour and realism. As the credibility of homoeopathic therapy is increasingly established we will see a shift towards trials of homoeopathy as she is practised, as opposed to trials in which the homoeopathic method is cramped by the methodological demands. These more realistic trials will be less rigorous in the strict sense, but they will give a clearer picture of the capabilities of homoeopathy.

More importantly, they will be of greater clinical relevance. Many rheumatic diseases, particularly RA, are chronic and the important thing is the long-term outcome, which cannot be assessed in a short-term study. Recent studies of conventional therapy have led to a mood of therapeutic nihilism[14,15] among rheumatologists. If homoeopathy is to become established as a major therapeutic option in the treatment of rheumatic disease, it must show long-term benefits. In addition to two 6-month double blind clinical trials of homoeopathy in RA, we are also carrying out a three-year study comparing outcome in patients seen at the RLHH with those seen at a teaching hospital rheumatology outpatients and a general hospital in a deprived area of London.

Development research: rewriting the repertory

As all practising homoeopaths are aware, there are great deficiencies in the homoeopathic literature. Most of the data is now at least a century old, much of it is of unknown provenance and questionable validity. It has been said that half of *Kent's Repertory* is inaccurate, the only question is which half! Most of the data in the repertories is not traceable to provings, but derives from clinical experience.[16]

Traditionally only prescribing features from striking clinical responses have been recorded, and the vital information which might be gained from failures or modest responses discarded. In addition there are problems with the repertorial method itself. Experienced homoeopaths generally do not prescribe on the basis of 'totting up', or even a 'weighted totting up' of repertory rubrics, but on the basis of a 'gestalt' – a characteristic constellation of features which they recognize as corresponding to a medicine.

The information technology revolution has provided a springboard for a quantum leap in terms of the quality and quantity of information on which we base our prescribing data. The Faculty of Homoeopathy and the Homoeopathic Medical Research Council have supported the development of a computerized data collection system adapted to the needs of homoeopathy.[17,18] This initiative has now reached a level of sophistication where it is capable of starting to deal with the complex problems of analysing homoeopathic prescribing.

Systematic outcome correlation

The method which we are currently evolving at the RLHH in response to the problems of improving homoeopathic prescribing is known as 'Systematic Outcome Correlation' (SOC) (box 3). This is an innovative

---

**Development research
methodology**

*Systematic Outcome
Correlation*

Question: Which medicine, selected on
which grounds, is associated with favourable outcome, and which not?

Method: Systematic collection of data on:
prescribing indications, prescription and
outcome within prospectively defined domain.

Investigates differential efficacy of
homoeopathic medicines. Systematic collection essential for internal control. Requires sophisticated database software.

Reference[19]

Box 3

method in which prescribing features used and ignored, prescription and outcome within a particular domain are linked and analysed. The 'domain' will normally be a diagnosis, but might also be a particular medicine or other variable. The main reason for defining the domain in terms of diagnosis is that most assessments are more or less diagnosis-specific.

It is vital that all data within the prospectively designated domain is recorded, because this allows 'internal control', in which comparison is made between the good and poor responders, so that it is possible to distinguish the effects of prescribing variables (medicine, indication) from other variables (e.g. disease severity)[19] (Figure 22.3). The use of standardized outcome measures, both objective and subjective, is also important. In our work on RA we are using a mix of traditional methods, such as VAS of pain and whole-patient-function measures such as the Health Assessment Questionnaire (HAQ) (Figure 22.4).

The method hinges on a large-scale, detailed and flexible database. We have adopted ABIES, a Xenix-based medical database system widely used in general practice, which incorporates the Read codes – a comprehensive system for recording medical data on computer which has recently been adopted by the British government as the standard for computer recording of medical data.[20,21] Read codes for all major homoeopathic medicines already exist; the heroic task of creating codes for the vast number of homoeopathic prescribing symptoms is being undertaken by Dr Jeremy Swayne. The number of codes required is so great that an expansion of the coding system from four to five digits is required to accommodate them.

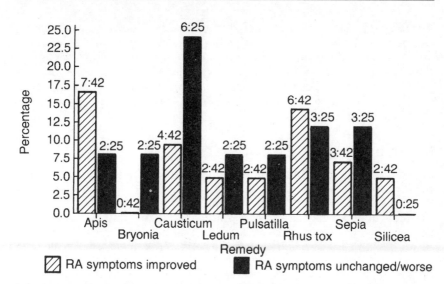

Fig. 22.3 Systematic Outcome Correlation, preliminary results. Response to treatment at three months in 67 consecutive RA patients seen at the Royal London Homoeopathic Hospital and treated with the eight medicines most commonly prescribed for this condition. The left-hand bar of each pair indicates good response, the right poor response. Note that the length of the bar is in terms of proportion so that 2:25 poor responses gives a longer bar than 2:42 good responses.[19] (Reproduced by permission of the *British Homoeopathic Journal*)

Are you able to:
Dress yourself, including tying shoelaces and doing buttons?
Open a new carton of milk or soap powder?
Open car doors?
Run errands and shop?

Responses to all questions are:
Without any difficulty
With some difficulty
With much difficulty
Unable to do

Fig. 22.4 Some typical questions from the Health Assessment Questionnaire (HAQ).

The analysis of the correlations in the data is at the present preliminary stage being done by traditional methods. But we intend to develop two analytical methods: multivariate analysis, and a rule-generating system. Multivariate analysis is a relatively recent statistical technique which allows the correlation between defined variables and outcome to be calculated.

Rule-generating systems are an advanced IT method in which the database is scrutinized by 'intelligent' software for associations between variables. The advantage of the latter method is that the entire database can be automatically scrutinized for any association, while multivariate analysis can only confirm or refute the presence of predicted correlations. In addition, a rule-generating system can detect constellations of prescribing features associated with particular outcomes, an approach which is closer to the way in which homoeopaths operate in practice than other methods.

Conclusion: more effort needed

Several high quality double blind clinical trials of homoeopathic treatment for rheumatic conditions have been published, and more research has been done on homoeopathy in this area than in any other. A variety of experimental designs has been employed, and we now have considerable experience of their drawbacks and advantages. Yet the total number of studies remains very small, all have been of relatively small scale, and none is immune from criticism.

There is a pressing need for more, and larger, studies of homoeopathy. In view of the increasing interest being taken by regulatory authorities, including the EC Commission, in homoeopathy, the highest priority is for further double blind controlled studies. Trials repeating previous work (but taking account of criticisms) and trials in other areas are required. We should move towards longer-term studies, and studies designed from the ground up with homoeopathy in mind, rather than simply adapting existing experimental designs. Development research aimed at improving the efficacy, reliability and range of homoeopathic treatment is also vital and should be conducted in harness with efficacy research. The problems raised by development research in homoeopathy are generating exciting methodological advances.

From the broader viewpoint, the priorities are to create a culture in the complementary therapies which sees research as a vital activity of central importance. And, secondly, that would-be researchers clearly define the problems they are addressing and select methods appropriate to their solution.

References

[1] Kumar, A., Jussal, R. A hypothesis on the nature of homoeopathic potencies. *Br Hom J* 1979; **68**: 197–205.

[2] Resch, G., Gutmann, V. Scientific foundations of homoeopathy. Berg am Starnberger See, FRG: Barthel & Barthel, 1987.

[3] Berezin, A. A. Isotopical positional correlations as a possible model for Benveniste experiments. *Med Hypotheses* 1990; **31**: 43–5.

[4] Del Guidice, E., Preparata, G., Vitiello, G. Water as a free electric dipole laser. *Phys Rev Letts* 1988; **61**: 1085–8.

[5] Gibson, R. G., Gibson, S. L. M., MacNeill, A. D., Gray, G. H., Dick, W. C., Buchanan, W. Salicylates and homoeopathy in rheumatoid arthritis: preliminary observations. *Br J Clin Pharmac* 1978; **6**: 391–5.

[6] Huston, G. Salicylates and homoeopathy. *Br J Clin Pharmac* 1979; **7**: 529–30.

[7] Dick, W. C., Gibson, R., Gray, G., Buchanan, W. Salicylates and homoeopathy. *Br J Clin Pharmac* 1979; **7**: 530.

[8] Gibson, R. G., Gibson, S. L. M., MacNeill, D. A., Buchanan, W. Homoeopathic therapy in rheumatoid arthritis: evaluation by double-blind clinical trial. *Br J Clin Pharmac* 1980; **9**: 453–9.

[9] Gibson, R. G. *et al.* The place for non-pharmaceutical therapy in chronic RA: a critical study of homoeopathy. *Br Hom J* 1980; **69**: 121–33.

[10] Shipley, M., Berry, H., Broster, G., Jenkins, M., Clover, A., Williams, I. Controlled trial of homoeopathic treatment of osteoarthritis. *Lancet* 1983; **1**: 97–8.

[11] Kennedy, C. O. Homoeopathy (letter). *Lancet* 1983; **1**: 482.

[12] Fisher, P. An experimental double-blind clinical trial method in homoeopathy. *Br Hom J* 1986; **75**: 142–7.

[13] Fisher, P., Greenwood, A., Huskisson, E. C., Turner, P., Belon, P. Effect of homoeopathic treatment on fibrositis (primary fibromyalgia). *Br Med J* 1989; **299**: 365–6.

[14] Scott, D., Symmons, D., Coulton, B., Popert, A. Long-term outcome of rheumatoid arthritis: results after 20 years. *Lancet* 1987; **1**: 1108–11.

[15] Rashad, S., Revell, P., Hemingway, A. *et al.* Effect of non-steroidal anti-inflammatory agents on the course of osteoarthritis. *Lancet* 1989; **2**: 519–22.

[16] Campbell, A. C. H. Rhus from provings. *Br Hom J* 1981; **70**: 179–82. Also other '. . . from provings' papers by Campbell, published in *Br Hom J*.

[17] Swayne, J. Joining the grown-ups. *Br Hom J* 1988; **77**: 235–44.

[18] Dempsey, T., Swayne, J. Thinking what we are doing. *Br Hom J* 1990; **79**: 82–99.

[19] Van Haselen, R., Fisher, P. Analysing homoeopathic prescribing using the Read classification and information technology. *Br Hom J* 1990; **79**: 74–81.

[20] *Br Hom J* 1991; **80**. The whole of this number is devoted to the impact of information technology on homoeopathy.

[21] Chisholm, J. The Read clinical classification. *Br Med J* 1990; **300**: 1092.

23 Experimentation in hypnosis: towards an adequate methodology

David Kidner

Summary

The growth of hypnosis as a therapeutic mode during the past century is reviewed together with an assessment of the relationship between hypnotherapy and scientific methodology. The characteristics of recent research into hypnosis are discussed, with particular emphasis on the drawbacks of employing conventional research methodologies in hypnosis research. In particular, the denial of subjectivity by much contemporary experimentation in the area is viewed as problematic, and alternative research paradigms which avoid this and related pitfalls are reviewed. It is concluded that while conventional research methodologies are of some use in hypnosis research if their ideological character is recognized, a more adequate understanding of hypnosis will also require the development of alternative research paradigms which can incorporate the contextual and relational aspects of hypnosis. Finally, some specific suggestions are made concerning the form which an adequate methodology might take.

Introduction

The use of hypnosis as a mode of therapy has a long and colourful history, with periods of widespread interest and activity alternating with intervals during which its use became dormant.[1] Undoubtedly part of the reason for this situation lies in the uncomfortable relationship between the intrinsically unobservable nature of consciousness and the requirements of the scientific worldview which has prevailed in the Western world over the past several centuries; a relationship which makes the scientific study of hypnosis both particularly difficult and especially valuable. For if hypnotic phenomena are notoriously difficult to study by means of conventional research methodology, they also raise fundamental questions about the ideology of scientific research; questions which are often insufficiently recognized within the scientific community. Thus therapeutic hypnosis, unlike conventional medicine, has had to develop without the support of a legitimating scientific context, and indeed has in many respects developed in spite of the existence of a tradition of scientific medical research. The issues which this chapter raises are therefore not simply those which concern the transposing of established research techniques to the field of hypnosis, but also those which are generated by the collision of a powerful, well-established paradigm with a field of study which is relatively undeveloped and poorly theorized, but which by its very nature suggests the limitations and incompleteness of the scientific worldview.

Modern hypnotherapy is usually traced to the well-known activities of Mesmer, which had a good deal in common with ancient healing traditions such as the laying on of hands and medieval exorcism. Mesmer seems to have possessed an excellent intuitive grasp of the power of expectation, and he used dramatic procedures and his own charisma to good effect. In keeping with the intellectual fashion of his time, however, he explained the healing process in physical, and especially electromagnetic, terms, enlisting the help of concepts such as 'stored cosmic fluid' and 'animal magnetism'; a theory which was discredited by the Royal Commission's report of 1784.[2] Although the members of the Royal Commission threw out the baby of hypnotic phenomena along with the bathwater of the theory of animal magnetism, Mesmer's work had inspired a number of followers, some of whom, more realistically, began to assign central importance to psychological rather than physical processes.

The influence of the French school of magnetism reached England during the 1830s, and among the foremost exponents in this country was John Elliotson, Professor of Medicine at the University of London. However, even Elliotson's prestige and the many successful cases published in the journal he founded were no match for the entrenched hostility of the Victorian medical establishment; Elliotson was forced to resign his post, and his findings were dismissed as fraudulent.[3] The dismissal of Elliotson's work can be seen as having a partly economic basis in that the affluent clientele of mesmerists represented a loss of income to conventional medical practitioners. However, there is no doubt that mesmerists, in implying that orthodox medicine was inadequate and incomplete, also threatened the monopoly which medicine claimed concerning knowledge of the origins and treatment of disease.[3]

The second major figure in the development of hypnosis in Britain was James Braid, a Scottish surgeon whose view of trance emphasized the importance of psychological factors such as concentration.[4] With Braid's death in 1860, interest in hypnosis fell dormant for several decades; in France, however, Charcot's experiments with women suffering from hysteria regenerated interest. Charcot's theory of hypnosis, in spite of, or perhaps because of, his narrowly scientific approach, was as misleading as Mesmer's, for by concentrating solely on the behaviour of his patients, he failed to realize that his observations were largely the result not of spontaneous displays of pathology, but of subtle physiological cues, his own prestige and the expectations held by his patients, his colleagues and himself.[4] Charcot's theory thus illustrates the problems that can arise when a phenomenon is studied in isolation from its context; an important point to which we will return later.

During the present century, the development of clinical hypnosis was due overwhelmingly to the work of one man. Milton Erickson's contributions to hypnotherapy are profound and various; he is perhaps best known for his many innovative techniques of hypnotic induction and for his emphasis upon allowing the creative resourcefulness of the client's unconscious mind to resolve problems, in contrast to the more traditional hypnotic techniques in which the therapist directly suggests the disappearance of symptoms.[5] Erickson's introduction of a less authoritarian, more permissive approach to therapy, together with the belief in the client's own unconscious resources as the basis of the healing process, are congruent with social changes which have occurred in this century, reflecting an increasingly individualistic ethos and a corresponding decrease in emphasis on power relationships. These changes are particularly marked with respect to gender roles; in the 1890s, when almost all hysterics were women and almost all doctors men, it is not surprising that the relationship between hypnotist and client reflected differences in power associated with both class and gender.

Today, however, the emphasis in hypnotherapy – especially that influenced by the Ericksonian tradition – is much more on the *facilitation* of healing in a largely client-centred therapeutic milieu. Indeed, Erickson's approach shared more than a few characteristics with that of Carl Rogers.[6] This significant change of emphasis, however, is less consistent with the ideology of orthodox medical research, in which the illness of the patient is seen in largely physical terms devoid of a subjective component, and in which curative influences are viewed predominantly in terms of external forces acting directly on the physical being of the patient, bypassing the person's subjective being.

The current antipathy between experimentalists on the one hand and Ericksonian practitioners on the other[7,8] can be seen to reflect a very basic conflict between two perspectives. On the one hand, pathology can be seen in terms of a mechanistic and dualistic metaphor in which the body is regarded as a malfunctioning machine and in which subjectivity is either irrelevant or misleading.[9] On the other hand, pathology may be understood as involving the whole person, and so subjectivity, accessed by means of an emphatic relationship between therapist and client, can be viewed as a royal road both to diagnosing the nature of the problem and to its resolution. Hence it is clear that the difficulties of bringing about a fruitful reconciliation between modern hypnotherapy and experimental methodology are not superficial. It is the encounter between these two traditions which provides the backcloth for this chapter.

Methodological problems in hypnosis research

As noted above, the concept of research into hypnosis is not one which has come easily either to hypnotists or to experimenters. Hypnotherapists have typically been more concerned with illustrating their techniques by means of anecdotes and case studies than they have with carefully controlled clinical trials, partly because the methodology associated with such trials is often incompatible with effective hypnotherapeutic procedures. Experimentalists, on the other hand, have usually forced hypnotic phenomena to fit the mould of conventional research methodology, and those aspects of hypnosis which cannot easily be accommodated by the experimental paradigm, such as the subjective experience of the hypnotized person, have frequently been ignored.[10]

In order to illustrate some of the problems associated with employing an experimental paradigm in hypnosis, consider an issue which has been central to the thinking of researchers in this area for several decades. This is the so-called state/non-state controversy, which revolves around the question of whether or not hypnosis can be considered to be a unique state of consciousness, distinguishable from so-called 'normal' consciousness. Some theorists, such as Barber[11] and more recently Spanos,[12] argue that hypnosis can be understood adequately in terms of social psychological processes without recourse to positing a separate state, and have supported this argument by attempting to show, with some success, that hypnotic phenomena can be produced in subjects who have not experienced a formal hypnotic induction. 'State' theorists such as Hilgard, on the other hand, suggest that reference to a separate state of consciousness, distinguishable from 'normal' consciousness, is necessary to explain hypnotic phenomena.[13]

It is interesting to examine the assumptions made by writers on both sides of this argument, and these usually include the following. Firstly, it is implied that 'normal' consciousness can be conceptualized as a single, uniform state which remains more or less constant in everyday situations. Secondly, any hypothetical state of hypnosis which may or may not exist is frequently assumed to result from, and only from, exposure to a hypnotic induction. Thirdly, it is often implied that for a 'state' theory to be valid, there must be minimal overlap and continuity between the two hypothetical states.

However, while it may be convenient from an experimental point of view to pose the issue in terms of separate states, clinicians have long recognized that certain 'normal' states of consciousness (for example, being absorbed in a book or being lost in fantasy) are in many ways similar to, and indeed overlap with, trance states. Thus the reified conception of consciousness which underlies the experimental comparison of groups which experience a hypnotic induction and those which do not may well be unrealistic. Ultimately, the state/non-state controversy is based on an unproductively adversarial view of research, and there is no doubt that both theories which emphasize social psychological factors in determining hypnotic behaviour and those which emphasize cognitive factors have grasped important aspects of hypnosis which need to be 'creatively synthesized' for a clearer understanding of hypnosis to emerge.[14] While many researchers have paid lip service to the importance of factors which are essential constituents of their opponents' approaches, they have not yet *integrated* these factors within their own theories, in part because to do so would imply a view of the person in which 'individual' and 'social' factors are more closely intertwined than many researchers are yet ready to recognize.

Furthermore, the experimental comparison of a group of subjects who have been exposed to a hypnotic induction – especially the rather inflexible 'standardized' variety usually employed in hypnosis research – with a group which has merely received suggestions that they will experience phenomena usually associated with hypnosis is unlikely to offer fertile conditions for any potential differences in consciousness to emerge, nor to reflect the diversity and contextually located nature of consciousness.[15] The experimental situation, with its necessary poverty of relationship and subjective meaning, cannot reproduce the situation of the hypnotherapy client, who is likely to be highly motivated and involved in a trusting and intense personal relationship. Thus the states of consciousness involved in these two situations may well be very different. Exposing subjects to a standardized induction, while convenient from an experimental viewpoint, does not offer the ideal environment for the development of an altered state of consciousness. Thus the researcher who uses a design which compares 'hypnotic' and 'non-hypnotic' groups is in grave danger of basing their research on an unrealistic view of the states of consciousness involved, and might well prefer a more individualized approach which incorporates feedback from subjects concerning their experiences during the session.[16]

A further problem with much experimental work on hypnosis is that the objectification involved in the laboratory excludes some of the most potentially significant aspects of the hypnotic relationship. (The alert reader will be able to detect the ghost of Charcot here.) It is important to recognize that group comparison designs are inherently insensitive to the diversity of individual responses, and so lose a good deal of information which is not expressible in terms of the particular experimental variables chosen. The experimental approach has its roots in the tradition of the physical sciences, in which an 'objective' scientist manipulates variables and dispassionately observes the results. The objectification which occurs in this process is thus not limited to the selection of certain variables from the many possible ones. It extends also to the hypnotist-experimenter, who becomes a purely rational 'funnel through which most of the important antecedent variables must filter',[11] and to the hypnotized person, who necessarily responds in a constrained and more-or-less predictable way to the stimulus variables to which they are exposed. If the hypnotized person is seen as possessing subjectivity, it is often viewed as a harmless byproduct rather than as an essential aspect of the person. The relationship between hypnotist and client, regarded as so vital by clinicians, is often avoided altogether by means of recorded inductions, or controlled for by the use of standardized procedures.

Here we come face to face with an apparent incompatibility between experimental methodology and the nature of hypnosis. As Shor has argued,[4] the requirements of the experimenter are diametrically opposed to those of the hypnotist. The former requires an 'objective' approach which minimizes subjective contact, while the latter would be likely to claim that a high degree of interpersonal trust and empathy, and an induction procedure which responds sensitively to momentary changes in the client's consciousness, are essential. It is perhaps not surprising, therefore, that non-state theorists question the existence of hypnosis as a recognizable state of consciousness, given that the laboratory setting and procedures are so inimical to the development of rapport between experimenter and subject. As Abeles has argued: 'The experimental method is an excellent approach for studying many things; it is not, however, appropriate for *everything*. Some phenomena do not survive its application; it is not fair to say that things which die on the dissecting table never existed'.[17]

A further problem which arises from the objectified viewpoint of the experimental laboratory concerns the nature of hypnosis, which is seen as determined largely by factors which exist within the hypnotized person rather than by characteristics of the complete social situation, which includes the subject, the hypnotist, and the cultural and interpersonal assumptions which they bring with them. Such psychologistic interpretations are based on the principle of 'drawing a generalization from the world of external observation, giving it a fancy name, and then asserting that the named abstraction exists *inside* the organism as an explanatory principle'.[18] A prime example of such an abstraction is the concept of 'hypnotic susceptibility' which is claimed to be a 'relatively stable' trait which is 'independent of the skill of the hypnotist'.[19]

While this approach should not be rejected as totally in error, it highlights some aspects of the hypnotic situation while ignoring others. This reflects an overly individualistic ideology common within psychology,[20] a stance which has clear limitations traceable to the reductionist preconceptions on which it is based.[21] Specifically, an overemphasis on individual susceptibility implies that it is meaningful to separate the hypnotic situation into various distinct components, and to ascribe greater importance to some of these components (those that lie within the individual) while paying only lip service to others (those which exist outside the individual). Thus the work of Hilgard and his colleagues, while demonstrating that *something* is reproducible over long time spans, does not show that those aspects of the hypnotic situation which are reproducible reside purely within the individual. They could more realistically be seen as aspects of the whole situation which are shared by the two testing occasions.[22] Thus the concept of hypnotic susceptibility serves to reproduce an experimental ideology which, by locating the phenomenon of hypnosis largely within the individual, perpetuates the notion of the scientist as external to and detached from the object of study. The experimenter, by means of an objective, dispassionate gaze, denies his or her own subjectivity as well as that of the subject.

This emphasis on the decontextualized individual is a feature common to much medical research. It tends to force us to perceive disease in terms of individual pathology, and implicitly denies the relation between illness and social context. It is a stance which complementary medicine in general, and hypnosis research in particular, will need to transcend if we are to offer real alternatives to conventional medicine. In the next section, we will examine some research methods which begin to fulfil this aim.

New directions for hypnosis research

In the previous section, some of the limitations of conventional hypnosis research were explored. How can we overcome these limitations, so that a fuller understanding of hypnosis can emerge?

It is clear that many of the problems considered originate in the various arbitrary splits which are implied by the orthodox experimental approach, and these must be recognized and healed if an adequate conception of hypnosis is to develop. Such splits include those between experimenter and subject; between 'hypnotic' and 'normal' states of consciousness; between the laboratory situation and the cultural and historical context from which it derives; and between the 'objective' viewpoint and everything which is denied by the concept of objectivity. In sum, recognizing the integrity of the phenomenon of hypnosis amounts to a radical challenge to current social scientific methodology, not merely a change in emphasis or a detailed tidying up of loose ends.

Some progress has already been made in the direction of including the subjective experience of the hypnotized person within our understanding of the term 'hypnosis'. A forerunner in this regard is Shor's 'phenomenological method',[23] which involves an interview after the hypnotic session in order to assess the individual's experience of hypnosis, using ratings on eight dimensions of experience. The multi-dimensional nature of this assessment is a clear improvement over the more usual unidimensional assessment of hypnotic depth, since the latter approach, while convenient from an experimental viewpoint, requires a simplistic notion of consciousness, and undoubtedly does violence to the varieties of experience encapsulated in the term 'hypnosis'.

Nevertheless, the phenomenological method clearly asks a good deal of the subject, who is required not only to remember experiences which occurred during the session, but to report them accurately and honestly. In this regard, Sheehan's Experimental Analysis Technique (EAT) has definite advantages. The EAT is 'primarily directed to the assessment of the individuality and distinctiveness of individuals' responses to hypnosis. It seeks to examine the ways in which individual hypnotic subjects pattern their personal meanings and responses to the suggestions that they receive, and purports to focus on the interaction between persons and context by examining these interactions in specific detail.'[24] Thus stated, the intention of this technique is congruent with the modern social psychological trend towards placing subjective meaning at the centre of explanation, and Sheehan's work is seminal in this respect. In order to achieve these ambitious aims, the EAT employs video playback of the hypnotic session, during which the subject is questioned by a third party in the absence of the hypnotist regarding their thoughts, feelings and behaviour during the session. The subject is encouraged to stop the tape at any time in order to elaborate on their experiences. A particularly noteworthy feature of the technique is that a greater degree of initiative is placed with the subject than is usually the case, and the stance of the experimenter is collaborative rather than directive, thus reducing the authoritarian overtones which have so often accompanied research in hypnosis.

Sheehan and McConkey[24] offer a good deal of material to demonstrate the effectiveness of the EAT in relating hypnotic behaviour to the subject's cognition and experience, and thus in fostering a more holistic account of hypnosis. However, the work of Sheehan, important though it is in breaking down the artificial barriers between experimenter and subject and between subjectivity and behaviour, still leaves untheorized and implicit the grounding relationship between the experimental situation and the cultural and ideological context which defines it. Sheehan has reported several attempts to 'humanize' the experimental situation by means of such strategies as attempting to establish a 'co-equal' relationship between subject and investigator, 'openly specifying the need for honest and frank communication' and attempting 'explicitly to promote personal, positive rapport'.[25] Such interventions within an experimental context which is otherwise orthodox surely only scratch the surface of a problem which is deeply embedded within the ideology of the experimental method. Sheehan himself recognizes this, remarking that 'the manipulations involved may have been too weak to alter the subject's recognition that he or she was in an unfavourable power relationship'. He also observes that this power relationship may be 'virtually impossible to undermine'.[25]

Such issues reach to the heart of social scientific endeavour. They suggest a fundamental incompatibility between the objective, controlling attitude of the experimenter, who remains fairly anchored to the assumptions of the scientific worldview, and that of the effective hypnotherapist, who needs to adopt a person-centred attitude which fosters a strong empathic contact with the client. The latter attitude has much in common with what Schactel has referred to as 'allocentric' perception – a viewpoint which embraces as fully as possible that which is being studied, and recognizes it in its entirety.[26] This represents a very different approach to that of the conventional scientist whose gaze categorizes, isolates and reduces to a predetermined format.[27] Schactel argues that the scientist '. . . looks at the object with one or more hypotheses and with the purpose of his research in mind and thus "uses" the object to corroborate or disprove a hypothesis but does not encounter the object as such, in its own fullness. This means that only those aspects of the object are deemed relevant which make it suitable for manipulation or control. . . . (In) their attempt to fit some object or phenomenon into some system, preconception, or hypothesis, one can often observe a blinding of themselves towards the pure and full being of the object itself. Perception, then, may become almost an act of aggressive violence in which the perceiver, like Procrustes with his hapless victims, cuts off those aspects of the object which he cannot use for his purposes'.[26] Relating Schactel's ideas to our central concerns, there is clearly a danger that the hypnosis researcher, in focusing on a few preselected, quantifiable variables, is in danger of losing sight of more subtle but no less significant aspects of hypnosis which escape the rather crude research paradigms currently available.

One way of avoiding this danger is to relate 'objective' indices such as observable behaviour or physiological measures to the individual's subjective awareness, which in turn will facilitate an empathic connection between experimenter and subject. This is the approach adopted by Ernest Rossi.[28,29] Rossi's work is thus essentially integrative in nature, and is an important step towards bridging the gap between the often mechanistic understanding of orthodox medical research and the more existentially oriented approach of many hypnotherapists.

The trend in hypnosis research away from a purely 'objective' stance towards a more holistic view of the person-in-context which incorporates subjective experience is one which challenges some important preconceptions of traditional research. The challenge becomes more explicit and threatening to a scientistic ideology when extended beyond the subjective experience of the subject to include that of the hypnotist-experimenter. Many hypnotherapists spontaneously experience trance when hypnotizing their clients, and Diamond has suggested that Sheehan's EAT could be used to explore the *hypnotist's* experience during an experimental or therapeutic session.[30] The ready availability of videotape equipment today makes the research possibilities emanating from this idea both practical and exciting. The use of the EAT in this manner will also facilitate detailed empirical investigation of the importance attached by many clinical hypnotherapists – especially those working within a broadly Ericksonian paradigm – to the necessity for the therapist to join with or 'utilize' the client's beliefs and momentary changes in subjective experience. Such an approach is in marked contrast to that of most experimentalists who, by using standardized inductions together with concepts such as hypnotic susceptibility, locate the responsibility for the outcome of the hypnotic session largely with the subject.

Research which includes the subjectivity of the experimenter among the variables to be studied will strongly challenge the present research tradition in hypnosis since, by deconstructing the assumption of objectivity, it will make explicit the values and interests which underlie the 'objective' stance of the experimenter.[31] While the inclusion of the subjective experience of both experimenter and subject is an important step towards a more adequate methodology (and, one might add, a more adequate epistemology), the development of a theory which incorporates the relational aspects of hypnosis still presents challenging problems. Throughout the history of hypnosis there has been a strong tendency to perceive the essence of hypnosis as existing *either* within the subject, as in Charcot's theory, *or* in the skills of the hypnotist, which was the view, for example, of Mesmer, and which today is the stance adopted by some of the more flamboyant neo-Ericksonians.[30]

Relational or systemic views of hypnosis, and for that matter of psychotherapy in general, have not been easy to formulate in the reductionist terminology of conventional social science, partly because they are less easily underpinned by psychophysiological and other 'hard' scientific evidence, which some social scientists feel the need to lean on to support their own less tangible concepts. That such relational theories are possible, however, is indicated by developments in areas other than hypnosis. In family systems theory, for example, relational concepts such as 'enmeshment'[32] and 'projective system'[33] are well established, and the therapeutic effectiveness of the therapies which draw on such concepts[34] constitutes a powerful argument for the development of relational or systemic approaches in other areas. Concepts such as 'rapport' and 'empathy' are widely considered among hypnotherapists to describe crucially important factors, but remain poorly understood and undertheorized. Diamond's survey[35] of research which emphasizes the relational dimension of hypnosis is a useful starting point for any investigator seeking to develop our understanding in this area.

Clinicians have been more insistent on the importance of recognizing and responding to the contents of clients' consciousness than have experimentalists, and this has been reflected in the increasingly common use of naturalistic, indirect approaches to induction. Conventional group comparison research designs have been used to study the relative effectiveness of direct and indirect induction techniques, and have demonstrated that while only highly susceptible subjects tend to be responsive to direct suggestion, both high and low susceptible subjects respond to indirect inductions which reflect moment-to-moment changes in the subject's consciousness.[36,37] Such findings are consistent with the reservations expressed above regarding the concept of hypnotic susceptibility, since they demonstrate that differences in responsiveness between high and low susceptible subjects diminish substantially if the hypnotist behaves empathically and flexibly. In other words, the concept of hypnotic susceptibility can be seen to be partly an artefact of the arbitrary constancy of the hypnotist's behaviour.

Such studies also demonstrate that traditional group comparison designs *can* be useful if the researcher maintains an awareness of the inherent limitations of such designs, and particularly if the variables concerned are selected carefully, with recognition of their origins and implications. Some researchers, however, may feel that the limitations of conventional research methodology[38] are such that alternative avenues should be explored. One such possibility is the use of case studies. The more intensive study of a single individual allows the investigator to be more responsive to the behaviour and experience of the person involved than would be the case with a group comparison design. A useful starting point is Nugent's methodological review of case studies published in the *American Journal of Clinical Hypnosis*.[39] It should be noted, however, that the more formal varieties of single case experimental design tend to make many of the same assumptions as traditional group comparison designs; in particular, they often subscribe to a rather simplistic view of the cause–effect relation between dependent and independent variables, and so may not adequately express the dialectical and systemic qualities of the hypnotic situation.

Nevertheless, in-depth investigation of particular subjects' performances can provide a much more detailed and sensitive understanding of the hypnotic process than can group comparison designs, and are better placed to explore subjective reactions to the experimental situation. Group comparison designs can often be supplemented with one or more case studies in order to elucidate the detailed processes and experiences which give rise to the general trends and relationships found, thus overcoming some of the objections to the group comparison approach. Even when considered in isolation from any larger scale research project, less formal case studies such as the many offered by Erickson,[40] although providing no basis for definite conclusions, are useful in indicating possibilities for more formal investigation.

Finally, the researcher needs to be aware of the relations among the social and historical context, the forms of trance which are observed, and the methods which are effective in inducing trance. Anthropologists who have studied altered states of consciousness cross-culturally[41] have recognized that an enormous variety of trance behaviours and experiences are possible. The assumption that trance can be a single, reproducible state of consciousness which can be isolated in a 'pure' form devoid of culturally specific features reflects a simplistic and misleading view of human nature.[42] For example, as noted above, directive approaches to induction may well have been relatively successful in Charcot's era. However, given the more egalitarian and individualistic ethos which exists in the Western world today, it is not surprising that permissive approaches are generally found to be more effective. Furthermore, the particular forms of trance noted by Charcot seem to be very different to those typically observed today. Thus to present the relationship between, say, hypnotic 'depth' and permissiveness of induction as an objective finding, implying independence from sociohistorical context, is to ignore the constitutive relation between context and the forms of consciousness and individuality which exist within that context.[43,44]

Similarly, the manifestations and incidence of disease processes can themselves be seen to reflect cultural and ideological contexts.[45,46,47] Smail has argued that such 'distal' factors are at least as important in determining the courses of both illness and therapy as the more obvious 'proximal' factors involving the immediate social and environmental circumstances.[48,49] Awareness of the whole spectrum of aetiological factors will allow researchers to develop a more realistic assessment of the potential effectiveness of hypnotherapy, as well as indicating the types of personal distress and illness which therapy might most effectively alleviate, and the forms of intervention which are likely to be successful.[32]

Sociohistorical awareness also needs to include a recognition of the assumptions and preconceptions made by the particular research paradigm which is being employed, so that concepts such as 'objectivity' can be seen as constructs which have evolved historically rather than as transhistorical universals.[50]

Conclusions

In this chapter we have reviewed some of the problems encountered in hypnosis research, and have considered a number of approaches and techniques which offer ways of overcoming these problems. What, then, are the major conclusions which this analysis suggests?

Firstly, effective research will recognize the essential contribution of subjectivity to our understanding of hypnosis. Sheehan's EAT is a useful technique in this respect.[24] Rossi's work[28,29] offers an important starting point for the researcher seeking to relate subjectivity and physiological functioning. It is essential that a form of therapy which seeks to empower individuals by enlarging the scope of their subjective action should be based on a research methodology which itself recognizes and incorporates subjectivity.

Secondly, the research strategy adopted should be sufficiently flexible to enable the researcher sensitively to pace the varying states of consciousness involved. For this reason, group comparison designs may often be less appropriate than case studies. Crude experimenter-centred instruments such as taped inductions are likely to be of particularly limited use.

Thirdly, the experimenter needs to be aware of the ideological framework of the experimental paradigm employed, and of the particular ideological baggage carried by the variables selected for study. For example, the concept of 'hypnotic susceptibility' implies that the hypnotic process is one which takes place largely within individuals, and so denies the relational and contextual aspects of the situation. By recognizing such issues the researcher will avoid being led unwittingly towards an unrealistic view of hypnosis.

Fourthly, the culturally and historically constituted nature of both states of consciousness and definitions of health and illness must be recognized. Illness and therapy are processes which can be usefully understood as both intrapsychic and culturally located, and thus an adequate account of hypnotherapy will incorporate ideological and contextual factors as well as psychological ones. For example, therapeutic efforts to increase a client's sense of confidence and personal power need to be tempered by an awareness of the *actual* power relationships to which the client is exposed in the course of their everyday life; and the models of therapy employed by the researcher will also need to embody this awareness.

Finally, effective research will need to recognize the systemic nature of the hypnotic situation, and it is likely that relational variables such as empathy will come to play an increasingly significant role in hypnotherapy research.

The points raised above indicate that traditional research designs may be of use if their assumptions and limitations are recognized, but that a thorough understanding of hypnosis and its therapeutic possibilities will also require the development of new approaches to research which transcend the convenient categories and divisions of conventional social scientific research. The nature of medical science cannot be divorced from the nature of the methodology which sustains and legitimates it, and so a more profound understanding of hypnotherapy will need to incorporate those features of context and relationship which have so often been denied in the past.

References

1 Fromm, E. Significant developments in clinical hypnosis during the past 25 years. *Int J Clin Exp Hypnosis* 1987; **35**: 215–30.

2 Pattie, F. A. A brief history of hypnotism. In: Gordon, J. E. (ed.) *Handbook of Clinical and Experimental Hypnosis*. London: Macmillan, 1967.

3 Parssinen, T. M. Professional deviants and the history of medicine: medical mesmerists in Victorian Britain. *Soc Rev Monographs* 1979; **27**: 103–20.

4 Shor, R. E. The fundamental problem in hypnosis research as viewed from historic perspectives. In: Fromm, E., Shor, R. E. (eds.) *Hypnosis: Research Developments and Perspectives*. Aldine Atherton, 1972.

5 Lankton, S., Lankton, C. *The Answer Within: A Clinical Framework of Ericksonian Hypnotherapy*. Brunner/Mazel, 1983.

6 Gunnison, H. The uniqueness of similarities: parallels of Milton H. Erickson and Carl Rogers. *J Couns Dev* 1985; **63**: 561–4.

7 McCue, P. A. Ericksonian hypnosis: a cautionary note. *Psychologist* 1988; **1**: 259–60.

8 Heap, M. Born-again mesmerism? *Psychologist* 1988; **1**: 261–2.

9 Sullivan, M. In what sense is contemporary medicine dualistic? *Culture Med Psychiat* 1986; **10**: 331–50.

10 Ward, C. A. The cross-cultural study of altered states of consciousness. In: Ward, C. A. (ed.) *Altered States of Consciousness and Mental Health*. London: Sage, 1989.

11 Barber, T. X. *Hypnosis: A Scientific Approach*. New York: Van Nostrand, 1969.

12 Spanos, N. P. Hypnotic behaviour: a social-psychological interpretation of amnesia, analgesia, and 'trance logic'. *Behav Brain Sci* 1986; **9**: 449–502.

13 Hilgard, E. R. *Divided Consciousness*. Chichester: Wiley, 1977.

14 Kihlstrom, J. F. Strong inferences about hypnosis. *Behav Brain Sci* 1986; **9**: 474–5.

15 Tart, C. T. A systems approach to altered states of consciousness. In: Davidson, J. M., Davidson, R. J. (eds.) *The Psychobiology of Consciousness*. New York: Plenum, 1980.

16 Sheehan, P. W., Perry, C. W. *Methodologies of Hypnosis: A Critical Appraisal of Contemporary Paradigms of Hypnosis*. New Jersey: Lawrence Erlbaum, 1976.

17 Abeles, G. Researching the unresearchable: experimentation on the double blind. In: Sluzki, C. E., Ransom, D. C. (eds.) *Double Blind: The Foundation of the Communicational Approach to the Family*. New York: Grune and Stratton, 1976.

[18] Bateson, G. Some components of socialisation for trance. *Ethos* 1975; **3**: 143–55.

[19] Hilgard, E. R. Hypnotic susceptibility and implications for measurement. *Int J Clin Exp Hypnosis* 1982; **30**: 394–403.

[20] Sampson, E. E. *Justice and The Critique of Pure Psychology*. New York: Plenum, 1983. Cushman, P. Why the self is empty: towards a historically situated psychology. *Am Psychologist* 1990; **45**: 599–611. Shweder, R. A., Bourne, E. J. Does the concept of the person vary cross-culturally? In: Shweder, R. A., LeVine, R. A. (eds.) *Culture Theory: Essays on Mind, Self and Emotion*. Cambridge: Cambridge University Press, 1984. Shweder, R. A. *Thinking Through Cultures: Expeditions in Cultural Psychology*. Cambridge, Mass.: Harvard University Press, 1991.

[21] Fourie, D. P., Lifschitz, S. Not seeing the wood for the trees: implications of susceptibility testing. *Am J Clin Hypnosis* 1988; **30**: 166–77.

[22] Diamond, M. J. Hypnotizability is modifiable: an alternative approach. *Int J Clin Exp Hypnosis* 1977; **25**: 147–66.

[23] Shor, R. E. A phenomenological method for the measurement of variables important to an understanding of the nature of hypnosis. In: Fromm, E., Shor, R. E. (eds.) *Hypnosis: Developments in Research and New Perspectives*. Aldine, 1979.

[24] Sheehan, P. W., McConkey, K. M. *Hypnosis and Experience: The Exploration of Phenomena and Process*. New Jersey: Lawrence Erlbaum, 1982.

[25] Sheehan, P. W. Contrasting research methodologies – humanism vs. standard method. *Aust J Psychol* 1982; **34**: 239–47.

[26] Schactel, E. G. *Metamorphosis*. London: Routledge and Kegan Paul, 1959.

[27] Levin, D. M. *The Opening of Vision: Nihilism and The Postmodern Situation*. London: Routledge, Chapman and Hall, 1988.

[28] Rossi, E. L. *The Psychobiology of Mind-body Healing: New Concepts of Therapeutic Hypnosis*. Norton, 1986.

[29] Rossi, E. L., Cheek, D. B. *Mind-body Therapy: Ideodynamic Healing in Hypnosis*. Norton, 1988.

[30] Diamond, M. J. It takes two to tango: some thoughts on the neglected importance of the hypnotist in an interactive hypnotherapeutic relationship. *Am J Clin Hypnosis* 1984; **27**: 3–13.

[31] Suppe, F. (ed.) *The Structure of Scientific Theories*. 2nd ed. University of Illinois Press, 1977. Polyani, M. *Personal Knowledge: Towards a Post-critical Philosophy*. London: Routledge and Kegan Paul, 1958.

[32] Minuchin, S. *et al. Psychosomatic Families: Anorexia Nervosa in Context*. Cambridge, Mass.: Harvard University Press, 1978.

[33] Skynner, A. C. R. An open systems, group analytic approach to family therapy. In: Gurman, A. S., Kniskern, D. P. (eds.) *Handbook of Family Therapy*. New York: Plenum, 1980.

[34] Russell, G. F. M. *et al.* An evaluation of family therapy in anorexia nervosa and bulimia nervosa. *Arch Gen Psychiat* 1987; **44**: 1047–56.

[35] Diamond, M. J. The interactional basis of hypnotic experience: on the relational dimension of hypnosis. *Int J Clin Exp Hypnosis* 1987; **35**: 95–115.

[36] Fricton, J. R., Roth, P. The effects of direct and indirect hypnotic suggestions for analgesia in high and low suggestible subjects. *Am J Clin Hypnosis* 1985; **27**: 226–31.

[37] Woolson, D. A. An experimental comparison of direct and Ericksonian hypnotic induction procedures and the relationship to secondary suggestibility. *Am J Clin Hypnosis* 1986; **29**: 23–8.

[38] Heron, J. Critique of conventional research methodology. *Comp Med Res* 1986; **1**: 12–22.

[39] Nugent, W. R. A methodological review of case studies published in the *American Journal of Clinical Hypnosis*. *Am J Clin Hypnosis* 1984; **27**: 191–200.

[40] Erickson, M. H. *The Collected Papers of Milton H. Erickson on Hypnosis. Volume 4: Innovative Hypnotherapy*. Rossi, E. L. (ed.) Irvington, 1980.

[41] Lambek, M. From disease to discourse: remarks on the conceptualisation of trance and spirit possession. In: Ward, C. A. (ed.) *Altered States of Consciousness and Mental Health*. London: Sage, 1989.

[42] Geertz, C. *The Interpretation of Cultures*. New York: Basic Books, 1973.

[43] Gergen, K. Social psychology as history. *J Pers Soc Psychol* 1973; **26**: 309–20.

[44] Sampson, E. E. *Justice and The Critique of Pure Psychology*. New York: Plenum, 1983.

[45] Kleinman, A. *The Social Origins of Distress and Disease*. Yale University Press, 1986.

[46] Shweder, R. A. *Thinking Through Cultures: Expeditions in Cultural Psychology*. Cambridge, Mass.: Harvard University Press, 1991.

[47] Levin, D. M. (ed.) *Pathologies of the Modern Self: Postmodern Studies on Narcissism, Schizophrenia and Depression*. New York: New York University Press, 1987.

[48] Smail, D. *Taking Care: An Alternative to Therapy*. London: Dent, 1987.

[49] Smail, D. Towards a radical environmentalist psychology of help. *Psychologist* 1991; **4**: 61–4.

[50] Keller, E. F. *Reflections on Gender and Science*. Yale University Press, 1985.

24 The evaluation of herbal medicines: an east Asian perspective

Kiichiro Tsutani

Introduction

Herbal medicine has long flourished in the eastern countries of the Eurasian continent. The 'test of time' has been used both by the public and by regulatory officials to determine therapeutic value in this part of the world. Herbal medicines which have been used over the ages are – or were – considered to have withstood the crucial test, the test of time itself, and to have 'proven' their efficacy and safety.

But in past decades, a new mood has developed with respect to the research and regulation of east Asian herbal medicines. New methods of evaluating the efficacy and safety of therapies have evolved in the West over the last half century. Gradually, these have been introduced to east Asia, where they have been employed increasingly by researchers and drug regulatory authorities to set regulatory standards, first for modern and then for traditional medicines.

It should be noted that the validation of therapeutic value cannot be made in a single study. Instead, validation relies on a series of studies ranging from non-clinical to clinical, including post-marketing surveillance. Appropriate legislation is crucial in helping regulatory authorities enforce and monitor the full verification process. Recently developed verification techniques, together with relevant laws, provide the new paradigm for reviewing the status and performance of traditional herbal medicine.

Traditional Chinese medicine with its variants in neighbouring countries is the dominant form of medical therapy in this part of the world. Introduced into Korea, Japan, Vietnam and other neighbouring countries over 1000 years ago, the original theories have been modified in accordance with each country's cultural and biomedical style. The Chinese themselves have played a role in disseminating their medical tradition through their migrations to and beyond south east Asia since the eighteenth century.

This chapter surveys recent developments in clinical studies and in the regulation of herbal medicine in China and Japan, two major countries in east Asia where herbal medicine is widely used. It describes the state of clinical studies, pertinent legislation in these countries, and discusses methodological, social, cultural, economic and political factors which affect the clinical evaluation of herbal medicine.

It is worth observing at the outset that China and Japan sustain not just one but a pluralism of medical traditions. In addition to traditional Chinese medicine and its variants, there are also a number of less well-articulated folk traditions. Chinese and Japanese folk medicines, however, interesting as they may be in their own right, will not be considered in this chapter.

China

1 Legislation

Law and provisions
As China is currently considered to have the most elaborate legislation on herbal medicine, it may be worthwhile introducing this legislation in some detail. It reflects the unique nature of herbal medicine and the research strategies of China.

The Law of the People's Republic of China on Drug Administration was enacted on July 1, 1985.[1] This is presently the basic law governing the administration of all drugs, including herbal medicines, in China. The law is aimed at guaranteeing the quality of drugs, improving their efficacy, assuring their safety, and safeguarding the physical health of the people. It is considered to adhere roughly to the same standard as corresponding laws in the West.

Pursuant to Articles 21 and 22 of the law, the Provisions for New Drug Approval were promulgated on the same day.[2] They contain general provisions and sections covering the classification and designation of new drugs, new drug research, the clinical investigation of new drugs, approval and production of new drugs, auxiliary provisions and annexes.

In Article 2 of this provision, the term 'new drugs' refers to 'drugs which have not been produced previously in this country', or to 'drugs for which a new indication, a change in the route of administration or a change of dosage form is to be adopted'. As defined here, new drugs are not only chemical entities derived from natural resources but also herbal medicines. This makes for a certain parallelism between traditional and Western drugs. The drugs are divided into two major categories with five classes in each, as shown in Table 24.1.

Two years later, on April 15 1987, a Supplementary Stipulations and Explanations of Issues Related to Traditional Chinese Drugs was appended to the provisions.[3] Unlike the law and the provision, English versions of which were issued together with the original Chinese text by the Ministry of Public Health (MOPH), only the Chinese version of this supplementary stipulations and explanations is available. It contains detailed stipulations on classification and data for application, material introduced and test cultivation, pharmacological and toxicological research, stability tests, and clinical investigation.

Traditional Chinese drugs
Since most of the traditional drugs consist of botanical materials, the title of my chapter uses the term 'herbal medicines' for the sake of convenience, although it is not strictly accurate. It should be recognized that some drugs referred to as herbal contain ingredients of animal and mineral origin. Other workers in this field in various countries have

Table 24.1 Classification of new drugs in China (1985)[2]

Traditional Chinese Drugs	
Class 1	Artificial imitations of traditional Chinese medicinal herbs: Newly discovered herbal drugs: Parts of a medicinal plant newly employed as a remedy.
Class 2	New dosage forms which cause a change in the traditional route of administration; Active principles extracted from natural resources and their preparations.
Class 3	New formulas of traditional Chinese drugs (including ancient formulas, confidential formulas, efficacious formulas and modified traditional formulas).
Class 4	Drugs for which a change in dosage form is to be adopted without changing the route of administration.
Class 5	Traditional Chinese OTC drugs for which a new indication is to be adopted.
Western Drugs	
Class 1	New drug substances and their preparations domestically initiated (including new chemical entities extracted from natural resources, new synthetic products and their preparations); New drug substances and their preparations reported in foreign literature but not approved by foreign authorities.
Class 2	Drug substances and their preparations which have already been approved by foreign authorities but no specification of which is found in a foreign pharmacopoeia.
Class 3	Compound preparations of western drugs: Combinations of traditional Chinese drugs with western drugs.
Class 4	Synthetic or semi-synethetic products of natural compounds known to be biologically active: Drug substances and their preparations which have already been approved by foreign authorities and whose specification can be found in a foreign pharmacopoeia: Drugs for which a change in dosage form or route of administration is to be adopted.
Class 5	Drugs for which a new indication is to be adopted.

encountered similar difficulty in providing strict definitions for 'herbal medicines', 'alternative drugs', 'traditional drugs', and other such terms. The classification provided in the provision may serve as a model for appropriate classification.

In the supplementary stipulations and explanations, examples in each class of traditional Chinese drugs are given. The gall stone of cattle artificially induced in the body, and the artificially drained gall bladder of bear (actually, the bile), are class 1, for example. Artificially fermented fungi are also class 1. Based on these official examples, it is presumed that drugs produced by biotechnology in the industrialized countries – callus formation methods, for example – may be considered class 1 as well. This applies as well to certain 'plants', such as ginseng, which are now produced in modern plant factories in several countries.

Non-single components extracted from plants, such as total flavone, alkaloid and glycoside, are considered class 2. Injectable forms of traditional Chinese drugs are also class 2. On the other hand, ingredients chemically purified from natural substances are covered by class 1 of Western drugs.

As used in this provision, the term 'traditional Chinese drugs' has an expanded meaning, as it applies also to drugs derived from 'non-traditional' materials and new production techniques. However, it can be observed that most drugs currently under study are either class 3 or 4 drugs, as these are easiest to develop.

Preclinical studies
The scope of new drug research in the provisions includes technical process, quality standard, preclinical pharmacological investigation and clinical investigation. The Investigational New Drug (IND) system was adapted from Western methods, i.e. before the clinical investigation, an application containing the required information specified in each category and class is to be approved by the drug regulatory authorities. The details of the requirements are indicated in Annexes 1 to 5 of the provisions. Annex 3 and Annex 4 show the list of required items with tables and remarks for IND and New Drug Application (NDA) covering the name of the new drug, constituents, and chemical, pharmacological, toxicological, pharmaceutical and clinical studies for Western drugs and traditional Chinese drugs respectively. Annexes 1 and 2 are application forms and Annex 5 contains the technical requirements for the pharmacological and toxicological studies.

When comparing the preclinical study requirements for Western drugs and traditional Chinese drugs in the provision, three major differences can be observed. First, recognizing the difficulty of chemically identifying all ingredients in traditional Chinese drugs, composed as they are of natural substances, the 'chemical structure or composition' of the drug is not required. Instead, data on 'physico-chemical properties relevant to its quality', and 'chemical and physical investigation on the active principle or active site' must be furnished.

Second, for traditional Chinese drugs, most of which consist of two or more natural substances and are considered to be combined drugs in the Western model, justification of the formula based on 'the theory and experience of traditional Chinese medical practice' is called for, in place of a clinical study.

Third, pharmacokinetics studies are not required for traditional Chinese drugs.

Clinical investigation

'Clinical investigation' is classified into 'clinical trial' and 'clinical verification'. The clinical trial is used for new drugs of classes 1, 2 and 3, while the clinical verification is used for classes 4 and 5. Clinical trials are usually carried out in three phases, clinical verification in a single phase. Clinical investigation of every new drug must be performed in at least three hospitals.

The definitions of each phase, however, do not completely correspond to the definitions of phases in the West. The premarketing phase consists of two phases (phase I and phase II), rather than the three phases of the West. Phase I in China has essentially the same objective as in the West, i.e. to explore possible toxic effects and determine a tolerated dose. Phase II is subdivided into two stages, the first being the 'controlled therapeutic trial' which generally uses at least 50 inpatients and adopts the double blind method as much as possible. The second stage is the 'extended controlled therapeutic trial', in which the double blind method is not generally necessary. The total number of cases in Phase II should not be less than 300, excluding the control group. Phase III in China consists basically of post-marketing studies which correspond to the phase IV studies of the West.

The sample size is stated in Article 12 of the provisions as follows. In clinical trials:

> 10–30 cases should be studied in phase I and not less than 300 cases in phase II; in addition, a control group should be maintained, the number of cases in the control group being dependent on the specialty of the treatment and statistical considerations.

And in clinical verification:

> not less than 100 cases should be studied in general; in addition, a control group should also be maintained, the number of cases in the control group being also dependent on the specialty of the treatment and statistical considerations.

Two points stand out here. The first is that the use of the control group has become mandatory. China came upon the notion of control groups early in its medical history but did not, until recently, make much use of controls. The first mention of a controlled study occurs in 1061 AD, in the *Bencao Tujing (Atlas of Materia Medica)*.[4] This Song dynasty text states:

> In order to evaluate the efficacy of ginseng, find two people and let one eat ginseng and run, and the other run without eating ginseng. The one that did not eat ginseng will develop shortness of breath sooner.

This is a classic model of the controlled study, and at the same time, a model of bioassay[5]. However, for the most part Chinese medicine did not benefit from this ancient example. Studies consisted, instead, of accumulated anecdotal evidence, and made no use of controls. Today's mandatory inclusion of control groups deserves to be recognized as a drastic and fundamental change in the evaluation of traditional drugs.

The second point worthy of note is that those factors usually considered in arriving at a sample size, such as difference to be detected, variance, type I and II error and possible drop-out ratio, were not mentioned in the provision. Instead, absolute numbers such as 100 or 300 are supplied. And although the highest statistical power is obtained when the control group has the same number of cases as the test group, special consideration with regards to treatment and statistics is given only to the number of cases in the control group.

This may reflect the underlying idea of the legislation – in order to give clinical investigators the clear and simple idea of a controlled study, exact numbers are provided. It may also be a reflection of the fact that the medical ethics of Chinese culture date back for such a long time, and may not be easily reconcilable to the idea of having a control group with the same number as a test group.

2 The guidelines for clinical investigations of traditional Chinese drugs

Overview of the guidelines
Along with the development of legislation, a total of 31 clinical pharmacological centres were established nationwide by the MOPH between 1983 and 1986.[6] Each centre was assigned a specialty in clinical pharmacology such as antibiotics, cardiovascular drugs, anticancer drugs, etc. The centres conduct clinical investigation, drug evaluation, post-market study, and so on. Eight centres are designated for traditional Chinese drugs.

One of the tasks of the centres is to develop guidelines for clinical investigations. So far, 15 draft guidelines for Western drugs and 48 draft guidelines for traditional Chinese drugs have been developed. Some of the guidelines for traditional Chinese drugs are published intermittently in *Acta Medica Sinica* in China. And in 1989, all 48 guidelines were compiled in a booklet by the MOPH[7].

Table 24.2 shows the headings of the guidelines. As the guidelines are not systematically ordered in the booklet, I have re-ordered them according to organ/ailment and diagnostic system. About half of them are for diseases as diagnosed by Western medicine. The rest are either for the *bing* (disease) or *zheng* (symptom-complex) as put forth by traditional Chinese medical (TCM) diagnosis.

The unique diagnostic system of TCM is already elucidated in several books in English.[8,9,10] Its major components include yin-yang, *wuxing* (five elements), *zang-fu* (viscera and bowels), and *qi-xue* (vital energy and blood).[11] The diagnostic system that uses the 'naked sense' observations of the physicians to reach therapeutic conclusions is called *bianzheng* (differentiation of symptom-complex).

Table 24.2 requires some explanation. *Bing* in TCM is either an entity defined aetiologically, such as ascariasis, or anatomically, such as carbuncle, erysipelas or haemorrhoids, or it is the most prominent sign or symptom of disease. While it is not easy, in English, to distinguish the *bing* of TCM diagnosis from the diseases of Western diagnosis, it is less difficult in Chinese as different characters are used. *Zheng* (symptom-complex), on the other hand, is a TCM entity which refers back to concepts specific to TCM, such as yin-yang, *zang-fu*, etc.

A brief explanation of three examples of guidelines with introductions to their major components may be useful at this point.

Guidelines for hypertension
In the guideline for hypertension, a Western diagnostic category, the entry criteria are the same as the WHO criteria for hypertension. But hypertension is further subdifferentiated into four traditional symptom-complex groups as follows: *ganhuo kangsheng*, exuberance of the liver-fire; *yin xu yang kang*, deficiency of yin with exuberance of yang; *yin yang liang xu*, deficiency of both yin and yang; and *tan shi yongsheng*, accumulation of phlegm-damp.

The phase I study employs 20 cases, preferably half being inpatients, with a test period of three weeks. The initial dose is one-tenth of the safety dose based on the subacute toxicity test, or the dose predicted as safe by group discussion, but not to exceed one-fifth of the safety dose. The total number of cases in the phase II study should be no less than 300, including 100 inpatients, and excluding control groups. Fifty cases each for the test and control group are required in one study. The use of randomized double blind methods is strongly recommended and the use of certain standard drugs, either Western or traditional Chinese, is also encouraged.

The endpoint is the reduction of blood pressure, but the evaluation standard for symptoms is also given in three levels: remarkably effective, effective, and not effective. The concept of quality of life (QOL) used in the West has yet to be adopted, but the evaluation of symptoms can supplement the reduction of blood pressure in determining the global usefulness of the drugs.

The phase III study aims at the evaluation of long-term efficacy and the monitoring of side effects.

Guidelines for stroke
In the guidelines for stroke in TCM diagnosis (the original Chinese for stroke – *zhongfeng* – means attack caused by wind), the entry criteria are the TCM diagnosis based mainly on objective symptoms. It is further subdifferentiated into nine symptom-complexes. It is recommended that modern medical diagnosis on the basis of a CT scan and a spinal fluid test accompany the TCM diagnosis. The phase I study requires no less than ten cases. The total number of cases in the phase II study should be no less than 200. No less than 50 cases are required in the control group.

Guidelines for deficiency syndrome of the spleen (pixu)
In the guidelines for deficiency syndrome of the spleen (*pixu*), the entry criteria for *pixu* are described in detail and are further subdifferentiated into six symptom-complexes. The Western diagnosis is also given. The evaluation standard is stated in detail based on subjective and objective symptoms, ending up with four categories as follows: clinically cured, remarkably effective, effective, and not effective.

Table 24.2 Guidelines of clinical investigation of traditional Chinese drugs (according to organ/ailment)

Organ/ailment	Diagnosis in Western medicine (disease)	Bing (disease)	Diagnosis in TCM Zheng (symptom-complex)
Cardiovascular	– cor pulmonale – hypertension	– pectoral pain with stuffiness	
Respiratory	– chr. bronchitis – acute pharyngitis – chr. pharyngitis – bronchial asthma – pulmonary tuberculosis	– heat in the lung in acute febrile disease caused by wind	
Digestive	– acute cholecystitis, cholelithiasis – peptic ulcer – viral hepatitis	– diarrhoea – gastralgia – haematemesis and tarry stool (bleeding of the upper digestive system)	– deficiency syndrome of the spleen – disharmony of the liver and stomach – disturbance of the spleen due to cold-damp, accumulation of damp-heat in the spleen – heat in the stomach, deficiency of yin of the lung – insufficiency of spleen with stagnancy in the liver – stuffiness and fullness in the chest and abdomen
Kidney and urinary	– chr. nephritis – urolithiasis – acute renal insufficiency	– oedema (acute nephritis) – dysuria (urinary infection)	
Neurological	– epidemic haemorrhagic fever – malaria	– stroke – blocking syndrome	– syncope and collapse
Infectious	– epidemic haemorrhagic fever – malaria		
Haemato and metabolic	– chr. aplastic anaemia – geriatric dis.	– diabetes (diabetes mellitus)	

Cancer	– primary bronchocarcinoma – primary hepatocarcinoma	
Surgical	– bone fracture – haemorrhoids	– lumbago and pain of legs – suppurative infection on body
Gynaecological	– inflammation of female reproductive organs	– dysmenorrhoea – menstrual disorders
Paediatric		– infantile diarrhoea – fever due to exogenosis infection (upper resp. infection)
Ophthalmological	– thrombosis of retinal vein	
Dermatological	– lupus erythematosus	– vitiligo

1 The grouping and ordering of guidelines is not in the original government document and is developed here by the author as an overview of the structure.

2 The disease and symptom-complex names under TCM diagnosis are stated using TCM terminology. Disease names of Western medicine in parenthesis appeared in the original guidelines.

It is stated that phase I study should be conducted on the basis of the Provisions for New Drug Approval and the Supplementary Stipulations and Explanations of Issues Related to Traditional Chinese Drugs. In the phase II study, the total number of cases should be no less than 300. Inpatients should be the major focus. The outpatient number should not exceed one-third of the total number of cases. Placebo or standard traditional Chinese drugs are to be used in the control group. The test period is from one week to six months depending on the type of disease.

3 Research status

Some issues in the guidelines
Although the law and the provisions are already being enforced, the guidelines are still in draft form. Certain points in the guidelines are difficult to understand. For example, the sample sizes for control groups are not clearly specified. Where subdifferentiation is stated, it is not clear whether the number of cases specified is for each subdifferentiation or for the total.

The meaning of the Western medical diagnosis for the clinical investigation of the *bing* and *zheng* of TCM diagnosis is also somewhat vague. The inclusion of Western categories may, from a clinical pharmacological point of view, have a number of conceivable aims: to ascertain comparability between test and control groups balancing the number and severity of Western medical diagnoses as background; to facilitate retrospective stratified analysis; to provide added description of the patient population.

Some parts of the guidelines appear to be inconsistent with other parts. For example, differences between the terms *linchuang zhiyu* (clinically cured) and *quanyu* (fully recovered) are unclear.

Actual conduct of studies along these guidelines may reveal strong points to be endorsed and weak points which will require revision. It will, however, take some time to make these distinctions.

Although laws and provisions do not state it clearly, a 'new drug' in China is generally considered to be one intended for commercial production.

Probably partly due to difficulties alluded to above, most studies published in Chinese medical journals do not seem to follow the guidelines. Most are conducted to validate the usefulness of existing drugs rather than to develop new ones. These studies re-evaluate traditional drugs or seek to clarify indications as used in TCM diagnosis in terms of the Western paradigm.

Ready-to-use form and traditional form
In China, there is no distinction between ethical (prescription) and OTC drugs. Commercially available traditional Chinese drugs in ready-to-use forms are called *zhongchengyao*, which is often translated as 'Chinese patent drugs'. It is estimated that since the establishment of New China in 1949, about 7000 brands of Chinese patent drugs have been approved by the drug regulatory authorities, either at provincial or central levels,

and currently about half of them are still on the market. Though accurate statistics are not available, it is estimated that half of the Chinese drugs used in China today are Chinese patent drugs. The rest are in classic dosage forms such as decoction, traditional pill form, etc. Chinese patent drugs are being re-evaluated, although the rate of re-evaluation is slow due to their complexity.

Chinese patent drugs are becoming more popular because of their easy administration, but the traditional decoction form is still thought to have the advantage of permitting prescriptions to be based on the individuality of the patient. Most such prescriptions are variations of standard formulae, but different substances can be combined as well, and doses of each can be varied.

In contrast to Chinese patent drugs, which are ready-made, drugs in traditional forms are tailored to the needs of the individual. Individual-oriented therapy, however, presents a variety of problems for group oriented evaluation techniques.

Acceptance of modern evaluation methods
There has been both acceptance of and resistance to modern evaluation methodology among practitioners of TCM. The old generation of TCM physicians is less supportive, the younger generation more so. This difference is due at least in part to the kind of education received. Older physicians were trained through the traditional system of apprenticeship. The young generation receives systematic education in TCM colleges, the curriculum of which covers both traditional and modern medicine.

Under these circumstances it is reasonable to expect that the basic concepts of modern evaluation methodology will be introduced not all at once but gradually into research on traditional drugs.

Search of the studies
In order to review the current status of the methodological aspects of the clinical study of herbal medicine in China, a preliminary search using Medline was conducted using the MeSH (Medical Subject Headings), covering the period of 1966 to October 1991. MeSH terms such as PLANTS, MEDICINAL; MATERIA, MEDICA; HERBS; PLANT, EX-TRACTS; MEDICINE, TRADITIONAL; MEDICINE, ORIENTAL TRADI-TIONAL; MEDICINE, CHINESE TRADITIONAL; DRUGS, CHINESE HERBAL were used to identify materials being studied. Terms such as CLINICAL TRIALS; DRUG EVALUATION; COMPARATIVE STUDY; RANDOM ALLOCATION; RANDOMIZED CONTROLLED TRIALS; SINGLE BLIND METHOD; DOUBLE-BLIND METHOD and PLACEBO were used to identify aspects of methodology.

A total of 148 studies were reported in China. Of these, 39 studies were retrieved by MeSH with either a double blind method, random allocation, randomized controlled study or placebo.

One major limitation of Chinese research was encountered. Out of 35 Chinese journals referred to in a MEDLINE printout, only two are in the field of TCM, namely *The Chinese Journal of Integrated Traditional and*

Western Medicine (*Chung hsi i chieh ho tsea chih* in the Wade system as used by MEDLINE, *Zhong xi yi jie he za zhi* in the Pinyin), and *The Journal of Traditional Chinese Medicine* in its English quarterly version (the original Chinese version appears monthly).

Most articles retrieved by MEDLINE are from the former journal. Its articles were incorporated into MEDLINE in 1985 and dated back to its first issue in 1981.

However, more than 50 journals in the field of TCM are published in China. At this point no computerized database exists in the field of the study of traditional Chinese drugs, although the Chinese plan to develop one. My group started to review the quality of clinical investigation in five major journals of TCM in China. The first randomized double blind study on traditional Chinese drugs may be the one on angina pectoris using drugs in injection form in 1983.[12]

After we have completed a chronological review we expect it will be easier to see that the elements of evaluation techniques – randomization, blindness and others – are gradually being introduced to China.

Japan

1 Kampo drugs

Historical perspectives
TCM is well known outside China, less through the translation of its medical classics than through the proliferation, in a variety of languages, of works for the layman. While Kampo medicine has not achieved anywhere near the same degree of international recognition, it is extremely popular in Japan. In fact, Japanese per capita consumption of herbal medicine may now be the highest in the world.

Kampo medicine is the Japanese variant of TCM. *Kam* or *Kan* means 'China' or '*Han* dynasty', as it was dating from this dynasty that Japan assimilated a large portion of Chinese culture. *Po* means 'method' or 'technique'. *Kampo* literally means 'Chinese method', although this term is restricted to use in the medical field. Since Chinese medicine was introduced into Japan more than 1000 years ago, it has naturally been modified to suit Japanese culture.

It was during the *Edo* period (1603–1868) that Kampo medicine underwent its unique development. Three factors were responsible.

First, the *Edo Shogunate* adopted an isolationist policy, which encouraged fermentation in Japanese culture. One powerful trend in some areas of culture in the mid-*Edo* period was the emphasis placed on the restoration of traditional values. Japanese Confucians idealized those periods of Chinese history when Confucianism was still in its original form. The same trend can be observed among Japanese physicians who idealized the practice of ancient Chinese medicine, and venerated Chinese classics in the field, particularly the *Shang Han Lun* (*Treatise of Febrile Disease*, third century).

Second, Dutch medicine was introduced through Nagasaki. During the

Edo period trade with the West was restricted to trade with the Dutch, and the Dutch, in turn, were restricted to the port of Nagasaki. This contact with the West was sufficient to bring new influences to bear on Japanese medicine. Physicians developed a way of thinking known as *shinshi jikken* (experimentation by him/herself), which placed value on experimental ideas.

Third, the endemic of syphilis, first introduced to Japan in 1512, created an urgent need for effective modes of treatment.[13] The form of TCM practised at that time was relatively ineffective in treating the disease. Consequently, Japanese physicians developed a practical system that directly related symptoms and treatment, bypassing the metaphysical concepts of Chinese medicine. This method is called *zuisho chiryo* (treatment according to symptom-complex).

These three factors helped shape Kampo as a variant of TCM.

The drugs used in Kampo medicine, incidentally, are known as Kampo drugs. Each Kampo drug is a formula usually consisting of 5–10 different herbs.

Modern features

New features have been introduced into the practice of Kampo. First, modern ready-to-use forms of the original formulae, most of which are produced in industrialized granular, powdered or other forms based on decoction, are widely used. Introduced in 1957, it is now estimated that more than 95% of Kampo drugs used in Japan are taken in ready-to-use form.

Most Kampo drugs are now used as ethical drugs in Japan. Since 1961, almost 100% of the Japanese population has been covered by the National Health Insurance (NHI). Forty three Kampo drugs for ethical use were included in the NHI Drug Price Tariff in 1976, joining a few predecessors. More Kampo drugs were included later, and now 147 Kampo drugs (as formulae) are available as ethical drugs. As these were already registered as drugs by the Ministry of Health and Welfare (MHW), their inclusion might be assumed to have been a matter of course. But it is worth remarking the rather unusual fact that their acceptance took place without clinical validation studies.

There were several major reasons for this. A strong lobby from the Japan Medical Association[14] took the position that Kampo drugs were suitable for the disease patterns of industrialized Japan, where chronic, degenerative disease and diseases of the elderly are prominent. Modern evaluation methods were viewed as insufficiently developed for use with Kampo drugs. Similar points were made by patient groups petitioning for Kampo drugs. In addition, there was strong lobbying from the Kampo drug manufacturing industry, anxious to enter this potential market.

Current use of Kampo drugs

After inclusion in the NHI scheme, the use of Kampo drugs doubled each year so that by 1990 it had reached JYE 162 billion (US$1·3 billion using the exchange rate of US$1 = JYE125) (Figure 24.1). A seventeen-

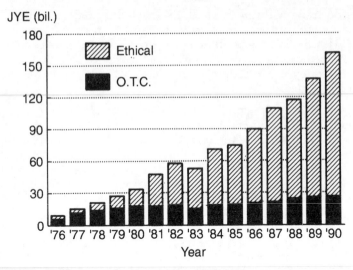

Fig. 24.1   Kampo drug production during 1976–1990.

fold increase in the use of Kampo drugs was reported during the period 1976–1990,[15] compared to a 2.8-fold increase in the use of pharmaceutical drugs over the same time. The annual use of Kampo drugs is now $10 per capita (Japan's population is 124 million), possibly the greatest expenditure for traditional drugs in the world. This constitutes nearly 3% of the total drug expenditure of Japan. Japan already has a problem with the overuse of drugs.[16] The per capita use of pharmaceutical drugs is US$390 as of 1990, also the highest in the world.

The top ten formulae of Kampo drugs constitute more than 80% of sales in the Japanese market. The leading formula is *Shosaikoto* (*Xiaochaihutang* in Chinese) consisting of seven herbs, developed in the third century, and sometimes called Minor Decoction of Bupleurum in English.

Among the reasons for this rapid increase in the use of Kampo drugs in Japan, one can suggest that their inclusion in the National Health Insurance scheme met certain health needs in Japan, both biomedical, which concerns the efficacy and safety of drugs, and cultural, which is to do with the country's history and its system of beliefs handed down generation to generation.[17]

2   Legislation

New Kampo drugs
Today, new Kampo drugs are regulated in essentially the same way as Western drugs in Japan. Unlike China, there is no independent major regulation for traditional drugs in Japan. They are regarded as a form of combined drug, and the same data required for new Western drugs is required for new Kampo drugs in the NDA. The time-consuming and expensive chronic toxicity test and special toxicity tests such as mutagenicity, carcinogenicity and teratogenicity depending on the

possible length of treatment and indications are applied to new Kampo drugs. Data for three phased clinical trials is also required.

However, because of technical and financial difficulties, subjecting new Kampo drugs to the same preclinical and clinical studies as Western drugs has had the effect of slowing down or completely preventing their development.

For the generic Kampo drugs, bioequivalency data is required, which again discourages development. Pharmacokinetic studies of Kampo drugs are difficult to conduct and bioassay methods are quite limited. This may reflect a government policy to limit the use of Kampo drugs until suitable evaluation methods are developed.

Quality control
There was an improvement in the quality control of Kampo drugs in the mid-1980s. After a report on poor quality control, the Advisory Committee for Kampo Drugs was established in 1982 in close association with the Pharmaceutical Affairs Bureau of the MHW. The Working Group on the Quality of Kampo Drugs was established and, three years later, a new regulation was issued by the Pharmaceutical Affairs Bureau setting standards for the manufacture and quality control of Kampo drugs.

This ensured that the quality of herbs used in each original formula would meet with precise standards. The regulations also called for quality monitoring of specific ingredients using at least two different chemically or physical methods to test them. (Generally speaking, no more than 30% of the active ingredients should be lost when finished products are prepared from standard decoctions.) Since October 1986, new Kampo drugs meeting these criteria have appeared.

Good Manufacturing Practice (GMP), a standard required of pharmaceutical drugs issued by MHW in 1976, is also applied to Kampo drugs. In addition, in 1988 the Japan Kampo Medicine Manufacturers Association drew up self-imposed guidelines that take into consideration the unique nature of Kampo drugs.

Re-evaluation of Kampo drugs
Since 1971, the MHW has been running a programme for the re-evaluation of all drugs marketed before 1967. In 1967 the Japanese government instituted a new policy requesting scientific evidence for the efficacy and safety of new drugs. Results of the first re-evaluation of ethical drugs approved prior to 1967 have been made public in several instalments since 1973, and those of the second re-evaluation of ethical drugs approved from October 1967 to March 1980, since 1988. Re-evaluation of more than 99% and 58% of the total number of the products has been completed in the first and second re-evaluations respectively. A new system to re-evaluate the efficacy and safety of all ethical drugs every five years was launched in 1988.

In the course of these programmes, Kampo drugs were one of two categories considered difficult to evaluate. The other was the Bio Response Modifier (BMR) for cancer.

BMRs became a major issue in the second cycle because of the huge use of them and questions as to their efficacy. Kampo drugs had never been subjected to re-evaluation procedures and became items of the new evaluation programme. Being aware of the rapid growth of the use of Kampo drugs, the small Working Group for the Clinical Evaluation Methodology of Kampo drugs was set up in 1989 in association with the Pharmaceutical Affairs Bureau, and in September 1990, the Examination Group for the Re-evaluation was also created.

Among the issues discussed in these groups were differences in diagnostic systems between Kampo medicine and modern medicine; group oriented evaluation *vs.* individual oriented evaluation; entry criteria and endpoint; and randomization, blindness and placebo formulation. Special attention was given to *Shosaikoto*, widely used for chronic hepatitis. It is estimated that this drug is employed by nearly 1 million Japanese. Guidelines for the clinical trial of this formula in chronic hepatic disorder were developed by the working group and issued in December 1991. The aim was to develop a model of clinical trials, to explore their feasibility, and to provide evaluation criteria for the quality of the study. Eight formulae, including *Shosaikoto*, were designated for re-evaluation by the MHW in February 1991. Results will appear in 1993.

Post-marketing surveillance (PMS)
The MHW has three major systems for the collection of domestic adverse reaction data. The first is the Adverse Drug Reaction Monitoring System. 2915 monitoring hospitals have been designated and requested to report cases of adverse reaction to the MHW. This is a 'voluntary' monitoring system. 1158 cases of adverse reaction were reported in 1990. Fifteen of these cases pertained to Kampo drugs.

The second data collection system is the Pharmacy Monitoring System formed by 2733 pharmacies. This system mainly collects data on cases of adverse reaction to OTC drugs. In recent years, about 400 cases have been reported annually. Among these, reactions caused by Kampo drugs are the most common, though most adverse reactions are minor, involving symptoms such as gastric discomfort and skin problems. Fifty cases were reported in 1989.

The third system is Adverse Reaction Reporting from Manufacturers. Several severe cases caused by *Shosaikoto*, including drug-induced hepatitis and pneumonitis, were documented at medical conferences and in journals and were reported to the MHW by the company responsible in 1990.

In addition, since 1988, the newly drafted Good Post-Marketing Surveillance Practice (GPMSP) has been used as a pilot scale for Western drugs dispensed in Japan. When new Kampo drugs are approved and appear on the market, this guideline will apply to them as well.

3 Research status

Search of the studies
A literature search was attempted using computerized databases of the medical literature in Japanese from 1975 until September 1991

(JICST7580 for 1975–1980 and JMEDLINE for 1981–1991). *Kampoyaku, Shoyaku, Shokubutsuseizai, Wakanyaku* were among the key words used in the search. A sharp increase in the number of papers was seen in the early 1980s, and currently around 1000 papers on Kampo drugs are produced annually in Japan (Figure 24.2). Half of these were studies using human subjects. But when using key words such as randomization, blind methods, placebo and so on, only 19 papers were retrieved.

A manual search was then conducted to supplement the computer search, and eventually a total of 59 controlled studies were found, the

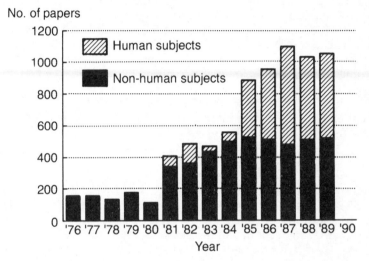

Fig. 24.2 Number of papers on Kampo drugs (data for 1990 is incomplete).

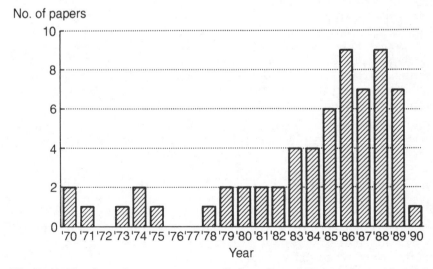

Fig. 24.3 Number of papers on controlled studies of Kampo drugs (data for 1990 is incomplete).

first appearing in 1970. The minimum requirement of the manual search was that the study had a comparative group.

Preliminary analysis of these papers revealed common problems of poor experimental design, lack of randomization, vague justification of dose setting, unclear entry criteria, lack of consideration for *sho* (see below), unclear endpoints, lack of appropriate follow-up, inappropriate handling of drop-out cases, inappropriate statistical analysis and insufficient experimental details to justify the conclusions. Details of the quality of these studies will be reported soon by the writer.[18]

Japan, unlike China, does not have traditional medical physicians. All Japan's 80 medical schools teach modern medicine, with the exception of a few which offer a short course of training in Kampo medicine as well.[19] Thus, most studies of Kampo drugs are based on modern diagnoses. Nevertheless a few investigators have an interest in the *sho*. The same Chinese character as *zheng* is used to describe *sho* in Japan, but the concept of *sho* in Kampo medicine is somewhat different from that of *zheng* in China. *Sho* is the therapeutic entity for which a specific Kampo formula is to be used. For instance, the *sho* of *Shosaikoto* is the specific symptom-complex for which Shosaikoto should be applied.

I will discuss two randomized clinical trials which gave consideration to the *sho*.

Example 1
The first was the multi-centre, randomized, double blind placebo controlled study of *Unseiin* for Behcets disease conducted in 1984–85. (*Unseiin*, or *Wenqingyin* in Chinese, developed in the sixteenth century, consists of eight herbs, and is sometimes known as Tang-Kuei and Gardenia Combination in English.)

Four points merit mention. First, this study is one of the first to use a placebo in granule form. There had been widespread concern that placebo preparation was impossible because of this drug's unique appearance, taste and smell.[20] More than ten test placebo formulae were developed and subjected to the sensory test. The duo-trio method was applied using 20 testers, including ten males and ten females. The formula was improved gradually, and in the end its appearance, taste and smell approximated true *Unseiin*. The blindness of the placebo formulae used in the double blind study was confirmed.

Second, in order to ensure accurate identification of drugs and to ascertain that the drugs studied were the same as those marketed, blinded chemical testing of the drugs was conducted. Special ratios of the true drugs and placebo were mixed, and measurement of leading ingredients which may reflect the potency of drugs such as berberine, baicalein, geniposide and paeoniflorin were made. These ratios were withheld from the chemists. After receiving the chemists' reports, the original chemical content was calculated using the ratio of mixture. It was planned that the results of this chemical study would be published in the article of the study.

Third, from the Kampo medical diagnosis of Behcets disease patients,

臨床試験調査表

TJW-59057A

薬剤番号	組	番
施 設 名		
担当医師名	署名	印
試験責任者名	署名	印

記入上の注意
○ ボールペンまたはペンで記入して下さい。
○ 訂正箇所には必ず訂正印を押して下さい。
○ 番号の付いているものは適応するところに○印をつけて下さい。

カルテ №		試験開始日 昭和　年　月　日	試験終了日 昭和　年　月　日

| 患者名 | | 1. 男　2. 女　年令　　才 | 体 重　　kg 身 長　　cm |
| | | | 生年月日 M.T.S　年　月　日 |

1. 入院（ 年 月 日 ）　2. 外来　3. 入院⇄外来　　罹病期間　　　年　　カ月

診 断　病 型　1. 完全型　2. 不全型
特殊病型　1. なし　2. 神経ベーチェット病　3. 血管ベーチェット病　4. 腸管ベーチェット病

既往症　1. あ り　2. な し（但し、現症に関係をもつもの）
（ありの場合）疾患名

合併症　1. あ り　2. な し
（ありの場合）疾患名

開始時漢方的症状

体 格	1.肥満型	2.普通	3.やせ型	舌	1.乾燥	2.普通	3.湿潤
血 色	1.あから顔	2.普通	3.青白い	舌 苔	1.厚い	2.薄い	3.ない
筋肉のしまり	1.緊張	2.普通	3.弛緩	小 便	1.近い	2.普通	3.遠い
腹壁緊張	1.強い	2.普通	3.弱い	便 通	1.便秘	2.普通	3.下痢
皮 膚	1.乾燥	2.普通	3.湿潤	手 足	1.ほてる	2.普通	3.冷える
脈 拍	1.強い	2.普通	3.弱い	汗	1.多い	2.普通	3.少ない
不 眠	1.強くある	2.弱くある	3.ない	不 安	1.強くある	2.弱くある	3.ない

＊前治療薬

薬 剤 名	投 与 量	投 与 期 間
	／日	年　月　日〜　年　月　日
	／日	年　月　日〜　年　月　日
	／日	年　月　日〜　年　月　日
	／日	年　月　日〜　年　月　日
	／日	年　月　日〜　年　月　日
	／日	年　月　日〜　年　月　日
	／日	年　月　日〜　年　月　日

患者の同意　昭和　年　月　日　1. 口 答　2. 文 書

＊ 前治療薬剤　・4週間以内の使用薬剤　但し、コルヒチン、免疫抑制剤、免疫調節剤、
金製剤、D－ペニシラミンについては、3カ月以内に中止した薬剤も記入のこと。

Fig. 24.4 Cover page of the case report form including the checklist of signs considering the *sho* of *Unseiin*.

several formulae are considered suitable for the different *shos* in the disease. But most physicians participating in the study had insufficient knowledge of Kampo medicine. Thus it was agreed that the entry criteria for the trial should be a modern diagnosis, but for the retrospective stratified analysis a special checklist was developed and included in the case reports (Figure 24.4). The items in the list are the signs which reflect the nature of the disease and the constitution of the patient. Having the physician who participated in the trial fill out the *sho* diagnosis was also discussed in the planning stages, but was not implemented as most participating physicians were untrained in Kampo medicine.

Lastly, there was a certain gap in the efficacy ratio between preceding open studies and the controlled study. Before the controlled study, several studies had been made showing a high efficacy rate. Most of the studies have one or a few patients who were successfully treated by *Unseiin*, and one open study with 30 patients reported a 60% efficacy rate, including slightly effective cases (30% excluding slightly effective cases).

One hundred and ninety two patients were employed in the controlled study, the results of which were negative. There was no significant difference between the outcomes for the two groups. The true drug efficacy ratio was 47% (23% excluding slightly effective cases), and for the placebo group, 41% (25%). Seven and six cases respectively were reported to have side effects in each group. A difference in the efficacy ratio was noted between previous open studies and this blinded study.

Retrospective stratified analysis was performed. Aside from the ordinary strata such as sex, ages, and severity of the disease, special strata were constructed from the special checklist that took into account the *sho* of *Unseiin*, with the traditional indications of the formula such as dry skin, red face, flushing at extremities, and so on. But this stratified analysis again did not show significant differences between the true and placebo groups. Several additional strata were constructed but all 'data dredging' efforts were unproductive. The study has not yet been published.

The points which can be learned from this study, in which I was involved, are as follows. A careful review of existing studies justifying large scale multi-centre randomized study is important. And the phased manner approach should also be adopted in clinical trials of Kampo drugs, i.e. from the exploratory small scale study including careful dose ranging and finding the condition to be treated, to the large scale confirmatory study.

Example 2
The second example was a multi-centre, randomized, controlled trial for diabetic neuropathy.[21] The efficacy of *Goshajinkigan* (*Niucheshenqiwan* in Chinese, consisting of eight herbs, developed in the third century, sometimes called Achyranthes and Plantago Formula in English), was evaluated using envelope methods. Mecobalamin (methyl vitamin B_{12}) was used in the control group. Ninety four cases entered the trial and eight cases dropped out. It is not clear from the paper which drop-out cases were from which group, but it is presumed that most were from the mecobalamin group, as the final number of cases for statistical analysis was 48 and 38 respectively.

Three points of interest emerge from this study.

First, there were different compliance patterns between test and control groups. A background analysis for checking comparability of the groups revealed that those who had the disease chronically were more compliant to *Goshajinkigan*. This was especially so among those who had suffered with the disease for more than 20 years. Eight finished the study in this Kampo drug, while only one in the control group finished. Second, multiple endpoints were used, i.e. 28 subjective signs, three objective signs, ten laboratory examinations. Besides global improvement rate assessed by the patients, efficacy assessed by physician, and usefulness which summarizes the improvements, efficacy and laboratory examinations were also analysed. Decrease in numbness was reported as a statistically significant difference between the test and control groups. But there was a problem of repeated statistical testing in the study. This kind of bad use of statistical testing was found not only in Kampo drug trials, but also more generally in clinical trial literature until very recently. The MHW issued guidelines on the statistical analysis of clinical studies in 1992.

Lastly, the more interesting point in the paper is that multivariate analysis was adopted to see the relation between the outcome and *sho*. The Hayashi's Quantitative Method I[22] was used. This is a modified multiple regression analysis giving dummy variables in categorical and ordered data.

The global improvement rate was used as a dependent variable; demographic data, subjective and objective signs were used as independent variables. It was found from this analysis that the more severe cases, involving moderate numbness, lower Broca's index, and aged between 50–69, with duration of less than ten years, had better improvement (Figure 24.5). However, while this is an interesting analysis it is still not clear whether this indicates the *sho* for *Goshajinkigan* or the general patient profile of diabetic neuropathy, since the corresponding analysis of the control group was not mentioned in the paper.

Having raised these two examples for discussion, let me say that my goal in criticism is to stimulate further improvements in the clinical trials of Kampo drugs.

Discussions and conclusions

1 Research and legislation

Very often herbal medicines are seen as so unusual that current research methodology is regarded as inappropriate for them. But I would maintain that so far as clinical evaluation is concerned, only two basic differences obtain between east Asian herbal medicines and modern drugs. The first is that herbal medicines consist of natural products. The second is that east Asian diagnostic systems differ from those used in modern medicine.

VARIABLE CODE (Factors)		Cases	RANGE Markedly improved ....Aggravated
Severity (before treatment)			
0	Asymptomatic	0	
1	Slight	4	
2	Moderate	17	
3	Severe	13	
4	Very severe	9	
Numbness (before treatment)			
0	Asymptomatic	1	
1	Slight	5	
2	Moderate	15	
3	Severe	11	
4	Very severe	11	
Control of diabetes			
1	Good	15	
2	Fair	18	
3	Poor	10	
Broca's index			
1	~ 79%	0	
2	80 ~ 89%	4	
3	90 ~ 109%	23	
4	110 ~ 119%	9	
5	120%~	7	
Age (years)			
1	~ 39	1	
2	40 ~ 49	4	
3	50 ~ 59	22	
4	60 ~ 69	8	
5	70 ~	8	
Duration (years)			
1	~ 1	0	
2	1 ~ 5	9	
3	5 ~ 10	6	
4	10 ~ 20	20	
5	20 ~	8	

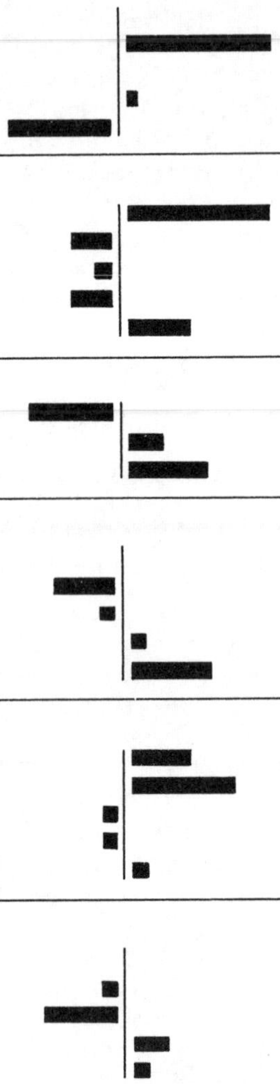

Fig. 24.5 Factors affecting efficacy in relation to the *sho* of *Goshajinkigan.*

These differences, however, need not affect evaluation methodology, which can be the same for both kinds of drug. In both cases evaluation relies on the same series of studies ranging from non-clinical to clinical, including post-marketing surveillance.

However, in order to enforce evaluation in this full range, clearly stated policies with the force of law are required.

For example, the Kefauver-Harris amendment of the Food, Drug and

Cosmetic Act passed in the US in 1962, by requiring 'substantial evidence' of drug effectiveness, boosted the wide use of evaluation methods such as randomization and blindness in drug development. The impact of appropriate legislation on clinical studies can hardly be overstated.

However, in some countries herbal medicine remains outside the scope of legislation. Some of these countries exclude herbal medicine because they have an extremely strong biomedical perspective which recognizes only purified compounds as drugs. Other countries have poor regulatory mechanisms which retard the development of legislation pertaining to drugs in general, herbal remedies included.

I hope that the above consideration of herbal medicine in east Asia can be of some assistance to these countries.

2 Different policies in the evaluation of herbal medicine

Returning to the comparison of China and Japan with regard to the evaluation of herbal medicine, it can be observed that while China gives strong support to the development of new herbal medicine, backed up by necessary legislation, Japan's main emphasis at present is on re-evaluation, basically a post-marketing study of already existing formulae.

China's elaborate legislation in this field may be attributed to the fact that previously its legislation was quite underdeveloped. During the cultural revolution, especially, many 'new traditional Chinese drugs' were marketed without appropriate evaluations. When Chinese officials decided to regulate all drug therapies, they availed themselves of information on legislation abroad without losing sight of the unique position herbal medicine enjoys in China, with its strong public and political support. The result was a unique and extensive body of law. Although many studies on herbal medicine do not yet adhere to modern evaluation methods, it can be expected that such adherence will come gradually.

In Japan, however, legislation plays a different role. Japanese legislation resembles the Kefauver-Harris amendment in the US, with its focus on chemically purified drugs. This may be the reason why Kampo drugs came to be re-evaluated last. Due to the nature of Kampo drugs, Western methods of evaluation developed for chemically purified drugs seeemed difficult to adopt.

One reason for the recent movement towards the re-evaluation of Kampo drugs may well be Japan's escalating national drug expenditure, paralleled in other industrialized countries. There have already been several efforts by the regulatory authorities to force national drug costs down. In 1983, for example, a vain attempt was made to eliminate vitamins and Kampo drugs from the NHI Drug Price Tariff. It is conceivable, however, that the result of widespread testing might, by establishing the efficacy of drugs, lead to an increase in their consumption.

3 Economic and disease pattern influences in the evaluation of herbal medicine

In China, with the exception of some tonic drugs, herbal medicine is still considered to be inexpensive in comparison to Western drugs. In Japan, the situation is reversed. Japan imports more than 90% of Kampo drug material such as bark, fruit, root, and stem from abroad, primarily from China. It is generally recognized in Japan that Kampo drugs are more expensive than Western drugs. However, almost no rigorous cost-effectiveness studies have been conducted in either China or Japan to date.

Different disease structures exist in the two countries. Though China's disease patterns are rapidly changing to those prevalent in an industrialized country, certain infectious diseases still prevail. Consequently there are guidelines for the clinical investigation of traditional Chinese drugs for malaria and tuberculosis. It is worth noting that guidelines for cancer have been developed as well, and may be applicable in both developing and developed countries.

There used to be little incentive for the Kampo drug companies of Japan to conduct scientifically sound studies. Kampo drugs were already on the market and already included in the National Health Insurance scheme. 'Risky' controlled studies which could yield negative results were therefore studiously avoided. However, the recently initiated re-evaluation programme is expected to lead to a greater quantity of such studies and to improve their quality.

In short, one can conclude that in addition to a constant biomedical need for clinical studies of herbal medicines, various economic, cultural and political needs come into play as well.

4 Acceptance of evaluation methodology and people's attitudes

A two-fold response to modern evaluation methods was seen in China, and in Japan as well, although there are no officially registered traditional physicians in Japan. In both countries there are 'modernists', strong supporters of modern evaluation methodology. These are countered by 'traditionalists', who oppose the application of such methods. Traditionalists emphasize the individual nature of diagnosis and therapy and dislike what they see as the cold, mechanical, and artificial aspects of such techniques as randomization and blindness. It may be argued, however, that traditionalists oppose these methods without fully understanding them.

A further question pertaining to the acceptance of medicines is who, in the end, is to be the final arbiter? Should it be patients, physicians or drug regulatory authorities?

The modern history of drug regulation shows that authority has been increasingly entrusted by the public to the drug regulatory authorities. This is based on an assumption that consumers – patients and physicians both – lack the means to evaluate the efficacy and safety of drugs. Only recently has this authority to evaluate drugs come under fire as 'paternalism', particularly by AIDS activist groups in the United States.[23]

There is an interesting similarity between the attitude of AIDS activists and that of many consumers of herbal medicine. In both cases significant numbers of people insist that they, and not the authorities, should decide upon the value of medicines they use. In the case of AIDS this is because the disease is life-threatening, the need for remedy urgent, and the process of verification slow. In the case of herbal medicine it has to do with other factors: the drugs consist entirely of natural (and therefore, presumably, trustworthy) products; they are used primarily on common diseases; their use derives from unique systems of diagnosis.

5 The unique character of herbal medicine in east Asia

Mixture of the individual-group relation and the different systems of diagnosis
As described above, the *bing* and *zheng* in China and *sho* in Japan are based on unique diagnostic systems. Some proponents of these systems claim that modern evaluation methods are inappropriate, but this is symptomatic of a misunderstanding about modern evaluation methods prevalent in east Asia.[5]

Differences in diagnostic systems have nothing to do with the randomization and blindness methods used to minimize bias in clinical trials. Techniques such as stratification used to minimize variability in a study are similarly unaffected by the diagnostic system used. They can be applied to any diagnostic system subjected to clinical trial.

The individual approach is always emphasized in east Asian medicine, and it is the case, as traditional practitioners assert, that a disease as diagnosed by Western medicine can be broken down into many subcategories by traditional medicine. It is less commonly recognized, but no less true, that the disease categories of traditional medicine can be subcategorized by Western medicine.

The whole issue of different diagnostic systems is often confused with the issue of individual-group relations. This may be because traditional diagnostic systems are more sophisticated with regard to symptoms than Western medicine.

It is useful in this connection to understand that the *zheng* and *sho* have layered structures. At the bottom of the structure, each patient has a different *zheng* or *sho* and is to be treated differently, whereas at the higher level each patient conforms to a population group. Theoretically, the clinical trial could be done at the higher level without serious deviation from the individual *zheng* or *sho* diagnosis.

The daily practice of medicine and clinical trials have purposes whose differences are all too often overlooked or misunderstood. The clinical trial is fundamentally group-oriented in certain diagnostic categories. Information derived from the study is applied, in treatment, with appropriate individual variations as becomes evident, for example, when the results of a fixed dose clinical trial are applied with variation of doses based on patient constitution and the conditions of disease.

Entry criteria and endpoints
The concepts of entry criteria and endpoints are not yet well recognized

in clinical trials in east Asian traditional medicine. Instead, the 'indication' is widely used. 'Indication' has two meanings for evaluation in clinical trials – entry criteria and endpoint. Specific endpoints could be formulated and stated in the research protocol on the basis of each diagnostic system. Specific concepts using suitable words would be used (in protocol and case report forms) depending on the medical education, traditional or modern, of the investigators.

There are two different kinds of endpoints in herbal medical research. The first are the endpoints of modern medicine, such as blood pressure for hypertension studies and blood glucose level in diabetic studies. If herbal medicine is applied to a modern medical diagnosis, the hard data employed for the evaluation of modern drugs should also usually be employed. In some cases, however, subjective and objective symptoms can still be appropriate endpoints, as in chest pain for angina pectoris and the symptoms of most psychiatric diseases.

The second kind of endpoints are the traditional medical endpoints. Aside from the conventional subjective and objective symptoms, the improvement of the *zheng* and *sho* could serve as major endpoints. It is this which may reflect the original strengths and advantages of east Asian herbal medicine. The recently developed concept of Quality of Life (QOL) is more closely related to such traditional targets of treatment. QOL endpoints resemble traditional notions of better 'balance' in the body.

The concept of 'usefulness' is often employed in evaluating therapy in east Asia. 'Usefulness' aims at an assessment balanced between the demands of efficacy and safety. For instance, in self-limiting diseases such as the common cold, the safety of the therapy is of greatest importance; serious side effects would be unjustified. In the case of life-threatening diseases such as cancer, on the other hand, some side effects will be tolerated for the sake of efficacy. Though this is reasonable and may reflect the idea of 'balance' prevalent in east Asian thought, it sometimes obscures the concept of a clear endpoint.

These two concepts, i.e. entry criteria and endpoint, are confused by most physicians and investigators in east Asian traditional medicine, a situation which would in all likelihood change if there were more opportunities to study modern evaluation methods.

If, despite all that has been said, one nevertheless strongly insists on the individualized nature of herbal medicine, there are alternatives to the conventional randomization of drugs besides literature control, historical control, matching, etc. The physician or hospital, for example, could serve as the unit of randomization to help derive comparative groups for evaluation. This may retain the individualism of herbal medicine, though at a cost in weaknesses of design and possibly inferior quality of information.

I have limited myself in this paper to describing the status of herbal medicine with regard to modern evaluation techniques in China and Japan, but I would like to add at this point that China and Japan are not the only countries in this region where such considerations apply. In Vietnam, the Republic of Korea (South Korea), the Democratic People's Republic of Korea (North Korea) and some south east Asian countries where overseas Chinese practise traditional medicine, similar issues are being raised in an effort to improve the quality of clinical trials of herbal medicine.[24,25,26]

Acknowledgement

The writer is a former medical officer responsible for the traditional medicine programme in the WHO Regional Office for the Western Pacific. The current chapter was written during his stay at the Takemi programme in International Health, Harvard School of Public Health. He expresses gratitude for the cooperation provided by Dr Xie Zhufan, the director of the Institute of Integration of Traditional and Western Medicine, Beijing Medical University and Dr Peter Goldman, Professor of Clinical Pharmacology, Harvard Medical School.

References

1 *Zhonghua Renmin Gongheguo Yaopin Guanlifa* (Law of the People's Republic of China on Drug Administration). Beijing: The State Council, 1984. An English version of the law can be found in Cui Yueli (ed.) *Public Health in the People's Republic of China*. Beijing: People's Medical Publishing House & Medical China Publishing Ltd., 1987.

2 *Xinyao Shenpi Banfa* (Provisions for New Drug Approval). Beijing: The Ministry of Public Health, 1985 (in Chinese and English).

3 *Xinyao Shenpi Banfa* (*Youguan Zhongyao Wenti de Buchong Guiding he Shuoming*) (Supplementary Stipulations and Explanations of Issues Related to Traditional Chinese Drugs to the Provisions for New Drug Approval). Beijing: Ministry of Public Health, 1987 (in Chinese).

4 *Bencao Tujing* (*Atlas of Materia Medica*), 1061. From bibliographical study the original text is considered to have disappeared. The extract is quoted in *Jingshi Zhenglei Daguan Bencao*, 1108. The photolithograph of this is published from *Kuoli Chungkuo Yihsueh Yenchiuso* (National Institute of Chinese Medicine), p. 140. Taipei: 1971.

5 Tsutani, K. Dentoyaku no Hikakushiken no Rekishi to Genjo (The history and the present status of controlled study of traditional medicine). *Igaku no Ayumi* (*Journal of Clinical and Experimental Medicine*) 1985; **132**(2): 103–6.

6 *Drug Administration in China*. This brochure describing the current status of drug administration in China was issued from the Ministry of Public Health in 1988, both in Chinese and in English.

7 *Xinyao* (*Zhongyao*) *Linchuang Yanjiu Zhidao Yuanze* (*Guidelines for Clinical Investigation of New Drugs* (*Traditional Chinese Drugs*)). Beijing: Drug Policy and Administration Bureau of the Ministry of Public Health, 1989 (in Chinese).

8 Unschuld, P. U. *Medicine in China: A History of Ideas*. Berkeley: University of California Press, 1985.

9   Sivin, N. *Traditional Medicine in Contemporary China*. Ann Arbor: Center for Chinese Studies, University of Michigan, 1987.

10 Wiseman, N., Ellis, A. *Fundamentals of Chinese Medicine*. Brooklyn: Paradigm Publications, 1985.

11 For the translation of TCM terms, I consulted Xie Zhufan & Huang Xiaokai (eds.) *Dictionary of Traditional Chinese Medicine*. Hong Kong: The Commercial Press, 1984.

12 Shan Ping, *et al.*, Huangyangning Zhiliao Guanxinbing – Yong Shuanmangfa Guangcha 110 Li Lingchuang Liaoxiao Fenxi (Analysis of the effect of *Buxus harlandii* on coronary heart disease by double blind method. Report of 110 Cases. *Zhong Yi Zazhi (Journal of Traditional Chinese Medicine)* 1983; **24**(5): 357–60.

13 Yamamoto, I. Nihon Kampo: Koho e no Shotai (Japanese Kampo medicine: introduction to Koho). *Kampo Kenkyu* 1981; **116**: 282–316 (in Japanese).

14 Yakazu, D. Takemi Kaicho ga Kampo Seizai wo Yakka Kijun ni Tosai no Ketsui wo surumade no Haikei (Background of the decision of inclusion of Kampo drugs in the National Health Insurance by Dr Takemi, President of the Japanese Medical Assocation). *Kampo no Rinsho* 1987; **34**(7): 442–7 (in Japanese).

15 *Yakuji Kogyo Seisan Dotai Tokei Nenpo (Pharmaceutical Industry Production Statistics Annual)*. Tokyo: Yakugyo Keizai Kenkyujo, various years.

16 Fukushima, M. The overdose of drugs in Japan. *Nature* 1989; **342**: 850–1.

17 Tsutani, K. Dento teki Iyakuhin ni taisuru Senshinkoku no Seifu, Seiyakusangyo no Yakuwari (Role of the government and the drug industry on traditional drugs in developed countries). *Rinsho-Igaku* 1988; **4**: 855–60 (in Japanese). Original English text presented at the Symposium on Pharmaceutical Development, Regulation and Ethics, 30 July 1987, Tokyo, appears in *Watashitachi-no-Kampoyaku* 1989; **41**: 68–77.

18 Tsutani, K. Current status of controlled trials of Kampo drugs in Japan (in preparation).

19 Yakazu, D. The role of education in the revival of traditional medicine in Japan. In: *Report of Regional Workshop on Training in Traditional Medicine, Manila, Philippines, 25–28 November 1986*. Manila: World Health Organization Regional Office for the Western Pacific, 1987.

20 Tsutani, K. Kampoyaku no rinsho hyoka ni kansuru ju no gokai (Ten misunderstandings in clinical evaluation of Kampo drugs). *Happy End* 1990; **52**: 29–41 (in Japanese).

21 Sakamoto, N. *et al.* Tonyobyo sei Shinkei Shogai no Toyo igaku teki Chiryo (Treatment of diabetic neuropathy with Traditional, Oriental Medicine). *Tonyobyo (Journal of the Japanese Diabetic Society)* 1987; **30**: 729–37 (in Japanese).

22 Takeuchi, K., Yanai, H., Mukherjee, B. N. *The Foundation of Multivariate Analysis* (pp. 345–346). New Delhi: Wiley Eastern Limited, 1982. The original article is: Hayashi, C. On the prediction of phenomena from qualitative data from the mathematico-statistical point of view. *Annals of the Institute of Statistical Mathematics* 1952; **3**: 69–98.

23 Edgar, H., Rothman, D. J. New rules for new drugs: the challenge of AIDS to regulatory process. *The Milbank Quarterly* 1990; **68**(Suppl. 1): 111–42.

24 *Report of Scientific Group on Herbal Medicine Research, Tokyo, Japan, 10–12 March 1986*. Manila: World Health Organization Regional Office for the Western Pacific, 1986.

25 *Hoi Thao Quoc Gia Ve Nghien cuu Cay Thuoc (National Seminar on Research of Medicinal Plants), Hanoi, Vietnam, 6–8 January 1987*. Hanoi: The Ministry of Health, 1987 (in Vietnamese and in English).

26 *Han Kuk ye ser eui Saeng Yak Yeun Gu ye kwan han Kuk Nae Yeun Su Hoi (National Workshop on Herbal Medicine Research), Suanbo, Republic of Korea, 19–22 April 1988*. Seoul: Natural Product Research Institute, Seoul National University and East-West Medicine Research Institute, Kyung Hee University, 1988.

25 Herbal medicines: research strategies

Simon Mills

Summary

A review of the particular requirements for investigating the efficacy of herbal medicines leads to the outline of a range of research methods which might be applied. The suggestion is made that cooperation between herbal suppliers and legislators in developing appropriate scrutiny will be in the public's best interest.

Who asks the question?

No review of the state of research into herbal medicines can be complete without asking what it is for. There are three groups who might be thought as having an interest in the results of scientific enquiry.

1 The public (patients and consumers)

An obvious point to make is that a great many people have already found herbal medicines effective,[1] and all those using them will have strong anecdotal evidence of their apparent benefits. Compared with the experience of most modern drugs the human use and approval of most herbal remedies is awesome. The requirement by the medical and scientific establishment for research to 'prove' that herbs are effective is not found among the population at large. It is almost certain that the recourse to herbal remedies as a popular option will outlive the current era of scientific inquiry.

There is also little interest in the questions that exercise scientists. There is perhaps a gut feeling that science is a sad substitute for the warm self-confidence of 'home-truths'; that perhaps the fact that 90% of all scientists in history are alive today is a reflection of an age out of touch with itself. Certainly the proliferation of scientific papers (1 million per year in 40,000 journals), the 'publish or perish' imperative that has developed, and the widespread fraud in articles uncovered by those such as Feder and Stewart at the US House Subcommittee on Oversight and Investigations, does not inspire confidence in the authority of science.

It is apparent that most ordinary mortals are, to use Popper's image, happy to accept that swans are white because all swans which they have seen are white. It was, after all, unnecessary for a long time to question the obvious impression that the sun rotates around the earth provided that its movements were charted as well as possible. (A recent survey in fact showed 37% of people in Britain still think the sun does move round the earth!)[2]

However, the public do want to be assured that someone is looking after them (and will pillory those who are seen to have failed – as witnessed by the furore over *Listeria* and *Salmonella* contamination in food in the UK in 1989). They therefore assume the questions are being asked by those who ought to do it.

2 Those speaking for the public

The public elects politicians to represent their interests but their real guardians in matters such as health care are the civil servants, expert and otherwise, paid to do the actual work. It is the experience of those who have debated the subject on the national scene that politicians, like most of the public, have a relatively detached view about both scientific arguments in general, and the demands for research proof in particular. As long as public safety is seen to be protected, then the public guardian will be seen to have discharged his duty.

The drive for evidence comes principally from the panel of medical advisors who help a politician declaim in this area. As best they may see themselves as facing, in herbal medicine, a fiendishly complex and possibly dubious and antiquated form of medicine with potential hidden perils for the unsuspecting public; at worst they are protecting an established, wealthy and powerful medical interest. The experience of such counsel is that it can be particularly harsh in its requirements for evidence.[3]

Nevertheless, in the wake of the thalidomide tragedy, the Medicines Acts 1968 and 1971 with subsequent Statutory Instruments have been developed as the major mechanism for screening what medicines are made available to the public. The discussions continue and the legislative landscape develops; it is to be hoped that positive contributions from those expert in the particular character of herbal medicines will after all be given due weight in determining legal controls on the availability of herbs.

3 Those using the herbs in practice

The development of medicine has generally been marked by a disinclination to subject acquired truths to the rigours of independent assessment. In medical history, periods of innovation and challenge have been occasional and brief, marking eras of cultural ebullience, such as the Ch'in and Han dynasties in China,[4] the Greece of Hippocrates, Dioscorides and Galen, and its renaissance in the Islamic era of the ninth to tenth centuries. By contrast there have been overwhelmingly long periods of apparently quiet acquiescence to orthodoxies formed often centuries, or even millennia, before. The modern era is unusual in the extraordinary level of research activity which has followed the marriage of medicine with rationalist science and technology.

Knowledge within traditional medicine has generally been in the form of received wisdom moulded to the individual needs and prowess of each practitioner. Such means of acquiring healing skills seem temperamentally suited to most practitioners, herbal and conventional, even today. Their interest in inquiry for its own sake, with secure truths up for constant possible refutation, is understandably secondary to their concern to survive in practice.

The community of those who practise herbal medicine has been no exception to this general rule. Only recently, for example, have practitioners in Britain become sufficiently organized to generate the impetus for stringent research from within their own circle.[5] Fortunately however, more are now realizing that an attitude of inquiry is an advantage in improving the performance of their therapy.

At its heart, research is a process by which it is possible to select, sort and clarify the information available about a healing technique, to answer the fundamental question: 'Is this treatment likely to make the patient well or not?'. As C. R. Rogers put it:

> Scientific methodology needs to be seen for what it truly is: a way of preventing me from deceiving myself in regard to my creatively formed subjective hunches which have developed out of the relationship between me and my material.[6]

It is quite possible of course that the herbal lobby might question the validity of the research forum, might play it only so far ('...render therefore unto Caesar the things that are Caesar's'), or might even call down a plague on its head, but it should at least have the strength to face the challenge:

> if what you say is so valuable and powerful then it should be able to stand up for itself in any forum.

The difficulty of questioning

There are, however, three practical problems in pursuing good clinical research.

1 To produce results carrying sufficient statistical weight is very expensive and laborious. Herbal medicine in the West can boast no teaching hospitals or research institutes, nor funding by a wealthy industrial sector. The necessary infrastructure is lacking.

  Neither can the costs of undertaking research studies be easily justified commercially; it is difficult to patent herbs and the size of the market is not comparable to that for conventional drugs.

2 Herbs are complex medicines, in fact, occupying an unusual position as being medicines with the characters of foods.

  Being a vast complex of pharmacologically active chemicals, the whole package will have different properties from that of any single constituent acting alone. Knowing the action of the latter will not itself be predictive of the effect of the former, particularly if the experimental evidence is based on work done on laboratory animals.

3 The application of herbs and their effect on the body is not always the same as usually understood for conventional medi-

cines. Clinically, herbal medicines are used more to evoke healing responses in the body than to attack symptoms and, although this is not a concept easy to put on a product label, it reflects a fundamental difference in emphasis.

How do you measure an experience?

The problem is of course most acute in assessing the clinical use of herbs. There is considerable doubt about the applicability of the conventional technological/engineering model of scientific pursuit and analysis to the healing event in general and to herbal practice in particular. To the extent that healing involves an element of purely human contact – the healer stepping outside his or her own position and into the life of the patient – it is not an event assayable by independent observers or cold analysis. Current medical research generally concerns itself only with measuring events and data divorced from the human being, ignoring the latter's immensely powerful forces for change and development in defiance of the clearest signs to the contrary.

These are problems generally aired in regard to medicine elsewhere, but it may be possible to illustrate the problem with specific examples from the world of herbal medicine. One might start with a question originally put by Molière and rehearsed by Bateson concerning a substance no longer used by medical herbalists in the West, but which is relatively well understood by many: 'State the "cause and reason" why opium puts people to sleep'.[7] One of Bateson's students replied triumphantly that it was because opium contained a sleep-inducing principle! The qualities of this substance have been very well investigated by medical science. For over a century the active constituents of *Papaver somniferum* have been known, as well as something of their effects on the body. It is established that *morphine* is both analgesic, depressive and euphoric, as well as tolerogenic and addictive, that it depresses the respiratory, vasomotor, coughing and vomiting centres in the brain stem, as well as ACTH and gonadotrophin secretions, yet stimulates the chemoreceptor centre and ADH production; that *codeine* has similar but lesser effect; that *thebaine* produces seizures in low doses; that *papaverine* potentiates morphine but also relaxes smooth muscle; and that *noscapine* suppresses the cough reflex. There is also a great deal of intriguing information about interaction with opiate receptors in the nervous system.

In spite of this information, however, we still understand most of the actual effects of opium itself from the personal testimony of Albrecht von Haller, Thomas de Quincey and others, as well as the diverse medical and social literature of anecdotal accounts of those observing in reality the complex effects of opium consumption and withdrawal.

To take an example more relevant to the modern medical herbalist: in the case of feverfew (*Tanacetum parthenium*), the British herbal profession was faced with a sudden media-induced public demand for an apparently effective migraine remedy without much personal experience of its use. In a short time an appreciable amount of research work was done in conventional medical and scientific settings on the pharmacological characteristics of the plant, including clinical trials.[8,9,10,11] In spite of this work the therapeutic character of the remedy has remained elusive for any practitioner not simply prescribing symptomatically, and trying to assess the most advantageous circumstances in which to use feverfew for any particular patient. Good clinical experience with case histories are still required. (Some clues are perhaps to be seen in its essentially vasodilatory – warming – effect. Most migraines are accompanied by vasoconstriction of blood vessels, a significant minority are not; the former often obtain relief by applying hot packs to the head and are probably more suited to feverfew than the latter.)

Towards a herbal research policy

Back to the human being

In spite of such misgivings, if the herbal lobby is being charged to provide reassurance to the consumer, then it will have to develop coherent and consistent new models of research which are appropriate to the material, but also with the authority to convince the public's guardians of their validity.

Of all the forms of investigation into the effect of medicines that convinces the authorities, there can be no substitute for full-blown clinical research. Unfortunately this is also the hardest, the most expensive, most fraught with ethical problems and the most demanding of infrastructural support.

Conventional clinical trials

Even with these difficulties, conventional double blind random assignment clinical trials can sometimes be completed. Recent papers, for example, have demonstrated clinical benefits of feverfew in migraine,[12] chamomile on wound healing,[13] ginger in seasickness,[14] garlic in lipidaemia,[15] and valerian in insomnia.[16] At Exeter we have started a trial to test the effect of a herb on the incidence of PMT in women, choosing 600 subjects from an initial field of 2000 volunteers. In such selective investigations the conventional methodology is very powerful and can never be ignored.

Fortunately there have been some considerable efforts in constructing appropriate methodologies of sufficient weight.[17] These generally rely on improving the monitoring of individual cases rather than comparing treatment and control populations.

Where n = 1

The main charge against single case studies is that they cannot credibly select out real effects from confusing variables, treatment effects from placebo effects, and so on. The following scenario for such research, however, shows both that it can have more credibility than might be supposed, and that it is not a soft option.

The criteria for validity of such trials have been well reviewed by Reason and Rowan[18]; they are challenging, even daunting. They include ensuring that the perceptive faculties of the researchers are constantly and clearly sharpened, providing as many points of view as possible, clarifying these perspectives, and recycling observed data around the researchers for checking and possible refutation. At stake is the need to ensure that, while denying the possibility of a truly objective view, we do not confine ourselves to the subjective, aiming instead to create a perspective which transcends the two.

Each observer makes a unique map of any territory, and all such maps are selective, idiosyncratic views of a phenomenon that cannot be devalued. To the extent, however, that maps are necessary for the exchange of information, the more that observers can submit their own maps for re-evaluation by others, the more likely that a real consensus, a common map, will emerge, and the better may outsiders grasp the nature of the territory portrayed.

Such a research design would draw data about a particular treatment from:

> The *patient*, acting as co-researcher and with uniquely intimate, though of course slanted, view of the internal landscape;
> The *practitioner*, with sufficient competence and clinical experience to provide both an informed and empathetic account of the encounter;
> A third person acting as *coordinator* and *observer*.

The account of each participant would be assembled individually, and then brought back for a case conference editorial discussion at a later date to cross-check and combine so as to produce a final report of the treatment. Each such report can be examined by the coordinating researcher or assistant, applying a form of inquiry similar to that proposed by Diesing in the social sciences.[19] In other words, themes of disturbance and incapacity are elicited, then used to construct the working case story, both steps being subjected to re-evaluation by all co-researchers. As each case is thus graphically characterized; it can be used for comparative purposes with other cases to see whether a pattern occurs and can be sustained.

Truth emerges from such an exercise as a consensus, with individual judgement constantly subjected and resubjected to scrutiny by others.

Inherent validity is, of course, no greater than when a number of people agree among themselves that 'all swans are white', but it can still be argued that this is a fair basis on which to base practical predictions and applications (it would be considered very sound intelligence in the business world). It has the advantage that all conclusions are based on real experiences and can more thoroughly be applied to meaningful clinical application.

Such an exercise would be best conducted in the environment of a training clinic, where there is likely to be a more overt climate of inquiry and debate, and extra administrative labour. It could allow for a useful database of reliable case histories to be assembled over the years, as both an educational and research exercise.

Another way to explore the action of a herbal remedy that is sympathetic to its claimed activity is to apply a different form of measurement of pharmacological effect, a different clinical pharmacology.

The measurement of transient clinical effects

Herbs have traditionally been applied in a qualitatively different way from conventional drugs. Whereas the latter are primarily designed directly to affect a specific disability without regard for the context in which that disability occurs, herbal remedies have been directed to supporting the individual's recuperative capacities, where the chief complaint is seen as only one feature in a wider pattern of disturbance. The character of the remedy reflects this broader, interactive and often supportive action. Its apparent clinical effect is not entirely measured by purely analytical investigative method, whether that be chemical fractionation, or clinical trial conducted on groups of patients rendered homogeneous by random assortment and by reference entirely to isolated symptoms.

The herbal practitioner insists on the uniqueness of the individual patient, and on the right to provide a unique mixture of remedies in each case. Apart from this objection to taking part in randomized blind trials, there is the impression that herbs to a significant effect are interactive with the patient, i.e. their actual effect varies with the nature of the disturbance treated. This impression is consistent with the view that many herbal remedies act to encourage self-correcting processes. Other traditional views of herbal remedies emphasize their primary influence on transient body functions, e.g. they are classed as diaphoretics, expectorants, circulatory stimulants, diuretics, digestive stimulants, laxatives and so on. In other words, contrary to common belief, most herbs can have almost immediate results on the body.

The requirement is to devise a process by which such approaches can be validated. Clearly conventional models for testing drugs are insufficient. Rather than aiming for conclusions about isolated pharmacological actions divorced from individual variation, it is necessary here to chart changes within individuals, using such parameters as are relevant, useful and non-invasive.

Emphasis shifts, too, from the isolated observation to the simultaneous recording of several parameters of change. Synchronous events mutually influence each other rather than act as causes or effects of each other; they are thus all equally related to each other and to the 'effect' that is observed from their operation. It is precisely this interdependence, this inductive relationship, that leads to their exclusion in conventional trials as distracting variables. Acceptance of these variables as important data is a key feature of such work and must therefore profoundly change the nature of the information gathered.

Instead of trying to eliminate all variables that might cloud the specific issue in question ('Is it drug A that reduces inflammation in this organ or other factors?', for example), the aim of the 'functional assay' as it might be called[20] is ideally to define all factors which determine the medicinal substance's influence on the course of disease ('What, in fact, is drug A actually likely to do in this individual?'). The task would in some ways resemble the homoeopathic 'proving'; in other ways take advantage of modern computerized and multilevel diagnostic techniques known as 'metabolic profiles'. Such information will, for example, be better suited to systems, rather than causal, analysis, and any conclusions drawn from it will be qualitative rather than quantitative; relationships are induced rather than causes analysed. The process will, not unfittingly, more resemble anthropological than conventional medical research. It could of course augment the collation of exhaustive case stories as described above.

The demonstration of transient effects will not in itself lead to predictable changes in pathologies, representing as these do the somatic accumulation of previous functional disorders. However, many clinical presentations are wholly functional (e.g. acute inflammations, asthma, migraine, digestive disorders, and the whole range of psychosomatic disorders) and it should be possible to draw useful implications from functional responses for the treatment of even the strictly pathological.

Thus it might be more valid to say that a herb, for example, in certain individuals at least, changed the constitution of phlegm, or urine, or altered circulatory activity to one or other tissues or over the body as a whole, rather than that it is statistically likely to be effective against bronchitis, urinary stones, or other disease state.

Medical audit techniques

Considerable information about the use of medicines can be had from questionnaires or records analysis. The data can be obtained from both consumers and suppliers of herbs in a number of contexts. Such material can be very useful for those determining policy or concerned with auditing performance or use.

However, the information provided suffers from one clear problem: it is very rarely subject to independent validation or review, so usually reflects partisan judgements. Its use in determining efficacy of treatment is therefore limited.

Nevertheless, in certain circumstances it can help cast light on apparent usefulness. We are currently involved at Exeter in a collaborative exercise with a centre in the USA to design a questionnaire-based instrument to improve the recording of patient progress under clinical treatment, taking into account quality of life and medical outcome criteria, and even the patient's own words (thematically assessed as above), along with conventional medical records.

Pharmacological and pharmacokinetic research

Something of the present state of knowledge of the action of plant constituents is reviewed in the section following this and it may be apparent that these raise specific questions. The following might be investigated.

1 In what ways are plant constituents likely to interact to affect bioavailability and action (obvious interactions are between tannins/alkaloids/saponins/minerals/complex carbohydrates)?

2 To what extent are activities of plant constituents localized to the digestive tract given that many of them are not absorbed into the body fluids; what physiological/pharmacological models are there to explain referred systemic responses to gut wall stimulation?

3 Is it possible to apply other new physiological models to improve the understanding of the effects of plant constituents (possible leads are cell-receptor function, neuropeptides and other transmitter agents, local controls of circulation and the inflammatory response, prostaglandins and lipid metabolism)?

4 What is known of hepatic action on plant constituents such as would help clarify the results of the 'first-pass effect' and enterohepatic recycling? (see later)

5 Following from the above, is it possible to assess what plant-derived constituents are likely to reach the systemic circulation? (An answer to this question is an essential requisite for meaningful tissue culture experiments, see later)

6 Is it possible to assess broadly to what extent plant variability affects median pharmacological and pharmacokinetic activity?

7 How do changes in pharmaceutical preparation affect the bioavailability of constituents? For example, do alcoholic tinctures and fluid extracts have significantly different actions from the aqueous extracts generally predominant in traditional practice?

Experimental research

Cell, tissue and organ cultures

As part of the modern move to find alternatives to animal experimentation, increasing attention is being paid to techniques for assessing the effects of drugs on cultures of cells, tissues and organs *in vitro*. Conventional drug research is switching in this direction for preliminary screening in drug discovery programmes, and there is a lesser move for at least initial toxicological testing.

The advantages are in the opportunity for the direct observation of the action of an agent on target cells with some reduced ethical difficulties (although the sacrifice of animals is often necessary to supply short-lived organ and tissue samples).

The problems are the limited application of such observations to the *in vivo* situation and the need to confirm any *in vitro* findings anyway; from the point of view of herbal research there is the additional problem that it is impossible at this stage to reproduce that balance of plant constituents that will actually reach internal tissues (after digestion, absorption, and the 'first-pass' hepatic effect). Difficulties are increased by the desirability of using tissues most closely mimicking the real situation, i.e. mammalian organ cultures (rather than the easier to culture amphibian tissues, or the less sophisticated cell lines).

Nevertheless, *in vitro* techniques could provide valuable supplementary information to other research, as in the following suggested projects:

(a) The influence of herbal extracts on epithelial tissue cultures (e.g. gastric, enteric and tracheal tissues; unfortunately the former two decline rapidly in culture). This represents a point of genuine tissue interaction with herbal remedies and might add much to pharmacokinetic research.

(b) Observations on the biotransformation of plant constituents using liver cultures (again short-lived, and a technically difficult operation, but one that is well established in conventional pharmacological research).

(c) Alteration in the migratory behaviour and internal metabolism of macrophages as a result of exposure to herbal extracts (much is made in herbal explanations of claims to improve resistance to infections by a general enhancement of defensive mechanisms; looking directly at macrophage response is an established screening technique).

(d) The influence of herbal preparations on microbiological cultures (direct antiseptic action for some plant constituents has been established, notably by Dr Belaiche in France, but there are still many questions remaining unanswered).

(e) Non-specific observations (as in gerontological research) on cell migrations, length of interphase, longevity and other pointers to *in vitro* cell health.

It would also be worth considering conventional screening techniques for the assessment of individual plant constituents, to be applied particularly where a remedy needed closer examination (e.g. for legislative purposes). The wider application of such findings would be limited, but they might provide useful peripheral information.

Animal experiments

There can be no doubt of the problems of using animals to support research into herbal remedies. Apart from the difficulty of applying findings to the human situation, there are extremely strong ethical objections from almost all those who support the use of herbal medicines, at least in Britain.

Nevertheless the subject cannot be dismissed entirely. In the first place, much phytotherapeutic research in Europe involves animal experimentation and the findings have entered everyday debate about the action of herbal remedies. Secondly, it is quite possible to devise trials that involve no pain or discomfort to the animals involved, as is the obvious practice in gerontological research (animals live longest when well treated). It is recalled that herbal therapy aims to support vital functions (in China the worth of any therapeutic practice is determined by how successfully its use appears to encourage a long and healthy life!). If the intention of any trial was to assess the effects of herbal medication applied in approximately therapeutic doses adjusted for body weight and metabolism, there can be little complaint that the animals would be harmed, and they are likely actually to benefit. Advice is that the Home Office in Britain, responsible for issuing licences for such research, would consider such trials as indistinguishable from keeping animals as pets, and no licence need be obtained.

Feasible trials might include observing behavioural and social changes after administering 'relaxants' and 'nerve tonics', monitoring the effects of posited 'adaptogens' on life expectancy, stamina and reproductive capacity, the effects of antimicrobial remedies on normal resistance to disease among large populations, and observing changes in digestive and urinary performance (as judged by changes in excretion, appetite and weight). As the common laboratory animal with a metabolism closest to the human being, the humble rat would probably be the creature of choice.

It might also be valuable to have the results of careful observations of the use of herbs in veterinary practice, where many of the limitations attending patient-practitioner interaction can be minimized.

Nevertheless, the net contribution of such trials to a useful understanding of the effects of herbal remedies on human beings is probably not sufficient to justify the risk of offending strong sensibilities on this issue.

Phytochemical research

It is also helpful to have information about the chemical properties of herbal medicines. This constitutes the bulk of research activity into medicinal plants so far, not least because of the interest of pharmaceutical companies in the possibility of finding new drugs or lead structures.

The analytical techniques developed in this research, such as thin-layer (TLC), high-pressure-liquid (HPLC) and gas chromatography, X-ray crystallography and nuclear-magnetic-resonance and mass spectometry can be applied to the standardization and quality control of herbal medicines. The TLC standards laid down in the new edition of *British Herbal Pharmacopoeia* show how it is possible to establish inexpensive standardization for commercial products. The use of the technique as a broader research tool, in quantifying sample quality for other research projects, as applied for example at the School of Herbal Medicine (Phytotherapy), is also worth noting.

The obvious drawback in such an approach is its tendency to provide only fragmentary insights into the action of the whole medicine. To be really useful there should be a way to link the chemistry and the pharmacology of plant constituents to the therapeutic action of the whole plant. In Exeter we are well advanced in the development of an expert database (EXTRACT), using relational software, that will seek to establish a network of structure-activity relationships for plant constituents in respect to the action of the whole plant. This will have important predictive and interpretive potential for future herb research.

Conclusion

In reviewing the prospects for validating herbal medicine in a doubting age, the first conclusion is that the job is overwhelming. The large number of medicines in use, the complexity of their pharmacology and the low financial gearing of the industry rule out an early overhaul by scientific scrutiny. The public is going to have to rely largely on the precedent of tradition in choosing to use herbal remedies for some time yet.

But choose herbs they will. The suppliers of herbal medicines and the legislators overseeing the supply have a common interest in working together to improve the level of knowledge available as best they can.

The industry and profession may thus consider adopting an integrated, moderate cost, intermediate technology, but rigorous and validatable research programme that really reflects the special character of the material. The projects should be able to be conducted in small clinics and laboratory facilities and without prohibitive capital investment. To screen out the wacky or time-wasting project, rigorous scrutiny of clinical trial protocol, or, better, actual protocol design, should be performed by specialists, such as we are blessed with in the Department of Mathematics, Statistics and Operational Research at Exeter.

In return for such endeavours the herbal industry and profession should expect more cooperation from the Department of Health and their European equivalents. We should have clear encouragement for investigation that is not necessarily identical to that appropriate to the proving of new synthetic drugs, and a declared willingness to include expert testimony from within the industry and profession in deliberations on the fate of herbal medicines. An undertaking of this nature will provide a strong incentive for the suppliers to invest time and finance in the necessary infrastructure for research activity.

At the end of the day, the wellbeing of the public depends on such constructive developments.

References

1 Herbs are patients' favourites. *J Alt Med* 1984; July: 1. This reports a survey of 2000 British people carried out by an independent research organization, RSGB. Twelve percent of those asked claimed to have used herbal remedies, more than any other alternative medicine, and of these almost three-quarters expressed satisfaction with that experience.

2 Jowell, R., Witherspoon, S., Brook, L. (eds.) *British Social Attitudes: Special International Report*. Aldershot: Gower, 1989.

3 *Alternative Therapy: Report of the Board of Science and Education*. London: British Medical Association, 1986. This inquiry heard almost no expert witnesses, allowed no cross-examination and was subject to no informed peer review. Not surprisingly its findings were largely inaccurate and its conclusions were hostile. Fortunately it was widely dismissed as biased by the media and public.

4 Read particularly: Needhan, J. *Science and Civilisation in China. Vol 2: History of Scientific Thought*. Cambridge: Cambridge University Press, 1956.

5 Notable is the activity at the School of Herbal Medicine (Phytotherapy) near Hailsham, and at the Centre for Complementary Health Studies, University of Exeter.

6 Rogers, C. R. *On Becoming a Person. A Therapist's View of Psychotherapy*. London: Constable, 1961.

7 Bateson, G. *Steps to an Ecology of Mind*. St Albans: Granada, 1973.

8 Hayes, N. A., Forman, J. C. The activity of compounds extracted from feverfew on histamine release from rat mast cells. *J Pharm Pharmacol* 1987; **39**: 466–70.

9 Heptinstall, S. *et al*. Extracts of feverfew may inhibit platelet behaviour via neutralisation of sulphydryl groups. *J Pharm Pharmacol* 1987; **39**: 459–65.

10 Murphy, J. J. *et al*. Randomised double-blind placebo-controlled trial of feverfew in migraine prevention. *Lancet* 1988; **ii**: 189–92.

11 Waller, P. C., Ramsay, L. E. Efficacy of feverfew as prophylactic treatment of migraine. *Br Med J* 1985; **291**: 1128.

12 Heptinstall, S. *et al*. Ibid.

13 Glowania, H. J. *et al*. The effect of chamomile on wound healing – a controlled clinical-experimental double-blind trial. *Z Hautkr* 1987; **62**(17): 1262–71.

14 Grøntved, A. *et al*. Ginger root against seasickness: a controlled trial on the open sea. *Acta Otolaryngol* 1988; **105**: 45–9.

15 Bordia, A. Effect of garlic on blood lipids in patients with coronary heart disease. *Am J Clin Nutr* 1981; **34**: 2100–3.

[16] Leathwood, P. D., Chauffard, F. Aqueous extract of valerian reduces latency to fall asleep in man. *Planta Medica* 1985; **54**: 144–8.

[17] See issues of *Complementary Medical Research*, the journal of the Research Council for Complementary Medicine in London, especially Vol. 1, No. 1, 1986.

[18] Reason, P., Rowan, J. *Human Inquiry: A Sourcebook of New Paradigm Research*. Chichester: Wiley, 1981.

[19] Diesing, P. *Patterns of Discovery in the Social Sciences*. London: Routledge & Kegan Paul, 1972.

[20] After Professor Manfred Porkert at the University of Munich.

26 Manipulation and low back pain: an example of principles and practice

T. W. Meade and A. O. Frank

Introduction

The purpose of this chapter is to illustrate the main principles and the conduct of randomized controlled trials (RCTs) involving manipulation using low back pain as an example. We have therefore not attempted a comprehensive review of back pain trials, whether these include complementary methods or not, though we summarize their findings. We have drawn extensively on one particular trial, not so much to emphasize its particular results as to illustrate in a practical rather than a theoretical way the main points about the design, conduct and analysis of these trials. We have not gone in any detail into assessment techniques other than RCTs because firstly, non-randomized comparisons are unsatisfactory for reasons considered later, and secondly because RCTs can and have been successfully carried out.

Manipulation is used by both orthodox and heterodox practitioners. However, trials involving complementary techniques do not differ in any significant way from trials of orthodox methods. Practitioners of some complementary techniques – dealing not just with back pain but with a wide range of conditions – sometimes claim that their methods are not suitable for assessment through RCTs. Their reason is, however, unclear, often illogical and certainly not convincing. Furthermore, as interest in complementary medicine grows, this approach may even be counterproductive since reluctance to use trials will rightly be viewed with suspicion by an increasingly sophisticated public and also by health service managers with expectations of firm evidence for what they spend their money on. Whether particular patients have personal preferences for complementary or orthodox treatments, they experience the same symptoms and illnesses from which they hope for relief. There is no fundamental reason why any complementary technique should not be compared with other complementary methods or with orthodox treatment.

Back pain

In almost every respect, back pain is an extraordinarily complex topic. It affects a high proportion of individuals – indeed, virtually everyone experiences symptoms at some stage. Wood and Badley[1] estimated that in the United Kingdom, 2.2 million people see their family doctor annually for low back pain, of whom 10–20% will be referred to hospital. In 1982 approximately 63,000 people were admitted to hospital for spinal pain (only 3% cervical) in England, Scotland and Wales.[2] Consequences for employment and provision of health care are enormous. Back pain is one of the commonest causes of inability to work through illness in the UK, with 46.5 million certified working days of sickness absence lost per annum in Britain in 1987–8 at a cost of more than £2000 million in lost output – greater than coronary heart disease and bronchitis combined. In 1988–9, this had risen to 52.6 million days – the largest single cause of sickness absence and 12.5% of the total. Such figures exclude the effects on individual patients, including housewives not in paid employment, and the costs of litigation. However, probably less than 10,000 operations are performed on the lumbar spine annually in the UK, the chances of any individual coming to back surgery being six times greater in North America than in Europe. Low back pain is a relatively small cause of permanent severe disability.[1]

Although some episodes of back pain can be attributed to known causes such as trauma, the original explanation for many episodes is still often a matter for speculation. This is not entirely surprising, since the spine consists of 139 joints, numerous bursae and a very large number of ligaments, virtually all being acted upon or supported by muscles. In addition, pain – which may arise from any of these structures – is a subjective symptom the perception of which is influenced by a range of personal, psychological and other characteristics. Back pain may be acute or chronic with treatment expectations ranging from complete relief to modest improvement only. It is hardly surprising that for a condition that probably consists of many syndromes whose causes and pathogenesis are poorly understood, a wide range of treatment and management methods should have evolved. As Table 26.1 shows, this has certainly happened.[3] The number and diversity of approaches in itself suggests extensive uncertainty about the effectiveness of different measures. Many of these, perhaps particularly among the group of physical treatments, have been devised on the basis of theories about the causation of back pain for which there is often little or no firm evidence. It is, however, not always necessary to know exactly how a condition arises in order to treat it successfully. Indeed, the aetiology of back pain is in many respects so poorly understood that it may only be by identifying successful treatments and considering ways in which these may have operated that causal mechanisms are eventually elucidated.

Non-specific low back pain (NSLBP) – i.e. that to which no definite pathological process can confidently be attributed – may occur at all ages, for differing reasons. Under the age of 25, congenital factors are likely to be involved, whilst disc lesions are more likely in early middle life. In later years, the aftermath of previous disc disease may be seen in the form of osteoarthritis (OA) of the facet joints.[4] In old age, OA may be compounded (particularly in women) by osteoporosis. There are many exceptions, e.g. injuries caused by overuse of poorly prepared structures during sport and in leisure at any age.

Most attacks of NSLBP are self-limiting and of short duration. Remaining episodes may require additional therapy, sometimes through hospital. A combination of the measures outlined (Table 26.1) may be used but even these more difficult problems are mostly resolved or greatly

Table 26.1 Therapeutic options in spinal pain

General measures
Strict bed rest
Local spinal support – collar, corset
Avoidance of aggravating factors, e.g. standing still, sitting, bending, and stooping, incorrect lifting, bad working postures
Adjustment of life style, e.g. avoid rushing about
Physical measures
Mobilization techniques/manipulation/traction
Manipulation under muscle relaxant or anaesthetic
Exercises
Postural training and self-care education
Proprioceptive strapping
Hydrotherapy
Soft tissue techniques – massage
Electrical treatments, e.g. interferential, ultrasound, pulsed short wave diathermy, laser
Transcutaneous electrical nerve stimulation
Acupuncture
Medication – oral
Pure analgesia
Non-steroidal anti-inflammatory drugs (NSAIDS)
Muscle relaxants, e.g. diazepam
Tricyclic drugs, e.g. amitriptyline
Medication – injection
Local steroid injection with local anaesthetic, or by epidural route
Dextrose-glycerine-phenol (sclerosant) into soft tissues
Long-term measures
Psychological assessment for: behavioural approach, development of coping strategies, depression or phobias
General toughening up exercise programme
Workshop assessment and treatment to assess: motivation and pain thresholds, standing tolerance, sitting tolerance, time-keeping and capacity for work

Modified from[3]

alleviated within a year. A few patients, however, fail to improve. They should be considered as 'failed conservative treatment' and require different strategies of management, occasionally including surgery.

Doctors trained to intervene in well understood processes may have difficulty in coping with spinal pain, where there are few objective physical signs or laboratory investigations to confirm the precise cause and severity of the complaint.[3] The availability of NMR and CT scanning in larger centres is gradually expanding our understanding of back pain[4] but the majority of people with minor symptoms will not have the advantage of these investigations; neither may they be helpful.

Manipulation has been defined as 'abrupt passive movement of a vertebra beyond its physiologic range but within its anatomic range'[5] although some would include active movements with the patient moving in one direction whilst the manipulator applies force in another. Different studies have often used slightly different definitions and varieties of manipulation. Chiropractors tend to use high velocity, low amplitude thrusts and physiotherapists Maitland mobilizations (generally, gentle passive movements within a structure's usual range of movement). Osteopaths are likely to use oscillatory techniques more frequently than chiropractors.

Although most patients are offered only physical methods of treatment, psychological aspects of management may for many be important from the earliest stage. For example, Fordyce[6] demonstrated that patients given precise instructions about the duration and extent of therapies did better than those given choices in the times of duration of their treatment. Thus, giving responsibility for the management of the pain to others seems in itself to be therapeutic.

Increasing emphasis on self-care in the management of low back pain within the constraints of limited budgets has led to the introduction of back schools,[7] where a comprehensive approach is adopted including (with varying emphasis) ergonomic advice, physical methods to increase the range of spinal movement and muscle strength, and psychosocial techniques.

General principles of RCTs

The first step is to be quite clear about the question to be answered. 'What is the most effective treatment for back pain patients?' is not a sufficiently precise specification for a trial. The general question has to be discussed in some detail so that it is eventually formulated in a way that identifies the different treatments or policies to be compared, the groups of patients considered eligible for the trial and the measures of progress or outcome to be used. This process also involves statistical considerations which will be dealt with in further detail later.

Randomization

Why should the evaluation of a treatment or policy be approached through an RCT? The reasons for RCTs are still not fully appreciated and are therefore worth setting out in some detail. The specific trial question eventually agreed upon involves a comparison – that is, the outcome in those who receive a particular treatment compared with the outcome in those who have received a different treatment (or who might be given the same treatment in a less intensive form). It is therefore essential to ensure that the two groups on which the comparison is based (usually two, but sometimes more) are, as nearly as possible, not only similar but identical in all respects other than the treatment in question. If they are not identical and if the ways in which they differ are associated with a tendency to a better or worse outcome, it is obviously not possible to be sure whether it is a treatment effect or the other differences between the groups that have been responsible for any contrast in outcome. Thus, it would not be surprising if high social class, associated as it is with higher levels of education, better housing and more support at times of illness, influenced the likelihood of doing well after a stroke. If the group that receives very intensive treatment after stroke is, on average, of higher social class than the group that receives less intensive treatment and if a better outcome is observed in the former group, was it the treatment or the social class composition of the groups that was responsible for the difference?

But there are major problems in establishing identical groups, other than through RCTs. It is possible to ensure that groups are comparable in terms of characteristics that can be specified and measured – for example, proportions of men and women, average age, social class composition – but there may equally be characteristics that cannot be measured or that are not even appreciated that may influence outcome. Random allocation of treatments is the means of ensuring that these unknown influences are the same in both groups.

Ethical considerations

The over-riding principle must be to provide the best available treatment for each individual patient. More often than is generally realized, however, it may be difficult or impossible to decide what the best treatment actually is. All too often, there is little or no objective information by which to decide and there are, unfortunately, instances where 'common sense', 'clinical impressions' and conclusions based on non-randomized comparisons are misleading. One of the best examples concerns the use of oxygen in premature babies. It was generally assumed that oxygen would help in prematurity and that it would certainly do no harm. It was not, however, until a trial had been carried out that the effect of intensive oxygen treatment in sometimes causing retrolental fibroplasia and blindness was demonstrated and appreciated.[8] Thus, apart from very rare occasions when the effect of the treatment is so obvious (as it was with penicillin) that a trial is clearly unnecessary, it is not only unsafe to assume that treatment must be effective – it may actually be against the patient's best interests to make this assumption.

If, therefore, the situation is one in which it is not clear that a common treatment is useful or where its value depends on an uncertain balance between beneficial and harmful effects, it becomes reasonable to make a comparison. For therapists who are personally convinced that a treatment is highly effective and involves no harm or inconvenience, it may be unethical to contemplate a comparison, though the example of oxygen in premature babies (and other examples) shows that convictions may be misplaced and even detrimental. In fact, the assumption that a treatment is effective when in fact it is not, coupled with the possibility that it may even be harmful, has rightly led an increasing number of people to agree that it may be unethical *not* to make the appropriate comparisons.

Indeed, the way in which ethical and responsible behaviour is often perceived may be quite the wrong way round. If a new drug becomes available, a doctor is free to prescribe it for all his patients even though information on its value and side effects is far from complete. But it is precisely these uncertainties that lead another doctor to use the drug in a way that helps to resolve them by using the drug in only half his patients, comparing their progress with a group treated differently. This approach, so many people conclude, immediately poses an ethical problem. Surely, though, it is the first doctor whose standards are more questionable. Sir Austin Bradford Hill pointed out[9] that it is the decision to make a comparison in the first place that may occasionally raise ethical questions. Once the decision to make a comparison has been justified, however, randomization is simply the technique that ensures the best possible information from the comparison. Randomization, as the word implies, means that the treatment the patient receives is determined at random and not according to any preconceived ideas or biases of the therapists, or of the patients for that matter.

Unsatisfactory methods

In the past, reliance has often been placed, for example, on comparing the outcome in patients treated by one doctor who uses a particular treatment with the outcome in the patients of another doctor who does not, or between hospitals only one of which has facilities for a particular treatment. 'Historical controls' have also been used, the outcome in patients treated after the introduction of a treatment being compared with the progress in patients treated at the same hospital before the method was available. All these and other similar approaches are flawed for the reason already considered – namely, possible differences between the groups in characteristics (besides the treatment), often coupled with different definitions of outcome in the groups studied and, in the case of historical controls, with other changes over time that may have influenced the natural history or management of the condition. Even where outcome is measured in the same way in different groups, intrinsic differences between them may well make any confident interpretation of the results impossible.

Numbers in RCTs

The numbers required in an RCT depend on several technical considerations. One is the magnitude of the difference in the outcome to be detected between the two groups. The larger the difference to be detected, the smaller the numbers required. Therapists and patients are unlikely to take much notice of results showing only small differences. It is therefore useful to consider how large a treatment effect needs to be to make it likely that the results will actually be translated into practice. But there is a danger in deciding on a large difference which, if established, would certainly influence practice, simply in order to minimize the numbers required. It would, for example, be easy to agree that a new hypotensive agent that lowered systolic blood pressure from 180 mmHg to 130 mmHg (on average) would be a major advance that most clinicians would want to take advantage of. The necessary trial would almost certainly not have to be very large in order to demonstrate such an obvious benefit. If, however, the observed reduction was from 180 mmHg to 150 mmHg, it would not be possible to say, based on the small number of patients studied, whether this was a true (and also useful) effect or whether the apparent difference was simply a matter of chance. Thus, deciding on the numbers required is often a compromise between setting out to demonstrate only very marked differences (which, unfortunately, are few and far between) and not running the risk of missing smaller but still useful effects.

Too small a trial is a waste of everyone's time, including the patient's who – in these circumstances – is being asked to take part in a study which has no chance of producing useful results. Given a reasonably accurate estimate of the numbers of patients available for a trial over a period of time, it may then be possible to estimate the size of any treatment effect that might be demonstrable with these numbers and a decision can be made as to whether it is worth proceeding. As a further word of warning, however, it is very general experience that estimates of the numbers of patients thought to be available for a trial nearly always exceed the numbers actually available, often by a considerable amount.

Required numbers also depend on the frequency of the endpoint or outcome. The higher this event rate, the smaller the numbers recruited into an RCT need to be. Outcomes may be categorical or continuous. An example of the former is heart attack. During a trial of (say) a drug to prevent this, each participant will either experience an event or not. In other words, only some participants actually contribute outcome events. Because heart attacks occur considerably more frequently in men than in women, a trial in the latter has to be substantially larger than a trial in men in order that the same number of events is eventually available for analysis of the results. An example of a continuous outcome is the severity of back pain (measured, for example, on the Oswestry scale). In this situation, all participants contribute since they all experience a change in pain severity, including – for statistical purposes – those whose pain is unaltered. In this respect, many trials of manipulation in back or neck pain enjoy an advantage over trials where categorical events form the outcome.

Finally, trial numbers depend on two formal statistical specifications. One is the significance level. For example, a result that is significant at the 5% level means that the observed difference would have occurred by chance only once in 20 trials. The second is the trial's power. A trial with 80% power is one that stands this chance of demonstrating a significant difference (at whatever level of significance is decided) if such a difference truly exists. The more exacting the significance level and power specifications, the larger the numbers required.

It is most unwise to embark on a trial without first consulting an experienced statistician about these and related points.

It should increasingly be the practice to keep a record of all the patients with the condition in question so that those who are eligible for the trial and enter it can be compared with those eligible who do not (and also, though less usefully, with those who are ineligible).

Outcome measures and 'blindness'

Another particularly important point during the planning stage of trials on topics such as back pain is to devise unbiased methods for measuring outcome. Drugs trials can almost always be double blind, neither the patient nor the doctor knowing whether active or inactive treatment is being used in any particular case. This makes it difficult or impossible for the doctor to be influenced by knowledge of the treatment when he or she assesses the patient's progress. In a trial concerned with the alleviation of pain, the doctor might be more inclined to record good progress if he or she knew the patient was taking an active compound. If this information is not available, the possibility of bias is avoided. However, there is the obvious problem in trials of the non-pharmacological management of back pain that both the patient and the therapist will nearly always be aware of the treatment group.

Three precautions can be taken. First, the therapist should not be involved in assessing outcome, as he or she will almost certainly be biased in favour of the treatment given. Secondly, the patient should provide the subjective information that is inevitably necessary to assess pain and disability in a setting removed from any actual or imagined influence of the therapist. For example, it is better to post questionnaires for the patient to complete at home than for the patient to fill these in while he or she is still in the hospital or department in which treatment was given. Thirdly, subjective measures may be complemented by more objective methods such as straight leg raising. Even though tests of this sort are usually of less interest to the patient than the subjective assessment of pain, they add conviction to results based on pain if they are in the same direction. As an example in another setting, changes in liver enzyme levels paralleled the decline in stated alcohol intake in patients being intensively counselled because of excessive consumption.[10]

Follow-up

High follow-up rates should be achieved. The longer a trial lasts, the greater the number of patients who may be lost to follow-up because they fail to re-attend or because they move away or for other reasons. If these losses are appreciable, they may result in a serious degree of uncertainty about the magnitude of any treatment effect if, which is not unlikely, those who are not followed up have tended to do worse than those who are. Furthermore, a greater loss to follow-up in one group than in the other may also introduce bias. For example, it might happen that one of the treatments is more unpleasant or difficult to comply with than the other and that those patients to whom this particularly applies do substantially worse than the patients in the same group who are not lost to follow-up. In these circumstances, it is possible that any difference in outcome in those who are followed up is not due to treatment but to self-selection of the patients in question.

Important though high follow-up rates are anyway, they are of particular significance when outcome depends on the difference between a measurement made initially and at the end of the trial. If either of these measurements is unavailable, there can be no result for that particular patient. For example, where (as for back pain) change in pain intensity is a leading outcome measure, it is essential to have findings initially and at follow-up.

Analysis

An accepted principle is that the main analysis of trial results should be according to 'intention to treat', i.e. that the patient is included in the group to which he or she was randomly allocated at the outset, regardless of whether or not this was the treatment actually received. Undue reliance on 'on treatment' analyses, i.e. according to the treatment the patient actually received, is unwise because of possible biases arising from the reasons for transferring from one treatment to another. If departures from randomly allocated treatment are infrequent, the problem does not arise. In general, 'intention to treat' analyses are likely to give a conservative estimate of the real treatment effect. In this context, it is obviously necessary to keep a systematic record of treatment actually received as distinct from intended.

Trials of manipulation for low back pain

As already indicated, the main purpose of this chapter is to set out and illustrate the main principles in RCTs of manipulation for low back pain, the unsatisfactory (and potentially misleading) nature of non-randomized comparisons having been summarized in an earlier section. Many of these trials were recently summarized in an overview which (though technically questionable in terms of both its methods and general conclusions) gives the main purposes of 30 randomized comparisons for low back pain and of five trials concerned with neck pain.[11] The conclusion of this overview, supported by an earlier review,[12] was that neither manipulation nor mobilization confers obvious short-term benefits although the situation may be different in the long term (see below).

Chiropractic and hospital treatment

The principles of RCTs are now illustrated by the trial of chiropractic and of hospital outpatient treatment for low back pain of mechanical origin, reported by Meade *et al.*[13]

The first step was to be specific about the general question as to whether chiropractic or hospital outpatient management is more effective for low back pain. Two approaches were possible. One would have been a 'fastidious' trial of a particular technique delivered in otherwise identical circumstances. Chiropractic could have been compared with either (a) a single non-manipulative treatment or (b) manipulation given by physiotherapists. In both cases, the number of treatment sessions, the time period over which they were spread and the settings in which they were given would have been the same. The second example, in particular, would have answered a very precise question – is there a worthwhile difference between chiropractic and physiotherapeutic manipulation?

When the trial was planned nearly ten years ago, these possibilities were ruled out for practical reasons. At the time, it would have been difficult if not impossible to arrange for chiropractors and physiotherapists to treat patients in otherwise identical settings, certainly on a sufficiently large scale. In addition, orthodox practitioners (doctors and physiotherapists) could not agree on the criteria for eligibility in trials of this kind or on the non-chiropractic treatment methods.

Accordingly, the trial was 'pragmatic', i.e. it compared the policies of chiropractic with hospital outpatient management rather than specific treatment methods, the decision about these being left to the chiropractors and hospital outpatient departments. This approach has the advantage of comparing what actually happens in day-to-day practice and is much less constrained by eligibility criteria or opinions on what constitutes the most appropriate treatment in individual patients. Its disadvantage is that it cannot precisely identify the component of chiropractic or hospital outpatient treatment responsible for any observed difference though, if there were a difference, this would be a powerful incentive towards further, increasingly 'fastidious' trials.

In making a choice between these possibilities, there is no absolutely right or wrong answer. Furthermore, there is no requirement to ensure that the number or duration of treatment sessions in a 'pragmatic' comparison are the same, particularly if these do actually differ in day-to-day practice. In fact, those managed by chiropractic did receive a greater number of treatment sessions which, in addition, were spread over a longer period of time. But these differences simply reflect the real life differences between chiropractic and hospital outpatient treatment and are part and parcel of the 'pragmatic' nature of the comparison made. The importance of 'comparing like with like' in a trial lies not in the treatments, which may be very different or quite similar (depending on the main objective), but in the composition of the two groups to which they are applied.

How was this comparability achieved? This is summarized in Figure 26.1. Patients were recruited from the chiropractic and hospital clinics to which they initially presented. Not surprisingly, there were marked differences between the groups at this stage, those presenting to the chiropractors being of generally higher social class than those presenting in hospital, for example, as well as differing in other respects. By randomly allocating patients eligible and willing to enter the trial from referrals to each type of clinic, the *treatment* (as distinct from the initial *referral*) groups were indeed very similar, so that any difference in outcome could only be due to treatment.

A refinement of the usual random allocation method, known as minimization, was used to enable the results to be analysed within various subgroups, as well as for all the patients recruited. Thus, it was possible to see whether results were the same for those with or without previous histories of back pain, for those with short or long current episodes, for those with severe or less severe pain at entry and for those randomly allocated to the two approaches within each of the referral groups. A previous feasibility study had already provided information on the

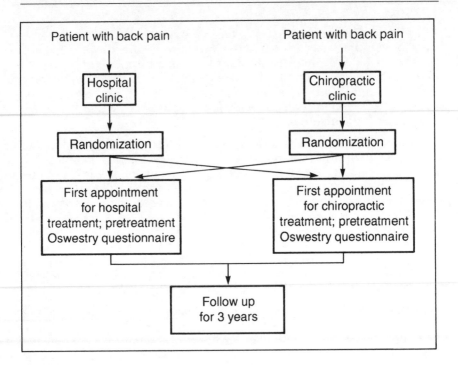

Fig. 26.1 Recruitment and follow-up.

numbers required. The main measure of outcome was to be change in the Oswestry pain disability questionnaire, a validated method based on the patient's record of the severity of pain and ability to carry out common daily activities.[14] Answers to this questionnaire range from 0% points (no pain, no disability) to 100% points (extreme pain, complete disability). To detect a difference between chiropractic and hospital outpatient management of 2% points on the Oswestry scale (at the 5% significance level, with 90% power) about 2000 patients would be needed – for example, a decrease in Oswestry score from 30% to 25% in one group compared with a decrease from 30% to 23% in the other. Differences of 2.5%, 3%, 4% and 5% points would require about 1200, 850, 500 and 300 patients respectively. In the event, 741 patients were recruited to the trial, thus enabling the detection of a difference of just over 3.0% points.

Figure 26.2 shows the main result of the trial. There was a significantly greater improvement in patients treated by chiropractic than in those treated in hospital, this improvement increasing with time and reaching a maximum two or three years after entry to the trial. Improvement was greatest in those who had had previous episodes of back pain and in those with the most severe pain. It was also greatest in those initially attending chiropractors.

In some of the participating centres (each centre consisting of a chiropractic and a hospital outpatient clinic), a record was kept of all patients with back pain who presented during the course of recruitment

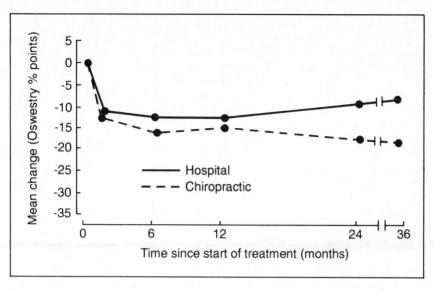

Fig. 26.2 The negative sign for changes in Oswestry scores means a fall – i.e. an improvement – reflecting the well-known tendency for back pain to improve spontaneously as well as any treatment effects.

to the trial. Many of the patients, particularly those presenting first to hospital clinics, were of course ineligible for the fairly forceful manipulation used in chiropractic on account of medical contraindications to management of this kind. After those who were so ineligible had been excluded, 47% of eligible patients agreed to enter the trial. The main reason that otherwise eligible patients did not enter among those initially attending chiropractors was that a high proportion wanted immediate treatment, having decided that chiropractic was their best option.

The experience of this trial illustrates the importance of considering the proportion entering a trial not in terms of all those with the condition but in terms of those who are eligible for the particular treatments under study. To take another example, by no means all patients who have survived heart attacks are eligible for trials of aspirin in preventing recurrence, since many patients cannot take this form of treatment because of indigestion that may indicate peptic ulceration and therefore a high risk of gastric bleeding. There is no point at which the proportion of those eligible and entering a trial automatically makes trial participants 'fully representative' of all patients to whom the results of the trial might be relevant. However, it is very unlikely that results based on those who do take part will differ *qualitatively* from those who do not, although they may differ *quantitatively*. In other words, the proportional benefit in those taking part may to some extent differ from the benefit in those who do not but it is rather – perhaps very – unlikely that there will be a harmful effect in those eligible patients who do not participate if, for example, a beneficial effect was demonstrated in those who do.

Biased recordings of answers to the Oswestry questionnaire were minimized by mailing these questionnaires to participating patients so that they completed them well away from actual or perceived influences of the therapists who had been treating them. In addition, the inclusion of more objective measures, such as straight leg raising (SLR) and lumbar flexion, made it possible to show that the chiropractic benefit demonstrated by the Oswestry questionnaire was paralleled by benefits in SLR and lumbar flexion. Furthermore, the self-exclusion of the patients initially consulting chiropractors who wanted immediate treatment almost certainly reduced the possibility that they would automatically record benefit from chiropractic simply because this would have been their prior expectation. In fact, the benefit due to chiropractic treatment was indeed greater among those initially attending chiropractors but this was probably because of characteristics (whether occurring in chiropractic or hospital referrals) that are more frequently seen in chiropractic patients and are associated with a greater response to chiropractic treatment, such as severe pain and a past history of back pain. In other words, it is the fact that severe pain and past episodes are more often found in patients attending chiropractors than in patients attending hospital, rather than biased outcome assessments, that explains the tendency for chiropractic-referred patients to do better than hospital patients as a result of chiropractic treatment. This is a complex and important issue set out in some detail to illustrate the precautions and cross-checks needed in analysing the results of trials where both patients and therapists know the treatment allocation and where biased outcome measurement is certainly a theoretical if not a practical possibility.

The tendency for the treatment benefit to increase with time also argues against biased Oswestry questionnaire answers, since bias would almost certainly have been more evident during or soon after treatment whereas the difference was greatest long after treatment had ended. The divergence with time also argues against a placebo effect, i.e. an effect unrelated to the specific management methods and due to non-specific care and attention. Again, an effect of this sort (which, incidentally, should not automatically be dismissed as unimportant) would almost certainly have been observed while treatment was still going on rather than long after it had ended.

Inevitably, there were some losses to follow-up, the proportions returning Oswestry questionnaires being 90% at six weeks, 84% at six months, 79% at one year and 72% at two years. As a result of re-doubled efforts, the response at three years was increased to 79%. At all stages, slightly fewer of those treated in hospital responded than those treated by chiropractors. This was almost certainly because those treated in hospital had done less well than those treated by the chiropractors but it is self-evident that assumptions of this kind – even when supported, as they were in this trial, by circumstantial evidence – are less and less necessary the higher the proportion successfully followed up.

Whatever conclusions different groups and commentators may have reached about this particular trial, there is no doubt that it has provided a major stimulus to the consideration of the 'fastidious' trials suggested by its results – is it chiropractic manipulation, chiropractic ergonomic advice, both or some other aspect of chiropractic that is responsible for the effectiveness of chiropractic in low back pain? – and that its experience will be valuable in now planning and conducting these further trials.

References

1 Wood, P. H. N., Badley, E. M. Epidemiology of back pain. In: Jayson, M. I. V. (ed.) *The Lumbar Spine and Back Pain*. 3rd ed. Edinburgh: Livingstone, 1987.

2 Wells, N. *Back Pain*. London: Office of Health Economics, 1985.

3 Frank, A. O., Hills, J. E. Spinal pain. In: Frank, A. O., Maguire, G. P. (eds.) *Disabling Diseases – Physical, Environmental and Psychosocial Management*. Oxford: Heinemann, 1988.

4 Butler, D., Trafimow, J. H., Andersson, G. B. J., McNeil, T. W., Huckman, M. S. Discs degenerate before facets. *Spine* 1990; **15**: 111–13.

5 Monograph for clinicians. Treatment of activity-related spinal disorders. In: Le Blanc, F. E. (ed.) *Scientific Approach to the Assessment and Management of Activity-related Spinal Disorders. Spine* 1987; **12**: 22–30.

6 Fordyce, W. E., Brockway, J. A., Bergman, J. A., Spengler, D. Acute back pain: a control-group comparison of behavioural versus traditional management methods. *J Behav Med* 1986; **9**: 127–40.

7 Klaber Moffett, J. A., Chase, S. M., Portek, I., Ennis, J. R. A controlled prospective study to evaluate the effectiveness of a back school in the relief of chronic low back pain. *Spine* 1986; **11**: 120–2.

8 Kinsey, V. E., Arnold, H. J., Kalina, E. E. *et al.* PaO$_2$ levels and retrolental fibroplasia: a report of the cooperative study. *Pediatrics* 1977; **60**: 655–68.

9 Hill, A. B. Clinical trials and the acceptance of uncertainty. *Br Med J* 1987; **294**: 1419.

10 Wallace, P. G., Brennan, P. J., Haines, A. P. Drinking patterns in general practice patients. *J Roy Coll Gen Pract* 1987; **126**: 86–94.

11 Koes, B. W., Assendelft, W. J. J., van der Heijden, G. J. M. G., Bouter, L. M., Knipschild, P. G. Spinal manipulation and mobilisation for back and neck pain: a blinded review. *Br Med J* 1991; **303**: 1298–1303.

12 Jayson, M. I. V. A limited role for manipulation. *Br Med J* 1986; **293**: 1454–5.

13 Meade, T. W., Dyer, S., Browne, W., Townsend, J., Frank, A. O. Low back pain of mechanical origin: randomised comparison of chiropractic and hospital outpatient treatment. *Br Med J* 1990; **300**: 1431–7.

14 Fairbank, J. C. T., Couper, J., Davies, J. B., O'Brien, J. P. The Oswestry low back pain disability questionnaire. *Physiotherapy* 1980; **66**: 271–3.

Section 4

27 An introduction to word processing as a research tool

David Aldridge

Summary

Word processing is a useful tool for the researcher. It is possible to prepare research reports and articles for journal submission. The word processor is also valuable for organizations wishing to produce newsletters and their own teaching material.

Introduction

Most of us recognize the need to be acquainted with modern methods of information technology. An important element in this technological realm is the microcomputer. For research purposes the computer is a valuable tool offering a wide range of capabilities to individuals and small organizations. Capabilities which, until a few years ago, were within the reach of institutional research departments only.

The microcomputer, small enough to sit on your desk top, can handle the tasks of word processing, data management and the calculation of statistics. In this chapter the use of word processing, or more accurately text management, will be discussed in terms of research needs.

The very terms 'text management' or 'word processing' raise the fear of too much jargon and obscure processes which I will attempt to avoid. However it is important to remember that one person's jargon is another's technical language. Making the computer accessible and usable has been a feature of most of the computer manufacturers. Manufacturers want to sell machines, and thereby people must want to use computers and feel that they can use such machines before they will buy. An obstacle to this use is that many of us are computer illiterate.

Hardware

First, to do any computing you need a computer. This is known as 'hardware', the actual physical equipment; i.e. a handful of stones, an abacus, a pocket calculator or a modern mainframe machine occupying a room. For the purposes of this chapter the basic hardware consists of: the part which does the computing (a microcomputer containing the 'chip'); a keyboard where you type in data; and a screen where you can see the effects of what you type. When you type into the computer it is important to have some means of storing that information electronically. This is achieved by using a disk drive in the form of what most people know as a 'floppy disk', or a hard disk. The main difference is that a hard disk is capable of storing more data. It has a larger memory capacity.

All computers will have at least one disk drive. Ideally a computer will have a hard disk drive to store the gathering sets of data and your written papers, and a floppy disk by which you load any new programs. These programs for the computer are referred to as 'software'. They are written for you to carry out specific tasks; word processing, statistical calculations, report printing and data management. By and large the measure of a computer's success is the ease by which you can accomplish your task, and the transparency of the hardware and software to that task. For instance, it is possible to write and produce an article without thinking too much about the actual computing and concentrating more on the task of writing. It is not necessary to have any knowledge of computer programming to use a computer.

Second, at the end of the process of document organization you will want to produce a hard copy of your work, i.e. on a piece of paper. This requires a separate printer. They come in a variety of forms and can print in black and white and colour. It is essential that the printer is compatible with your computer and that the software programs you wish to use will support your printer. It is possible to buy printers which produce high quality documents which do not look as though they were produced on a computer.

When buying a computer and the associated software it is a good idea to see what other people are using in your organization or within your work group so that you can share information or contribute to the same production. Not everyone needs to have the same computer. It is possible to have a compatible word processing program which will exchange information between differing types of computer. You must, however, have a disk drive which will read a floppy disk from another computer.

Modern computers are such that it is possible to have a computer which is started simply with one switch. Such a machine is being used for the preparation of this chapter. To print a copy of the chapter all that has to be done is to switch on the printer which is connected to the computer and select a command on the computer screen which says 'Print . . .'. Providing there is paper in the printer then things should go smoothly.

Getting started

Many of us have started our home computing lives with the Amstrad word processor. My experience of writing papers on an old 'sit-up-and-beg' typewriter was that I had to spend more time and Tippex correcting the pages than I spent in the act of writing. The Amstrad word processor offered an immediate form of word processing which allowed me to write unhindered. The whole equipment came as a package of computer, screen, printer and word processing software for the price of a portable electronic typewriter. A paper returned for correction on a Friday morning could be corrected, headings rearranged and posted by lunchtime.

Although my typing skills were only marginally improved at first, I did have the ability to correct mistakes before printing them on paper.

Furthermore, the word processor gave me the opportunity to lay out papers with correct margins both to the left and right, and above and below the text. Whereas formerly typing would often run off the page, with the ability to 'word wrap', any words which did not fit on the line were automatically sent to the line below. When it was necessary to insert or remove a paragraph in a document there was no need to retype the whole section, and a new copy could be reprinted already adjusted within minutes.

There are some important lessons for the would-be computer initiate to be learned from this pioneering machine. First, the technology was old and slow according to the state of the art computer wizards. However, its hardware and software were compatible and worked with the flick of a switch and the insertion of a plastic diskette. For the needy it offered relatively cheap available word processing (then about £500). That it was, and still is, used extensively by reporters is a measure of its applicability. Similarly, the teaching profession took it to heart for the production of teaching materials which could be readily updated and amended. Powerful state of the art technology does not always mean the best solution.

Second, the Amstrad was reputedly difficult to use. Actually, it wasn't. It was certainly different from what many computing specialists were used to. The essential point was that it did, and still does, the job which people required of it, and did it easily and well. Enough for this author to produce a book, a research report and two papers in four months (78,000 words). Word processing is a relatively straightforward task but it does require some dedication to learning. Most programs will offer an easy beginners' level suitable to produce satisfactory documents.

For the purpose of this and the following chapters it is assumed that the researcher is a relative novice to computing. The question of hardware I shall leave to the individual user, concentrating instead on the software, i.e. the program designed to carry out the particular task required. Rather than recommending the all-singing all-dancing computer which acquires laboratory data, analyses that data according to set parameters and writes a report which it circulates to all the registered members of your particular working group, I shall concentrate on specific document preparation tasks. In this case it is that of writing papers and preparing reports. It could well be extended to the preparation of teaching material.

If the reader is considering purchasing a computer, the task oriented approach is the ideal position from which to start. First, know exactly what you want to do. Second, find the appropriate software to carry out that task. This will suggest the machine requirements to run that software. Beware of mixing activities on one machine. The person writing papers and technical reports may not be the same person who wants to write membership reminders, prepare a training manual or handle statistical data. They may all want to use the machine at the same time. In addition each new activity will take time to learn.

Word processing

Perhaps the most important tasks for the researcher, after writing the necessary begging letters for research grant support, are writing reports and research papers. For preparing such papers the word processor is more than a sophisticated typewriter. While typed text is handled expertly, there are many powerful features available to the most basic of word processors. These are often referred to as writing tools.

Outlining

An important writing tool which has emerged in recent years is the outliner or thought processor. In preparing to write a document we usually have some idea of a structure to that document, and main headings, albeit provisional, which we want to include. These headings will in turn have subheadings, and these subheadings will beget text. This text often starts life as little notes and jottings as the headings are thought up. Such notes can be attached to particular headings and subheadings. Preliminary ideas can then be saved within an emerging structure. As the structure becomes refined into the framework for the document then the ideas can be expanded upon as fully written text. For some researchers, sadly, this has replaced the beer mat, or back of an old envelope, and pencil method.

The outliner provides a means of moving and organizing such initial headings and text when the structure of the paper becomes clearer. For example if you are preparing a report there are certain sections that you must include. It is possible to type these into the outliner and mark them as headings. The description of the contents of these sections can then be marked and attached as subheadings, and sub-subheadings. Any relevant 'body text', i.e. the general paragraphs of writing under these headings, can be typed in when necessary.

An essential feature of the outliner is that text can be hidden, or collapsed, so that only the headings and subheadings are visible on the computer screen, giving an overall view of the structure of the document. It is then possible to move the whole or a part of a section to another location until a satisfactory structure emerges.

These outlining tools are sometimes sold as separate 'thought processors'. A powerful word processor can incorporate such a feature allowing you to structure your document before you begin the actual detailed writing.

For the novice writer preparing a paper, this is probably the most effective tool. The initial problem in writing is always that of structure. Most scientific reports or papers for publication require a title page, an abstract, an introduction, a review of the relevant literature, the hypotheses and experimental method, the results, a discussion of the findings, references, tables and/or figures and perhaps an appendix (see Figure 27.1). These headings as sections can then be subdivided into subsections; for example, subjects, selection procedures, entrance or exclusion criteria, and statistical methods. Where no such standard

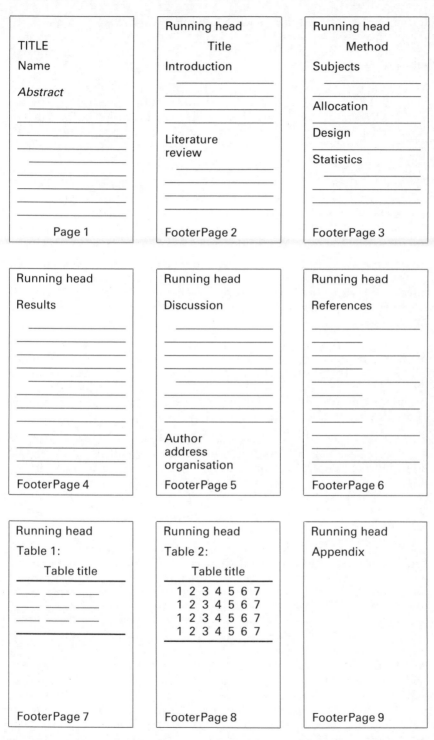

Fig. 27.1 A format for the structure of a paper for publication.

format exists the outliner provides a useful working tool as an aid to planning and editing writing.

Dictionary

Most quality word processors include a spelling checker. When you have typed in what you require you can scrutinize the typing for spelling errors at any time. This spelling checker also sorts out any typing mistakes. Spelling checkers are based on dictionaries of between 50,000 and 150,000 words. They can be used to check individual words, single paragraphs or complete documents.

These dictionaries are never wholly satisfactory, and it is possible either to purchase specific dictionaries for your profession or develop your own dictionary within the word processing program. For a given group of practitioners they can develop a common technical dictionary providing they have the same word processing software.

What these spelling checkers cannot do is distinguish when you mean to use 'form' but actually type 'from'. They simply compare what you have typed with a fixed, or developed, dictionary. Some offer alternative spellings of words when they find a word which is misspelled or they do not recognize it.

Extending this principle further, it is possible to have a thesaurus as part of the word processing capabilities or working as a separate program. While this can be a very useful aid to writing, it can also distract from the writer's style. There are also 'style checkers' available which generally comment upon length of words, length of sentences and repetition. These can be a hindrance as much as a help.

The manufacture of word processors for large international markets provides other-language dictionaries. For those publishing in international journals a useful adjunct is an American dictionary for use with an English language word processor which can be used to scrutinize the text for words like 'color', 'behavior', and 'center'.

Formatting

Given that you have typed in your material and scrutinized it for spelling mistakes and grammatical errors, the next step is to prepare the work for submission to a journal or your sponsors. Journals have requirements for their papers prior to submission. These are usually found under 'Instructions for Authors'. *Complementary Medical Research* is relatively relaxed in that it states simply that the manuscript should be typed and double spaced (the width between the typed lines) with wide margins (the spaces between the edge of the text and the edge of the paper). Illustrations should be on separate pages and references must follow the Vancouver style for formatting. Other journals state specific margin widths and other reference formatting styles. As a writer you will have to instruct the computer that you wish your document to be structured in a particular style, which is a relatively easy task on modern word processors.

The setting of margins comes under the general heading of page management. When you want to produce teaching material, for example, and this has to be bound together it is possible to specify margins and then a little extra, known as a 'gutter', to allow for the paper taken up in the binding.

The main principle with word processors is that the typing of text and the appearance of text are separate activities. You can therefore type away to your heart's content, and then rearrange that text until it appears as you wish. In theory. The critical issue here is to use a software program and computer which give you an exact replica on the screen of what you have typed. The typewriter did this. You saw immediately what had been typed complete with failings. Not all computers and word processing programs print what you see on the screen.

When you type it is also possible to alter the typeface within your document. With a typewriter the typeface was invariably fixed unless you had the benefit of a daisy wheel or golf ball which could be interchanged. The modern word processor and software allow typefaces, or 'fonts', to be interchanged. It is also easy to change between plain text, *italic* and **bold** text, each adding emphasis where necessary.

Within your document you will also wish to apply a standard format to the paragraphs. Within this chapter each paragraph has its first line full out, with a half line space above. These formats can be altered as you wish. Quotations can be set into narrow patterns and presented in another typeface. This is particularly useful for presenting tables where the typeface, or font, is often simpler.

At the top of this page, you will find a chapter heading or book title. This is known as a header (see Figure 27.2). At the bottom, you will find page numbers. This is known as a footer. These footers and headers can be designed by you to run throughout your document and are easily incorporated. They provide a standard format throughout your article or report. This collective format of typeface, paragraph setting and page headers/footers can be saved as a 'Style' in some word processors and applied to all your documents, thereby giving a coherent image. Such a facility is very useful if you are writing a series of research papers, publishing teaching documents from within your own professional organization, or presenting material regularly to a publisher.

When writing research documents it is important to include references to other work, or additional notes for clarification. These are referred to as 'footnotes' or 'endnotes'. Each footnote must have its citation marker in the text and then the footnote placed either at the foot of the page or at the end of the document. This location and marking of footnotes is an automatic process in most modern word processors. It is possible to choose the type of marker, either a simple raised number[1] or another form.§

---

[1] See what I mean, a superscript, i.e. raised number, like this . . .
§ . . . or a marker, like this.

header section:

Title section:	FROM OUT OF THE SILENCE

Summary:	David Aldridge is a research consultant within the medical faculty of the University of Witten Herdecke. His work is to discover and develop research methodologies appropriate for conventional and unconventional medicine. Currently this work includes a survey of complementary health care delivery in Europe, co-editing a reference book of research methods for novice researchers with George Lewith, developing methods of single case research design which include the multivariate analysis of time series data, developing a complex systemic model for the emerging field of psychoneuroimmunology and preparing clinical research studies with the department of music therapy.

Quote:	"Art does not reproduce the visible, rather it makes visible. Formerly we used to represent things visible on earth, things we either liked to look at or would have liked to see. Today we reveal that reality that is behind all living things, thus expressing the belief that the visible world is merely an isolated case in relation to the universal, and there are many more latent realities" Paul Klee.

Body Text:

This article is concerned with developing appropriate research strategies for understanding human behaviour; i.e. how we make sense of ourselves and others.

*I*n medical research most of the modern initiatives for that research have come from the field of natural science. It is my contention that such research when applied to the study of human behaviour is partial and neglects the important creative elements in the process, and practice of healing. This is not to deny the scientific, rather to emphasize the aesthetic such that both may be considered together. Unfortunately the tension of understanding both elements of human understanding results in one or the other being denied. Such is the current situation in modern medicine. However, the continuing problems of chronic illness and human suffering urge us to go beyond our partisan beliefs and look again at how we know as well as what we know[2]. This is literally the art of re-search.

The problem facing the clinician is that he must often mediate between the personal needs of the patient and the health needs of the community. These needs are informed by differing epistemologies. Similarly there is often a split in medical science between researchers and clinicians. One group seeing themselves as rational and rigorous in their thinking, the other as sentimental and biased or reductionist and inhuman. Neither of these stances is true, each perspective has something to offer. However, the predominating ideas in published medical reseach are those of natural science as informed by statistical data.

The science of statistics developed in eighteenth century France as part of the centralised apparatus of the State. "Statistics" as the science of state was the empirical numerical representation of the resources available to the State and formed the components of a new power rationality. Health care then became, as it is now, a political objective, as well as a personal objective. Health is seen as the duty of each member and the objective of all. Individual needs are subsumed within the goals of the collective, the private ethic is informed by the public ethic and objective empirical data are the means by which goals are assessed. These data are related to the economic regulation of health care delivery (health as commodity); public order (the regulation of deviance), and hygiene (the quality of food, water and the environment).

footer section:	page 1

Fig. 27.2 Page set-up.

When additional footnotes are inserted in the text, the numbering of the footnotes can be set to be automatically updated. In the word processing program used to prepare this chapter a portion of the screen is then reflected in the portion of the screen reserved for the footnote and the writer can then type in the necessary note. This facility is of great importance for scientific documents where references must be clearly and precisely formatted.

It is possible to have reference formatting tools which work alongside the word processor. Essentially they allow the writer to insert references within the prepared text and format those references in the style suitable for specific journals. For example, in this book the reference style is known as 'Vancouver' where the references at the end of the chapter appear in numerical order according to the numerical citation markers as they occur in the text. For example, here are references Vancouver style:

1 Altenmüller, E. Brain correlates of cerebral music processing. *Eur Arch Psychiat* 1986; **235**: 342–54.
2 Barlow, D., Hersen, M. *Single Case Experimental Designs: Strategies for Studying Behaviour Change.* New York: Pergamon Press, 1984.
3 Bateson, G. *Steps to an Ecology of Mind.* New York: Ballantine, 1972.

And here are the same references in the Harvard style (author-date style):

Altenmüller, E. (1986) Brain correlates of cerebral music processing. *Eur Arch Psychiat* **235**: 342–54.
Barlow, D., Hersen, M. (1984) *Single Case Experimental Designs: Strategies for Studying Behaviour Change.* New York: Pergamon Press.
Bateson, G. (1972) *Steps to an Ecology of Mind.* New York: Ballantine.

With a reference database and bibliography maker it is possible to reformat your documents according to the journal style of your choice or according to your own wishes. Such a database can work within your word processor, giving you access to compiled lists of papers for in-text citation and then formatting the appropriate bibliography according to a preferred style. The details of any papers which are ready can be entered into such a database, with annotations, compiled and then cited in any written work. Colleagues with the same program can also help to build up a shared library of papers. The advantage of this tool is that the writer can easily keep track of any articles and quickly search through the database for references. For those involved in teaching it is possible to provide a regular commentary on current papers being read within your group, and then make these references available for use in a paper (see Figure 27.3).

Editing

Once you have written your text then it is easy to feel satisfied with a job well done, and thankful that the main portion is out of the way. You should be so lucky. It is almost an inevitability that some revision will

- Bailey L. The effects of live music versus tape-recorded music on hospitalized cancer patients. *Music Therapy* 1983;**3**(1):17–28.

  The effects of live music versus tape recorded music were assessed on 50 cancer patients. Each subject listened to 25 minutes of music. The patients listening to live music reported significantly more changes in physical comfort and improved mood state.

- Bason BT and Celler BG. Control of the heart rate by external stimuli. *Nature* 1972;**4**:279–280.

  Human heart rate can be varied over a certain range by sympathetic and parasympathetic control by entrainment of the sinus rhythm with external auditory stimulus. An audible click was played to the subject at a precise time in the cardiac cycle. When it falls in a critical range then the heart rate can be increased or decreased up to 12% over a period of time up to 3 minutes. When the click is not within the time range of the cardiac cycle then no influence can be made.
  This paper is important for supporting the position that music therapists meet the tempo of the patient in order to influence their musical playing.

- Bonny HI. Music and consciousness. *Journal of Music Therapy* 1975;**12**(3):121–135.

  Helen Bonny has achieved renown for her use of guided imagery and music. This is basically a psychotherapeutic technique where the patient is encouraged to explore the images invoked by listening to music.

- Bonny H. Music listening for intensive coronary care units: a pilot project. *Music Therapy* 1983;**3**(1):4–16.

  This study was designed to test the effectiveness of programmed taped music in reducing stress for the patient in a coronary care unit. Four selected programs of music were chosen by the investigator and played to the patient through earphones or "free field" from a tape recorder by a nurse.
  The scales used were: a relative severity of illness scale issued at the time of music administration to gather an immediate measure of the patients condition, physiological measures were pre and post test measures of heart rate, emotional condition rating scale, and nurse observation.
  Results: A significant reduction in heart rate when sedative music was played. Possible improvement in pain management as palliation. Staff also felt music helped mellow their own irritability with the patient and provided a pleasant environment.

- Bonny H and McCarron N. Music as an adjunct to anesthesia in operative procedures. *Journal of the American Assocation of Nurse Anesthetists* 1984;**Feb**:55–57.

  Music serves as a distraction from painful procedures and reduces anxiety. A brief clinical paper describing the use of a taped music programme in a hospital setting.

Fig. 27.3   Reference database compiled as abstracts.

have to be made. Editors often require additions and clarifications, or more significantly, deletions. Colleagues will advise you on areas which require elaboration, or on matters on which you inadequately expressed yourself. Sometimes they will remind you that some things in your text are best left unspoken. Others will suggest that perhaps the first paragraph of section five really ought to be in the preface to the report and that the Table you spent hours preparing really could better be relegated to the Appendix. This is the process of editing.

Search and replace

After writing a document you may find that certain words or phrases are not used consistently, or that you may wish to add extra explanatory text. This is when you can use the search function of the word processing programming. A simple command like 'Find' will enable the computer to scrutinize your document for the word or phrase you ask it to find. With a long document this saves time as it searches for all examples of that word.

In addition, there is often a feature called 'Search and Replace'. For example, it sometimes occurs that the words complementary medicine, alternative medicine and unconventional medicine appear in a paper. For the sake of consistency it is often better to use one term alone, e.g. 'complementary medicine' in England, 'unconventional medicine' in Germany. The 'Search and Replace' command can be used to find all examples of 'alternative medicine' and change them, manually or automatically, to 'complementary medicine'. This can also be used when the writer perhaps has unwittingly used a jargon word and needs to replace it with another word or phrase.

Where the writer often uses phrases, addresses or paragraphs then it is possible to build a specific glossary. A glossary is a collection of terms to be inserted into a document. For example, in the letters folder stored in my computer I have a specific addresses glossary with the addresses of particular journals and colleagues with whom I frequently communicate. This means that their addresses can be quickly inserted in a document. Within a technical writing folder it is possible to have particular paragraphs stored as a technical glossary. This function is exceptionally good for the production of standard text in letters regarding ethical requirements in clinical trials and patient consent forms. It is also a good facility for preparing invoices.

Contents

In the preparation of a long document it is advisable to prepare a table of contents. Advanced word processors offer this facility. The writer goes through the text on the screen and marks the words to be included in the table of contents. Using a simple command from the keyboard, the table of contents is then compiled complete with relevant page numberings (see Figure 27.4). On some computers it is possible to link several small documents together to produce a bigger document and have the pages automatically numbered beginning at 1 in the first document running through to the end of the last document. With an outlining tool

Summary 1
Introduction 1
Getting started 4
Word processing 6
Outlining 6
Dictionary 7
Formatting 8
Editing 11
Search and replace 12
Contents 13
Mailmerging 13
Graphics 13
Printing 14
Conclusion 15
Figure One:
      A format for the structure of a paper for publication 16
Figure Two:
      Page set up 17
Figure Three:
      Reference database compiled as abstracts 18
Figure Four:
      Table of contents automatically generated from head-
      ings 19
Figure Five:
      A graphic imported to the word processor 19

Fig. 27.4   Table of contents automatically generated from headings.

as mentioned above, it is possible to generate a table of contents from the outline structure.

Allied to this process is the compilation of an index. Essentially the routine is the same as creating a table of contents with certain elaborations for the compilations of nested terms in the index. Anyone who has ever attempted to compile an index by hand will appreciate the benefit of such a writing tool.

Mailmerging

For many of us, a maddening feature of word processors has been the ability to mailmerge. Whenever you receive through the post an obvious standard letter personalized with your name and address, then it has been 'mailmerged'. What happens in this process is that a letter for general circulation is written with specific codes embedded for the insertion of names and addresses. Then a list of compiled names and addresses is merged with the letter inserting the specific names and addresses in place of the codes. Such a feature is valuable for organizations wishing to send out hundreds of membership reminder letters compiled from their membership database, or to circulate selective members for particular committee meetings or regional symposia.

Graphics

Although this chapter is about the management of text, it is possible to include graphics in many word processed documents. Although the graphic elements must be produced in another program they can be easily introduced into the document (see Figure 27.5). Some word processors include a graphics handling ability, or supply a separate program with the word processor.

Modern technology has accelerated at such a rate that the user who wishes to incorporate photographs into his or her work can do so using a piece of equipment called a scanner. This is an extremely valuable tool for any organization wishing to prepare teaching material. Furthermore, the scanner can be used to 'read' already typewritten or previously published materials. Using this equipment a central organization can archive its previously printed material, or documentary material from other sources not yet prepared for the computer.

As word processing becomes more accessible then the producers of the software have progressively offered more features. One of these is the ability to compile tables. This really is a boon to the researcher. An extension of this ability is the possibility of preparing text as columns. Most of us type our pages as one column, and this is the format for most books. However, journals regularly organize their pages into two

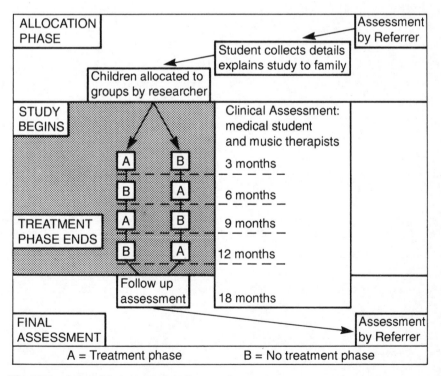

Fig. 27.5   A graphic imported to the word processor.

columns. Newspapers vary their format even more. For those organizations who wish to publish newsletters as well as papers, and teaching material, then the ability to organize text in multiple columns and include graphics is an essential feature.

Conclusion

Word processing is a relatively easy task to learn. Some modern computers are friendly to the user in that their operation is largely transparent. Once installed they require only that you switch them on, and with simple pointing actions using a hand-held device called a mouse, you can select the activities that you need. The entry of text is the same as typing, and documents are easy to prepare. Where word processing becomes complicated is when the user requires complicated page layouts with graphics inserted into the pages. This requires dedicated learning.

Before buying a computer to prepare your text, go and see what other people use, what they produce and ask what problems they have. Then be very precise in knowing what exactly you want to produce, who is going to produce it and who is going to develop the necessary skills to make full use of your investment in equipment. It is tempting to believe that 'desk top publishing' has been brought within the reach of many of us. This is not so. What we can do is prepare, change, store and print simple documents like research papers with the minimum of extra effort.

28 An introduction to electronic data management as a research tool

David Aldridge

Summary

For data to become information it must be structured. The personal computer offers varying ways to structure data and relate sets of data together. For researchers and practitioners wishing to maintain their awareness of current clinical research, the personal computer can provide access to electronic databases of the published literature. For researchers wishing to analyse their data, statistical analysis programs are available for the novice user.

Introduction

In this chapter we deal with the problem of data management. There are three general sections: databases, spreadsheets and statistical analysis packages. Spreadsheets and statistical analysis packages themselves are based upon a base of carefully organized data which have been subjected to further calculation and manipulation. The objective of all these data management programs is to convert raw data into information for the user. Before embarking upon any project which handles data it is important to think through these critical questions:

(a) What is the purpose of this data?

(b) Who is going to use this data?

(c) What sort of questions will the user ask of this data to fulfil the purpose outlined in (a)?

(d) How can this data be presented to others?

(e) How can this data be protected from unauthorized users?

Many of us first buy a computer to perform the task of word processing. However, the historical use of the computer has been to store, organize, and retrieve data. For these purposes the concept of a database was introduced. Data refers to anything that can be recorded as text or as numbers. Therefore, a telephone directory containing names (text), addresses (text and numbers) and telephone numbers is a primitive form of database; and of course you don't need a computer to use it. If you were to set about compiling such a directory you may well need a computer. In addition if you wanted to look for a particular family name in several regions of a country, then thumbing through a set of directories would take time. If these directories were computerized as an electronic database you could search the database for particular names and retrieve the information quickly by simply typing in keywords for searching.

Databases can provide opportunities to store and retrieve data quickly.

Most clinicians and researchers have a filing system which itself is a database, and no doubt they find their way around it quite quickly when they need to find information in a hurry. If they have a system which works already and fulfils their requirements then there is no need to computerize it. If they want to rearrange the way in which they store and retrieve data, perhaps to make a regular audit of work, to issue a standard letter to a particular group of patients or select a particular group for research, then it is worth while considering using a computer. In addition, it is possible to send data from a database to another software program for statistical analysis. What a computer cannot do is organize disorganized data, hence the questions suggested in the first paragraph.

The efficacy of any database reflects the way in which the person who constructs the database organizes their data and the understanding they have of that data. While some modern database programs are relatively easy to use and help the user to structure their data, there is no substitute for having clearly defined purposes for use of the data, a knowledge of the data itself (i.e. what it means) and a careful plan of the data to be collected. For example; the Complementary Medicine Index issued by the British Library Medical Information Service at Boston Spa was created by librarians who had no prior knowledge of database development. What they did have was a personal computer, enough money to buy 'off the shelf' computer software for database construction, and most importantly, a specialist expert knowledge of what an effective bibliographic database can do. To construct a new database they organized their data according to an existing database structure that covered other medical information and which they used as librarians on a daily basis. An expert knowledge of the data and the structure between elements of the data is essential for constructing an effective data management system.

A database, then, is a structured form of organized data. This organized data can be a set of patient records, a list of research papers, an inventory of herbal preparations or a list of employees and related personnel. Each database will comprise several components.

1 Data categories

If we take the example of a patient record we can see how a simple database is constructed. The categories involved in the simplest of databases would be:

Surname
Forename
Street address name and house number
Name of the town
Name of the region in which they live
Area code number
Telephone number
Date of birth
Date when registered, and
Name of their health practitioner.

Each of these categories is called a field, and these fields are either text fields (names), number fields (house numbers and code numbers) or date fields (date of birth, date of registration). (It is also possible to have a visual field for the storage of pictures or a sound field for the storage of music.)

All the fields for this one patient when considered together are called a record. All the patient records collected together are called a data file or table (see Figure 28.1). The above structure would give a basis for a simple database which could handle one file at a time; i.e. patient records. These systems are usually called 'flat file systems' or 'file managers' and they work like a card index. It is easy to adapt such a structure to contain more information fields. Such systems are also useful for creating bibliographies of references as mentioned in the last chapter.

However, the data structure is a little restricting and inflexible. You may want to store along with the name of the general practitioner the corresponding address and telephone number. This would involve typing on each record the same details for every patient with the same

A common data matrix structure for a database

| | | fields | |
	name	date	address
	patient 1	Brown	13.3.1991	High Street
records	patient 2			
	patient 3			

A common data matrix structure for a spreadsheet program

| | | fields | |
	column A	column B	column C
	row 1	cell A1	cell B1	cell C1
records	row 2	cell A2	cell B2	cell C2
	row 3	cell A3	cell B3	cell C3

A common data matrix structure for a statistical analysis program

| | | fields | |
	variable 1	variable 2	variable 3
	case 1	120	80	79,5
records	case 2			
	case 3			

Fig. 28.1

general practitioner, and should that practitioner change address then each separate record would have to be altered. The solution to this problem is to have two files; one for patients, one for practitioners, with a common linking field, i.e. name of practitioner. By having the name in both files then a relationship is made between files, hence the term 'relational database'.

Relational databases have been developed rapidly in the last five years. Essentially they are composed of user-defined lists (patients, patients' families, practitioners, referrers, medicines, disease classifications) which are cross-referenced one with another. These relational databases provide the most flexible way for the management of complex clinical data. However, they are not easy for the novice to use from scratch, no matter what the advertising literature or computer specialists say to the contrary.

2   Modification of data

It is important that data once entered can be modified. With a paper file it is possible to add a new record by inserting the sheet of paper in the correct alphabetical order. To remove a patient record you would simply take out the corresponding sheet. Similarly, patients may change their address, change their practitioner or leave the area. When purchasing a database system it is essential to know how easy it is to modify the data and the structure of that data once it is inserted.

3   Storage and presentation of data

For most patient data there would be a standard format for that data; a patient registration form, for example. This enables data to be entered and checked easily and collected systematically. Most modern databases provide an easy method of entering data which can be formatted to appear on the computer screen like a data entry form. There are also routines which can be built into such entry procedures which alert the operator to mistakes in data entry.

When we construct a database we are concerned with getting the data in, and, of equal importance, getting the data out again at a later date. To this end database programs have a way of formatting data as reports in varying configurations. Data from one record can be presented on the screen in the format in which it was entered, or a list of all the people living at the same address can be presented. It is also possible to construct a data field which is derived from calculations based on other fields; e.g. cost of medicines consumed by a group of patients of a particular age, number of patients seen in a month, number of articles published on a specified topic in a given year.

As word processors have become increasingly complex in their ability to present text, then databases have also developed to present their data in a form suitable for publication.

4   Ordering and retrieval of data

The ordering of data in a database is called indexing. The data can be ordered on a number of indexes (indices). Alphabetic ordering of names is one such way. Patient record numbers is another. Using the practitioner's name would also provide another index. Complex database systems allow for the use of particular key words. These words form an index which allows for a faster search of a large database and also means that the database does not take up so much space on the computer's storage device. When we want to retrieve data, and display that data according to certain criteria, i.e. all patients over age 65 living in the north of the city who have Dr Smith as their general practitioner, then we are using indexing for the purpose of retrieval. It is such complex tasks, where data is retrieved according to differing criteria, that are the strength of computer databases. Our physical paper file of patient records can only have one order; in most cases alphabetical, although it is possible to create a cross-reference. Generally a paper file only allows the user to find one thing at a time. With a computer database the data can be searched using aggregates of specific criteria as requested by the user.

5   Rules relating data

An extension of the relational database is the expert system.[1] The 'expert' refers to the human expertise which lies within the database. While a database contains data sets which can be related, an expert system can propose decisions based on data weighted for importance and rules which relate those data together. An abstract example of such a rule is:

> IF a configuration of symptoms is present
> AND these symptoms constitute a known pattern of a disease
> THEN there is sufficient grounds to classify the subject being
> considered as belonging to a definite diagnostic class.*

There is the potential in such systems to give each piece of evidence a weighting such that the classification can be given a defined probability.

Certain symptom groupings, in conjunction with particular laboratory tests and a known patient history, may suggest a diagnosis or clinical hypothesis. An expert system can suggest such diagnoses or hypotheses on interrogation, suggest further tests which will confirm hypotheses and give an indication of why the suggestion was made. This does not remove decision-making from the practitioner, it merely presents a broad platform of knowledge available to that practitioner.

The Centre for Complementary Health Studies at the University of Exeter, England, is currently compiling an expert knowledge-based system (EXTRACT) which will provide annotated information about the chemistry, pharmacology and therapeutics of medicinal plants, and their constituents, from a range of sources. This knowledge-based system is attempting to compile what is at the moment fragmentary

* IF it walks like a duck AND talks like a duck THEN it is a duck.

information and assemble it in a form which makes sense to the researcher. Knowledge base, in this sense, is the specific sets of information regarding medicinal plants and their properties, and the way in which they relate to each other as rated by an expert, or panel of experts.

In practice

A system, once it has been designed, should be able to handle differing requests to view the data in many ways. A well-designed system will allow anyone with authorized access to the information to find information easily according to their needs; this is sometimes termed the 'user interface'. When a program is termed 'user friendly' it means that this interface is accessible to a novice user and that interrogation of the database can be carried out using natural language commands without specialist computer knowledge; simply type in the words of the categories for which you are looking.

A clinical database should allow standard information to be entered only once. Ideally it will integrate with a previous paper or card system so that the new replaces the old, and the former users understand what data is being collected. It is important to develop a system which secretaries and administrative staff can use with a minimum of training. As with word processors discussed in the previous chapter, good software should be 'transparent' to the user. If a system is being developed then it should be better than the current paper system and facilitate the administrative processing of new patient records, for example. In addition there should be a straightforward way to facilitate the retrieval of important clinical information for administrative and research purposes. Although the database is electronically stored there must be a way of providing a paper copy of information which is contained within that database.

Medical record systems can be adapted to produce automatic reminder letters for immunization, recall to the clinic for particular tests or warnings for incompatible medicines according to predetermined criteria. An important use of such systems is that they can form the basis for a practice audit. For complementary practitioners the use of an international disease classification system as well as their own classification system can provide the basis for a continuing comparative research project within therapeutic modes and between groups of practitioners. Databases can be so constructed to consult standard tables when a recognized word is typed in a given field; a disease can be automatically classified using an international system or esoteric system, or a questionnaire answer can be automatically weighted.

A database can also be constructed such that specific data is requested at different phases of the patient's career; i.e. at referral, registration, first clinical contact, subsequent contacts, when the treatment is completed and at follow-up. Additionally specific sex or age-related data can be requested; i.e. cervical smear tests or developmental tests.

Examples of bibliographic databases

Some databases come already constructed and these are of particular value to the researcher interested in reviewing the published literature. The Medical Information Service of the British Library has access to over 200 databases, some 50 of which address medical and biological bibliographic data. They produce a regular index to specific topics in complementary medicine, and also offer a service which searches for user-specified topics. One of the databases which they search is the MEDLINE database compiled by the American National Library.

MEDLINE is an electronic version of the published bibliographic database *Index Medicus*. Each **record** in the database is a journal paper, some of the **fields** of which are

author field:	Vincent, S.
author field:	Thompson, J.
title field:	The effects of music on the human blood pressure
source field:	Lancet
date field:	1929
volume number field:	1
issue number field:	(March 9)
page number field:	534–537

Abstracts of articles are often included, as is the address of the institution producing the research. Of particular importance is the use of keywords for a special index. Using this index the computer searches accurately and quickly. It is possible to search on a free text basis, i.e. simply look for a word and the database will produce all records containing that word, but this method is slow. The speed of searching using particular keywords is vital if you are using an 'online' database.

An 'online' database is an electronic database which you access through a computer via a telephone link. The telephone services which give a weather report, details of airline flight timetables or, more importantly, cricket results, are all examples of an 'online' database. An electronic bibliographic database like MEDLINE gives the user the opportunity to search for information providing they are registered users of the database. There are various vendors of such databases and there are varying registration charges. Most important is the 'online' charge itself. It is costly to use a telephone link during the day to browse through a database of literally thousands of articles, hence the need for an index and speed of searching.[2] Furthermore, if you then download those references with their abstracts to your own computer there is an additional charge.

If you are thinking of providing a library service to a professional group and wish to use various 'online' databases then you will need several pieces of hardware to search 'online'. First you will need a computer, and a printer to retrieve, store and print out information. Second, that computer will need a telephone connector and a modem. A modem is a device which allows you to communicate with another computer at a remote site. This remote site will be where the master database is situated. To make this hardware contact between the user and the information source requires a telecommunications software package compatible with sender and receiver.

The vendor of the database will then supply you with a password which allows access to their database or, more often, databases. Access to more than one database is essential, as different databases store different information from a varying spread of literature sources. There are respective databases for medicine, complementary medicine, psychology, social science, education, cancer reports, chemistry, and toxic chemicals, to name a few among many. Some vendors give a password free of charge, the hidden costs are in the online charges. These vary from vendor to vendor and it is important to ascertain what these are before you search.[2] It is also important for organizations to know who in the organization requesting the service will pay for the search costs.

What you pay depends upon the nature and volume of information you request. Abstracts of the papers you find in your search will cost more than citations alone. Citations alone don't provide enough information. It is possible with some services to request photocopies of the papers which are found in the search. The British Library, for example, offer this service, but each photocopy itself comes at a cost.

For the individual user faced with the complexities of a medical database with no clearly defined set of keywords, the best way of searching is to use a librarian experienced in computer searching. The librarian should be skilled enough to ask the correct questions which will limit the search. However, librarians, no matter how skilled, cannot be expected to work miracles. Much time can be saved by asking yourself questions about the limits of your search: what languages do you want to include, do you want animal or human studies, what is the age range of your study, do you want studies of both males and females, and what years do you want to cover or are you willing to place a limit at 50 citations? If you are making a review of the literature on the treatment of asthma using acupuncture, your question will have different search parameters to that of an update on current therapeutic developments in asthma therapy.

Once you have the basic limits of your search you will need to know the terms on which you will search. It is at this juncture where you must study the index of the particular database or enlist the help of a librarian. A common method for structuring a search is to use a previously published example of research which typifies what you are searching for, in this case: Aldridge, D., Pietroni, P. The clinical assessment of acupuncture for asthma therapy. *Journal of the Royal Society of Medicine* 1987; **80**: 222–4. Library experts are helpful and save both time and money. They can often ask the simplest questions to which we as researchers are blind, or refer us to databases which we are unaware of.

The British Library provides a comprehensive information service offering computer searches on the main medical and paramedical databases[3,4] and monthly printed indexes for complementary medicine, occupational therapy, physiotherapy, rehabilitation and terminal care. In addition, there is a MEDLINE monthly update service for maintaining current awareness on specific topics from alcoholism and anxiety to schizophrenia and smoking. The faculty of medicine at the French University of Montpelier has compiled such an international 'online' literature service for acupuncture documentation (ACUBASE).[5]

When a database is published as hard copy and made available directly to the user it is known as an 'offline' database. Examples of 'offline' databases are the printed versions of *Index Medicus* and telephone directories. There are no hidden charges once the printed copy of the database has been purchased, and the user can search and browse at will. However, the searching of such a database, often involving several volumes, can take considerable time. With the advent of information storage on floppy diskettes and compact disks that situation has changed dramatically. It is possible to buy from a commercial vendor a copy of MEDLINE recorded on a compact disk, or the topic-related indexes (including Complementary Medicine Index) published by the British Library in floppy disk format. Most vendors have back copies available covering previous years, and each diskette contains one year of citations.

For compact disk databases, once the registration fee is paid, a new compact disk is sent every month with current information of newly published articles. The hardware required is a microcomputer and a compact disk player with the appropriate search software which is supplied by the vendor (some vendors also have a charge which includes the compact disk player). Searching in this manner allows for a relaxed browsing of the literature and is particularly useful for novices. The discovered citations and their abstracts can be printed out as required. The only disadvantage is that at the moment the databases available on compact disks are limited. With new technological developments it is possible in the near future that even small groups will be able to compile and distribute their own databases using this medium. Already several libraries publish their catalogues this way.

A further recent development is the publication of monthly compact disks which contain the current contents of journals as complete articles, photographs and letters. For example, a commercial service is available which sends the contents of over 300 of the most consulted European medical journals to registered users for them to browse and copy at their leisure. The cost is lower than that of buying all three hundred journals, and certainly saves library space. However, the sticking point is that there is a copyright charge levied by the publisher for each copy of the article made by the user. This copyright charge, while ensuring the survival of the journal, escalates the cost of the service.

It is essential when using any such database to have a clear idea of how the data is to be used so that it becomes information. There is a potential data explosion where people have access to vast sets of data. It is possible to generate long lists of citations and then find that the cost of obtaining the papers themselves is prohibitive. Furthermore, making sense of the contents of those papers can itself be a lengthy research task. This glut of data poses as many problems as an absence of data. The key to the solution of the problem is in the organization of thinking necessary for solving the task in hand. Preparation of research in the careful formulating of the research question will help avoid later confusions, and discipline in structuring the search for bibliographical data helps to prevent gathering too much data.

In the last chapter, personal bibliography databases were mentioned. These are a valuable aid to the researcher or a group of researchers. It is possible to download citations from an online database onto floppy diskettes and thereby construct specific libraries of citations according to particular topics. These can then be copied onto other floppy diskettes and shared with colleagues. Most database programs of this sort allow the user to enter details of conference proceedings, monographs, unpublished reports, newspaper cuttings and personal notes. When writing a subsequent paper, details from such a database can be cited in the paper and the paper references automatically compiled according to a particular journal format.

Security

The storage of data in computers has caused much concern in that personal data is potentially accessible to unauthorized viewers. When various fields of data are stored together then it is possible for a viewer to have quite a detailed picture of a person's private life. With the computerization of patient records containing psychological, medical, familial and social data, each entered at different sources by differing persons, then there is always the potential for a loss of privacy. Paper systems, although cumbersome, repetitious and often lacking in coordination, do have the advantage that they can be locked away safe from prying eyes. Their very faults, that they are personnel-dependent and slow, are their strengths for protecting privacy. With electronic databases it is possible to have rapid access to large stores of personal private data, and to corrupt that data.

If the user has a computer which stands alone on the desk, and that computer is not connected to a network of any sort, then the possibility of others having access to stored data is no greater than a filing cabinet being invaded, or a room being broken into. The information can be stored on a floppy diskette which can be removed from the machine and kept in a safe place. The computer can be switched off and locked. For added protection a password can be used to prevent other users having access to classified information.

Most problems occur when several computers are linked together on one site, and several users have access to documents or the same database; hence the various legislations for the protection of personal data. Passwords are often the commonest source of data protection. These are issued to authorized users and can be changed to apply to particular documents and activities only, or for particular time periods varying from minutes to months. Needless to say, the very idea of a password has spawned a breed of computer enthusiasts dedicated to breaking such protection devices, although small organizations have little to fear. Sensitive information can be stored on removable devices which are then locked away, but this means that access to such information is dependent on someone being able to put the relevant disk in the computer.

Spreadsheets

The spreadsheet is a particular class of data management. Its simplest form is that of a data matrix of rows and columns. It has been actively embraced by the business community who have been influential in developing easy to use software, as in the example of wordprocessing.

Data is spread out in a sheet before the user. Particular cases (*records* in our database terminology) are arranged in rows, and the columns of the spreadsheet correspond to the fields of those cases. In essence this is a simple data matrix (see Figure 28.1). Each particular row would be a patient and the corresponding column would be a field belonging to that patient; i.e. registration number, name, address, date of birth. These fields can be extended further to include laboratory or clinical test data. The space where each row meets a column is called a *cell*; row A column 1 is cell A1 (**record** A **field** 1).

The advantages of a spreadsheet is that it can be set up to make calculations based on information in those cells or range of cells, and store that data as a separate field for each record. For example; each patient record may contain scores for separate parts of a health questionnaire. These scores can then be totalled, or weighted with a particular constant, to produce a composite score for the whole questionnaire. The calculation of such a score can be automated such that when the row of scores is completed then the calculation is made. This is achieved by writing a simple formula which says 'add column 1 to column 2 to column 3 and divide by 3 (or whatever number is appropriate) and record the result in column 4'. For a particular treatment group (rows A4 to M4) it would be possible to compute the average score and record it in a separate cell in the data matrix, and then compare that score with the average score of a control group (rows N4 to Z4).

Such data matrices can be printed out directly as tables or sent to a word processor and incorporated in reports. The formatting of such data is very sophisticated, and with modern computing also allows data to be presented graphically in various ways. Most spreadsheet programs have the facility to present data as histograms, bar charts, pie charts, scatter graphs and line graphs.

As spreadsheet programs handle data matrices and have the capacity to make calculations upon the data which they contain, there has been a parallel development in the statistical procedures which can be applied to that data using such programs. However, while it is possible to make quite advanced calculations on data using a spreadsheet program it is generally easier to use a specialized statistics package for the analysis of data. Many spreadsheet programs are arranged to work with database packages so that they can import and export data between each other. It is possible to buy spreadsheet packages which double as rudimentary databases.

For initial data entry in research studies, spreadsheet programs are a useful tool in arranging and manipulating data prior to statistical analysis in that they are flexible in the way in which they allow the input and transformation of data. If researchers do use a spreadsheet to input data, it is important that the spreadsheet program is compatible with the program which they will use for the statistical analysis of that data.

Statistical analysis programs

Modern statistical analysis on a microcomputer is a relatively straight-forward process providing that the researcher understands the underlying structure of the data. Data can be entered into a matrix of columns and rows rather like a simple spreadsheet. Usually the rows of the matrix are the records (cases, patients or subjects) and the columns are the fields corresponding to those cases (i.e. patient variables).

Once the data is entered and the data saved as a file in the computer then various statistical procedures can be performed from the simplest of descriptive statistics to the most complex of regression analyses and time series computations. While the possibility of statistical analysis for computer novices appears as a boon, this benefit must be moderated by the knowledge that such programs will find correlations even within randomly generated data.

A recent development in statistical analysis, particularly for the business world, is that of exploratory statistics using graphics.[6] With refined and complex graphing techniques it is possible to present numerical data relating to several variables in graphical form. This allows changes in one variable, or set of variables, to be seen in relation. While this exploratory analysis can be informative, particularly when we are dealing with many variables and wish to make hypotheses which are grounded in empirical data, it can be confusing for the novice user and itself demands an underlying knowledge of the data.

Word processing programs have encouraged us to produce high quality documents in terms of formatting and presentation. Databases are capable of being formatted such that their contents can be represented in varying report formats. Spreadsheets in the business community are sold partly in terms of their ability to present data graphically. This graphical presentation, which often includes three-dimensional graphing with varying colour codes, can be as obscuring as it can be clarifying. So too with statistical packages. Too much information in a graph is confusing, and three dimensional presentations work counter to accurate judgement by encouraging visual illusions. For comparative studies simple histograms and line graphs allow the viewer to compare profiles of data.

Most statistical programs for personal computers have been developed from a mainframe parentage. They are easier to use than their parents and usually come with quite comprehensive handbooks as documentary support. If you are investing in a powerful program it is worthwhile attending a training course in the use of the program. Several companies offer a series of courses which cover an introduction to the program, and then various statistical approaches (descriptive statistics, time series analysis, multivariate analysis).

There are a range of general statistical programs available. Most of them offer a data editor which can sort and transform data, descriptive statistics, parametric and non-parametric tests and a graphics or charting package. There are other programs which have been developed for specific data analysis methods; distribution free non-parametric analysis, time series data analysis and analysis of variance.

When buying such a package it is important to know what statistics you wish to use. Not all packages will provide what you want; some packages are better for general statistics than others, while some packages may specialize in complex multivariate procedures, analytic graphics or high quality output. The essential questions to ask are:

(a) What statistical analyses do I wish to use?

(b) What statistical packages are available which can perform those analyses?

(c) Do I have hardware which is compatible with that software package to analyse data and print out results?

(d) Is my software and hardware compatible with my colleagues' such that we can compare and check our results?

(e) Does the software supplier offer an advice 'hotline' if I have difficulties, and regular updates of the package?

(f) Does the statistical package have a pedigree; i.e. has it been used before in the scientific community?

Ease of data editing, sorting and transforming play an important role in the use of a statistical package. If you cannot enter the data easily then it is likely that you will be discouraged from using the package. If the package itself does not have a good data editing facility it should at least be able to import data from a spreadsheet where data can be formatted prior to analysis. Do not be sidetracked by exotic graphing routines. If you require complex charts then it is possible to buy a separate charting program at a later data. Most researchers wish to present their results for publication so it is important to be able to export your findings and charts from the statistical package to a word processing program. Finally; ask colleagues which programs they use, contact a local computer user group and if possible prepare a set of data for analysis and make a test run; or, if you are planning to buy an expensive package, take a set of data to your software dealer.

When using a statistical program it is advisable to save any raw data matrices as a security back-up copy of the original material for the researcher, but also as a copy for validation by other researchers who can scrutinize and analyse the same data.

For the researcher wishing to use a computer for research purposes I can recommend the following software packages.

Literature database

EndNote: A reference database and bibliography maker. Niles & Associates Inc., 2000 Hearst Street, Berkeley, California 94709, USA.

For the clinician or researcher who needs to write and prepare papers this is a marvellous program. I use it daily and would not wish to be without it. It is an invaluable working tool.

First, it is a free text database program. That is, it specializes in storing, managing and searching for data, which in this case are literature references. This database of literature can be collated as separate personal libraries, and as a master library. Small libraries can be converged from the references of colleagues to form a larger subject library. It is therefore ideal for a group of people working together.

Second, it is a bibliography maker. As you write you can refer to your literature references and insert a special marker for that reference in the text, gradually building a list of references. When the paper is complete the program will scan the completed paper for those reference markers and compile a bibliography for you. Furthermore, it will insert the appropriate citation markers according to the journal style for which you are writing (numerical, author/date, alphabetical) and format the bibliography in the journal style you are choosing.[7,8] Finally, it will make a copy of your original paper complete with citation markers and a printed bibliography at the end of that paper suitable for the journal style of your choice.

Traditionally the collation of references was done by writing details of books and papers on card to form card indexes. This could also contain cryptic comments and notes referring to other files. This program works in the same way. The advantage that it has over a card index is that it can sort through all your references very quickly, word by word, and provide you with a list of those papers you have been looking for. There is a facility also for storing abstracts of papers. This is extended by a 'note' facility which also stores text and can be used for items like 'You can find this item in the folder marked "Computers: Literature databases" in the cupboard down the corridor'. Both note and abstract sections can contain about 3000 words each.

Most databases have a section for typing in keywords and this program is no different. Words not occurring in the text can be typed into this section. This is useful when you have found a paper about a specific clinical problem, and it also proves to be a very good example of a research method, or you later want to use it for teaching purposes. You can then type into your note or keyword section, 'teaching' or 'research methods'. Several months later the program can be asked to display the references you have marked 'teaching'. You can just as easily do it manually by putting the same papers in a folder marked 'teaching material'. But when several papers have more than one function, i.e. they are interesting methodologically, theoretically, discuss personality profiles of cancer patients, provide details of immunological status, and are useful for teaching purposes, then it becomes expensive in terms of paper and space to store several (thus illegal†) copies of the same article.

Recently I made a literature search using a computerized medical database for articles dealing separately with medical education and systems theory. It was possible to store directly the 300 references which I needed in this EndNote program, as the program is formatted to import data from online databases.

The EndNote program works on an Apple Macintosh and is very easy to use. It can be adapted to meet your specific requirements and also works with word processing programs as a disk accessory. For example, when I write an article in my word processing program (Microsoft Word 4) then I can open a reference library of stored articles on the screen as I write and search for particular references. That really is computing which meets the needs of the user. Highly recommended.

Statistical packages

Unistat III. Statistical package for IBM-compatible computers. Unistat Limited, PO Box 383, Highgate, London N6 5UP, 081–883–7155.

The III in Unistat III indicates that the statistical package has a lineage. From quite modest beginnings the package has developed into a very useful research tool offering a wide range of statistical routines.

The personal computer lends itself to statistical computing. For those of us who spent time with the University mainframe computers, the calculation of statistical data was often a complex and difficult process. Not so with this user-friendly program, principally for the way in which it handles the raw data and graphically displays the results of analyses.

To compute data it is necessary to log the data into the computer. This is achieved in Unistat by means of a spreadsheet. This initial part of the package is a major feat of computing in that it is simple to use and understand from an excellently produced handbook. An essential stage of any statistical analysis is assurance for the user that they can easily manipulate their data.

The statistical routines are comprehensive. This package will meet the basic statistical needs of any organization needing a wide range of descriptive statistics and there are also the standard parametric tests that are generally required, the non-parametric tests which feature in every good textbook and comprehensive regression and anova routines.

Once the data is statistically analysed it is important to be able to see clearly the results of that analysis. This Unistat does very well indeed. There are excellent plotting facilities which can be printed out in the form of hard copy on a range of standard printing devices. For those who need to handle data regularly in the same way then there is 'record/playback' facility which records the keystrokes that you make

---

† Only one copy of an article per person is allowed for individual research according to copyright regulations.

while handling the data. This routine is then recorded and can be applied to similar sets of data.

Overall, a solid dependable package which offers most of the routines a researcher could wish for. Such a software package with a wide range of routines, combined with a facility for the easy management of raw data, at a very reasonable price and capable of being run on readily available hardware makes this an ideal basic statistical package for clinical research.

The producer of this software is also open to feedback about the package which has led to its varying modifications. The user can therefore be secure that the package has been tried and tested at the workface. It is well worth trying the demonstration package available from the producer to see for yourself. Highly recommended.

MultiStat by S. M. Day. A general purpose statistical package for the Apple Macintosh. Biosoft, 22 Hills Road, Cambridge CB2 1JP, UK.

Biosoft are renowned for their range of scientific software. They have developed a range of products suitable for the analysis of scientific data, and this statistical package is a part of their excellent catalogue. The appeal of the Apple Macintosh range of computers is ease of use, particularly for the novice to computing. All software produced for the machine is expected to conform to certain operating principles such that the user feels at home in different programs; each program has a common series of commands. This is of particular value in a statistics package where the user may feel in a very strange world indeed.

Multistat is an extremely valuable piece of software for the novice and for the experienced user. It is extremely simple to use and to understand. It has none of the pretensions of the larger statistical packages developed for business users. What it offers is a good solid ground of statistical procedures supported by an excellent manual.

The method of data entry is rather crude, relying on data being entered as a series of columns. This is sufficient for most purposes. It is possible to import data from spreadsheets (e.g. Microsoft EXCEL), which is a valuable feature. I entered data as a text file from another statistical package quite easily. Once the data has been entered then it can be transformed logarithmically, trigonometrically, squared or raised to a given power, ranked and sorted. There is a range of descriptive statistics, as would be expected.

The statistical tests include most of those needed in a basic program: the Student t test (paired and unpaired); analyses of variance which extend the Student t test to more than two cases and also include the Kruskal Wallis technique and the Friedman procedure, simple and multiple regression, and proportion tests.

Perhaps the most commonly used test of probability for psychology students is the chi-square statistic. This program provides an unbelievably easy method of calculating this statistic for 2×2 contingency tables or larger. Just as importantly, it offers the Fisher exact test when numbers are unavoidably small for such a contingency test. The

Mcnemar test for handling data from before and after experiments is included, as are the Wilcoxon signed ranks test and the Mann-Whitney U test. Whereas the regression tests provide correlation coefficients for parametric data, the Spearman correlation coefficient offers a non-parametric equivalent, as does the Kendall correlation. Finally there is the Kolmogorov-Smirnov two sample test which can be applied to two sets of data to discover if they are similarly distributed. While appearing to be quite a modest array of tests, such a program would provide the ideal support for any individual or group wanting an introduction to statistics and could play an important role in medical training courses where an understanding of biomathematics is necessary.

There is a graphing facility which allows the user to make a quick appreciation of the data. However, this facility is rudimentary, as the author of the program acknowledges, and the suggested procedure for visually presenting results is to export the data to a graphics package. This could be the self-same spreadsheet software used to edit the data in the first place. Multistat would then be essentially a series of subroutines within a spreadsheet.

I have no hesitation in wholeheartedly recommending this package; it is unpretentious and does what it claims to do. I was recently asked to carry out a statistical analysis of a small educational project which evaluated students' assessments of their own knowledge of neurology, and the assessment of their tutor. This was a simple problem for a 2×3 contingency table. However, a computer program costing far in excess of Multistat could not calculate ready tabulated data. With Multistat, all that was necessary was to call the appropriate statistic from the menu of statistical tests, type in the numbers and see the results expressed as a statistic of probability.

It is well worth writing to Biosoft at the above address to obtain a catalogue of their software for both Apple and IBM-compatible computers.

Systat Version 5.0. Systat Inc., 1800 Sherman Avenue, Evanston, Illinois 60201, USA.

I must confess to a dread of statistics, which is rather embarrassing for an academic who tries to pass himself off as a research consultant. Occasionally, when the buck can't be passed on to someone else, or I'm feeling particularly brave, I flirt with the notion of becoming fluent in 'statistic'. This flirtation is usually accompanied by a dream where some strange alien being (yes, an American) has invented a computer and all I have to do is type in my results and the computer will do the rest. Out come fantastic graphs of highly significant correlations at stunning levels of probability and power.

For those of you with psychological leanings this potential pathological daydreaming of omnipotence, completely unfounded in reality, can be traced back to my adolescence. Having passed maths 'O' level a year early at school, I was eligible to start a course in calculus. After one lesson I decided that mathematics was all too much, and began a crash course in woodwork. For me woodwork was a blessing and a hardship.

It could only be studied in the break after school dinners, a time usually reserved for the illicit ciggy behind the bike sheds. Ever since then I always think of maths as something I can't do, and woodwork as something I can do instead of smoking. Come to think of it, I made a wooden ashtray stand.

Many modern statistical packages for the Apple Macintosh set out to fulfil my dream of the all-singing, all-dancing statistics package. They are designed to have a maximum impact on the business world which demands excellent graphics tools and presentation methods for reports and slide shows. Into this world have stepped the mainframe statistical package producers whose former products were only accessible to statisticians, students forced to take elementary courses in statistics, or people who hadn't passed 'O' level woodwork.

Systat has a long pedigree of development. It is available for a number of hardware platforms and the recent development for the Macintosh is an attempt to break into the potentially lucrative business market where the main demand is for the analysis of multivariate statistics. The program has many strengths; the graphing facilities are very good indeed and come with their own handbook which has an invaluable section on the presentation of graphical data. Incorporated in this part of the package is the concept of exploratory graphics which allows the user to see the data plotted in three dimensional space, to rotate that plot of data around three axes at determined speeds and in user-determined degrees. These plots of data do not stand alone but can be accompanied by statistical analyses of the same data.

The statistical routines themselves are extensive and easy to apply if you understand the relationships between the variables in your data set. Each statistical routine is called from a menu by clicking on the appropriate icon. Each icon has submenus. This system of icons and submenus is an elegant solution to what could be extreme complexity. Statistical analyses can be instantly linked to graphical presentations of results. While the exploratory graphics can suggest relationships which you have not previously thought of, these relationships can be completely spurious. Each particular section of statistical procedures is accompanied by examples in the accompanying handbook, although the reader cannot rely upon such brief explanations. Admittedly the handbooks do contain further references, and this is where the going gets rough as you probably don't have the requisite statistics paper to hand when you are in the middle of analysing a set of data.

All in all, this is not a program for beginners but is useful for statisticians and researchers. I cannot say that it is excellent as my review version contained a few bugs: the program did not like to load with any anti-virus INITs installed, some of the box graph routines did not work, the axes labelling was not diagonally off-set as described in the handbook, it was impossible to do a simple chi-square without a tabulation of the raw data, and the data editor was slow and unforgiving. Furthermore, and I must admit this is something which is particularly irritating to someone who works on a restricted budget; first you need at least 4MB of RAM (which for most users will mean buying additional memory chips for their machine); second, it is advisable for the production of bigger graphs to have a bigger screen than what was, and probably still is, the standard Macintosh screen; and third, the print output is at its best quality if the user has a laser printer. While the program gives a reasonable output on a desk jet printer, for large scale graphics it is necessary to import to a word processor. The enlargement of graphs then leads to both a distortion of scale and a distortion in the printing of dotted lines. In a complex line graph this spoils the whole appearance which defeats the purpose of having a graphics capability incorporated within the program.

If you are a 'power user' with large scale multivariate calculations, or need a comprehensive package with time series analysis with the possibility for 'add-on' statistical routines, and have the hardware, Systat is a very useful piece of software. However, it may be advisable for the user on a limited budget to discern exactly what they require in terms of statistical processing, whether or not their money may be better spent consulting a statistician, and then to purchase a series of exact solutions to meet their needs.

The Macintosh User Group has a number of contacts in the UK who are interested in medical computing and statistical solutions. They can be contacted at Macintosh House, 11 South Parade, Summertown, Oxford OX2 7JL. I recommend them as a valuable source of information, advice and support.

Conclusion

Electronic data management depends upon careful organization of data. If you are compiling or searching a database, or producing an expert knowledge system, the same organizational structure and relational rules are necessary. Most packages have a similar matrix format of rows and columns. How those rows and columns are related one to another depends upon particular sets of rules for analysing the data. Generally, if you understand the structure of your data, and the way it relates together, i.e. the meaning of your data, the management of that data and its subsequent analysis should be relatively straightforward. Where you are not sure of the relationships between sets of data then a statistical analysis package will assist you in this understanding by presenting correlations between data. It must be remembered that these relationships are only hypothetical and can be an artefact of the statistical procedure.

A most valuable form of electronic data management is the electronic library database which helps the researcher keep aware of published research material or allows access to research archives. Specialist library services are available to help researchers and it is advisable, as in the case of statistical analyses, to call upon the advice of experts in the field.

Modern medicine in Europe is trying to bring databases and expert systems together so that they have a common ground. In this way information and expertise can be shared beneficially. Complementary medicine could also organize itself such that common data sets are organized to facilitate further research and the sharing of expertise.

References

[1] Chytil, M., Engelbrecht, R. *Medical Expert Systems*. Wilmslow, Cheshire: Sigma Press, 1987.

[2] Hewitt, P., Chalmers, T. Perusing the literature: Methods of accessing Medline and related databases. *Cont Clin Trials* 1987; **6**: 75–83 and 168–77.

[3] Roberts, D. A new information service for occupational therapists. *Br J Occup Ther* 1988; **51**(10): 353–4.

[4] Roberts, D. Current awareness in the paramedical sciences. In: Hewlett, J. (ed.) *Keyguide to Information Sources in Paramedical Sciences*. Poole: Mansell, 1990.

[5] Deshays, C. *Guide pour L'Indexation et L'Interrogation d'Acubase*. Nimes: 1987.

[6] Wilkinson, L. *SYSGRAPH: The System for Graphics*. Evanston, Illinois: SYSTAT Inc, 1989.

[7] Aldridge, D. Single case research designs. *Comp Med Res* 1988; **3**: 37–46.

[8] Aldridge, D. A phenomenological comparison of the organization of music and the self. *Arts in Psychotherapy* 1989; **16**: 91–7.

29 A guide to preparing a research application

David Aldridge

Summary

There are several stages to preparing a research application. Careful thinking about clinical practice and the allocation of time for research is essential. Statistical decisions are best made before data is collected.

Introduction

The state of novice researcher can reduce even master practitioners to exasperation; few of us are trained in research methods during our clinical careers. Perhaps one of the keys to successful planning is to ask crucial questions early in the research process. Here then are some considerations which a research methodologist would bear in mind.

I shall assume that the researcher has already gone through the preliminary stages of having a good idea which appears to be completely original and potentially world-shattering when written on the back of an envelope. The next stages of writing the ideas down for colleagues to criticize and making overtures to funding agencies are far more gruelling.

If you wish to do research then it is a continuing struggle to maintain that first flush of excitement against what may seem unreasonable odds and what at times seem to be tiresome practical details. These challenges are the ones which curb our worst excesses and in the end facilitate our research. Research takes a great deal of personal motivation.

It is important to find some form of personal and professional support which is constructive but critical. In addition, it is possible to work as a group to support each other, share varying skills and to teach each other about research methods. It is important to bear in mind that research is greedy for resources. First there is money, which is presumably why you are considering some form of grant funding. At the end of this paper you will find a section about costing.

Second is time. It is essential to plan your own time very carefully as a researcher. Before the research and during the progress of the work, even in preparation, it is important to have time to think about what you are doing. It is also vital to read research literature thoroughly and perhaps with a different approach to the one which is used to scan journals for articles of interest. If you are a clinician who wishes to research concurrently with practice then you may have to consider drastically reducing your clinical practice or working with a restricted range of patients. The activity of research thinking and planned reading, while appearing as a luxury to colleagues, may mean a change in attitude to working for the clinician who constantly has to be seen to be 'doing'. At this stage it is useful to consider how long a period you want to spend on your research project, and then set a target date for the end of that period.

Finally, your immediate family and friends may not quite share your single-minded commitment to advancing the cause of modern scientific endeavour. Apart from research eating into recreation time, those sudden flashes of inspiration or extended thoughts concerning methodological conundrums can occur at weekends or in the evening when you begin to relax. Sometimes spouses do not appreciate the riddle of formulating an algorithm for multiple variables measured over a time series, especially if this occurs over dinner.

Research is a serious activity and cannot be tacked on to other activities. If possible find some specialist advice either from a colleague who has researched in the field you are considering, from a known expert in the field, or from the funding agency you intend to approach. It is at this stage that statistical or methodological advice must be sought, not after data is collected.

Purpose of the enquiry

It is important to state research questions precisely. The questions must be clear and simple. This process of clarifying your own emerging questions so that they can be understood by others is a vital stage for your work, and for finding funds. To a certain extent the purpose of the study will help define the target audience for your work. This will in turn influence the research methods you use.

If the purpose of your work is to satisfy your own curiosity as an individual or group of practitioners, then that methodology may be developed in a way which is totally idiosyncratic to your clinical practice. Your work may be seen as the development of a research methodology appropriate for your particular way of working. This could be extended to the arena of your clinical peers to whom you wish to validate a set of hypotheses about your common practice. They may demand that certain restraints are imposed. For example, in working as research consultant with music therapists, their demand of me was to find research methods appropriate to their clinical practice, not to adapt practice to research restrictions.

Those of us who have been through the academic research mill have often been fortunate enough to satisfy our own questions within the guidelines of a particular research discipline. What we may need to develop within complementary medicine is an agency which can offer such impartial supervision and guidance.

Most clinicians when they do research are attempting to convince someone of the validity of their approach. Either they are trying to convince other practitioners, or licensing authorities, journal editors, consumer or patient groups and insurance companies who provide reimbursement. It is important in the planning stages to discover what evidence these groups will admit as valid. Results are not persuasive to everyone. These audiences will have different sets of knowledge and may need to be educated to your approach. For example, a group of complementary therapists using natural medicines to treat cancer patients were enabled to gain government funding because they negotiated, through their research methodologists, an appropriate single case methodology with the government's scientific representative.

Similarly, not all investigators can demand the same confidence from those audiences. An application from a research institute with a proven track record will inevitably stand a better chance of gaining research funding from an organization which has supported them in the past.

What we have to establish within the community of complementary medical research is a platform of methodological expertise which both meets our own demands and those of sponsors. Our present trap is that for some studies we need funding for developmental studies of appropriate methodologies which will identify a common core of critical variables and appropriate methods. Sadly, such developmental funding is not part of the current research climate which is more concerned with 'productivity' in the short term. Long-term, or 'blue skies', research is not adequately supported.

In addition, there is always a political climate to research funding. Whenever we attempt to coerce, cajole, exhort or stimulate people to behave in a particular way then we are behaving politically. When that behaviour challenges an orthodox way of working, or demands an alternative means of practice which may alter health care delivery in terms of financial allocation, or threatens to remove some of the exercise of power from a monopoly agency, then we are entering a political arena.

It is important then to be able to see the purpose of what you are doing and why. In the field of complementary practice it is important to state where such practice could be used within a current health care framework, and how such a practice fits in with orthodox practice. In addition it is important to show where the proposed work will improve research expertise, current clinical practice or have an educational component.

Once these broad understandings have been considered then it is time to provide more details of the intended study.

Aims of the study

The aims of clinical studies are multivarious. The exploration and generation of hypotheses, the refinement of those hypotheses, the discovery of the optimal use of a therapeutic regimen, the safety of that regimen or the active ingredient in a composite therapy are common aims. Similarly, complementary practitioners often want to make a definitive demonstration of their therapeutic regime in comparison with another regimen or to demonstrate feasibility or efficacy in a particular setting.

Such clinical trials usually pose two radically different types of problem which demand differing types of solution and different methodological considerations.

The first is an explanatory trial. In this approach we seek information which will give us answers to scientific questions often at the biological level. Such trials are closer to laboratory conditions and may have no pragmatic consequences. The questions asked in these trials are more concerned with causality and the natural history of disease, the development of medicines and the refinement and application of techniques.

The second type of trial is a comparison of treatments as applied in practice. This is a pragmatic trial. In such a trial treatment conditions would be optimized and our purpose would be to make a decision about which treatment modality to use. In these trials we can incorporate factors other than the biological or psychological. These factors might be concerned with cost, efficacy, ease of use, acceptability by the patient, possibility for inclusion in general practice. Such trials are related to the context of the treatment approach and provide answers concerned with feasibility, but not necessarily answers which are explanatory; i.e. the treatment works but nobody knows why.

Both can be combined, but with extreme caution. In the interests of simplicity it is better to understand what you are attempting, and then ask yourself if you are taking on too much. Rather than attempt an overly complex study it may be possible to work as a research group of practitioners satisfying interdependent aims. In this way of working, practitioners can work cooperatively with colleagues developing differing sets of answers which answer a common question.

For example, in the music therapy research mentioned earlier, some therapists concentrated on developing methodologies which showed physiological changes during and after the process of therapy (explanatory trials), others were concerned with clinical outcomes (pragmatic trials), and all were concerned in the theoretical debate, based on experimental observation and clinical expertise about how clinical improvement was effected.

It is in the aims section where you will state your hypothesis (or hypotheses) to be tested.

Pilot studies

It really is important to make exploratory or pilot studies, but not as an easy option. By attempting to try out our ideas in practice then we can see the pitfalls and the possibilities of what we are attempting. Some of these pitfalls can be avoided by asking expert opinion beforehand. Unfortunately, the pressure of research sponsors can be for precocious results, and evidence that something is being done for their money. Exploratory trials and critical developmental thinking are often sacrificed to such impatience.

Pilot studies are not any easier to construct methodologically than later trials. Definitive studies cannot be generated from poorly thought out exploratory studies. As much statistical and methodological thinking must go into the pilot studies as the larger study. Data must be carefully evaluated in a series of sequential experiments. These are the platform for the future work.

The question always remains of when to stop piloting and when to begin a definitive study. The main objective in any clinical trial is to find a feasible, effective and tolerable regime which is easy to understand, is easily administered, has an evaluative index which demonstrates the identified clinical change, and cooperative clinical partners. Once you have such an approach then it is time to try it out. In an application for research funding it is important to link any pilot work to an overall developmental strategy with some clear indication of a future definitive study.

Background to the study

In your preliminary thinking you will have begun to understand the gaps in present knowledge. You will then need to say how your study will begin to fill these gaps and contribute to that knowledge. This understanding is based on your own clinical knowledge and that of other practitioners, but is based predominantly on reviewing the clinical literature.

Reviewing literature can be a research study in itself. It demands a great deal of application to search, collect and read the relevant material. However, it can bring much satisfaction. By reading of other research endeavours over the years we can gain a sense of the community of research practitioners in medicine who too have been excited by ideas, and attempted to demonstrate those ideas in practice.

There are numerous databases available for searching the literature. These searches are made easier and cheaper by your being clear about what categories you wish to search under, in what range of publications, published in which languages and over what period of time.

For example, by disease: *inflammatory bowel disease*; with the following factors: *family factors, immunological, histological, epidemiological, psychological*; published in *English, German and French*; during the last *five years*.

A good librarian is of invaluable help in preparing a literature search. A search facility may be available through your professional organization, but now there is a new service being offered by the British Library. For a basic fee of £10 for 50 references, plus 25p per citation thereafter, the BL will search the literature for you from their vast database. Apply to the Medical Information Service, British Library, Document Supply Centre, Boston Spa, Wetherby, West Yorks LS23 7BQ. Have your keywords already identified when making the request. The British Library are also able to supply the articles you select, at £3.69 inclusive of VAT per item (regardless of number of pages). This is the same price for individuals and libraries, but some libraries may pass on an additional handling charge if they negotiate the transaction for you.

It is then possible to make an extended search from the reference sections and bibliographies of those collected papers. Then you have to read the papers critically, make notes and write up the conclusions. This is where you find that your writing skills may have become a little rusty.

Literature too can also act as a pilot study of ideas where your work builds upon previous studies. It is always an advantage to contact the authors of studies to ask how they would further their work. In journal papers not everything is revealed about the trial in terms of practical details; i.e. it may be an elegant study when reported but difficult to carry out in practice. By looking through the literature with a critical eye it is possible to see exactly what is needed as a next step in your own therapeutic discipline in terms of clinical practice or research methodology. It is also possible to see the mistakes of others and construct a trial which builds upon what has gone before.

Clinical literature is not solely confined to journal articles and books. Some articles quote eminent authors and they are worth contacting, particularly for unpublished material which they may be willing to show you.

Design of the study

In this section you will say what research strategy is to be used. Will you use a laboratory style explanatory approach or embark upon a survey? Are you using a controlled trial with randomized or matched controls, or are you carrying out a series of related single case designs? Are you attempting to describe a service within a hospital setting or is this a formal trial of a therapeutic procedure? This is where your methodological musings and debate must leave the heady heights of discussion and appear on paper. It is important to give a detailed account of the research design you intend to use, and some indication of why you are using that design.

It is possible to be innovative in clinical trials design. The Research Council for Complementary Medicine in its original application form emphasized that 'Studies should not conflict with the best practices in the complementary discipline involved; they should be planned so that the major sources of error and bias are avoided; provided that this rigour is sought, they need not conform to the traditional patterns of clinical trials methodology'. What then are the major considerations for avoiding error and bias, and how do we show that rigour is being sought?

Selection of subjects for the study

It is important to describe the class of patients who are to be included in the study. If you are studying a particular disease then it is important to define a subclass of patients who are suitable for that trial. This will mean giving discrete criteria for patient inclusion and exclusion (e.g. by age, gender, chronicity, previous treatment). Beware of defining this group too narrowly such that they become unrepresentative. The study which accepts a broad spectrum of patients has a generalizability and persuasiveness that is essential to influencing a target audience of practitioners. Although hand-picking patients may be desirable in statistical terms there is a trade-off between efficiency and generalizability. If your purpose is to demonstrate the efficacy of your approach with the aim of influencing applicability in general practice, then choose carefully over a broad range of patients.

If you are conducting a controlled trial you will have to say what criteria are being used for control selection.

There is also a further subclass of patients: those who complete the trial, i.e. those you actually gather data about. Withdrawals give rise to serious difficulties, especially if they occur during the treatment regime. People leave trials because they are frightened of what is going on, they may believe that they are not receiving an important life-saving medication, the regime or data collection may be tedious, the medicine may taste nasty or the procedure is painful. Some patients do not see the point of the study after a while and somehow their commitment to research does not match that of the researcher. Some patients at follow-up are found to have left the area. Some patients die. Some researchers call this process one of 'patient attrition'.

While withdrawals may throw important light on a particular practice and provide useful information it is always better to structure such a possibility into the trial if you believe this is going to happen. A careful pilot study should give some ideas about whether a treatment regime can be sustained or not.

Another important consideration is that of sample size. This is why it is emphasized that statistical thinking is vital at this stage of the study, not after data has been collected.

If groups are to be compared then decisions will have to be made about randomization of subjects to groups, how many patients are needed in those groups to achieve statistical significance and, more importantly, what is the power of those statistics? It is vital that appropriately sized groups are chosen in clinical trials designs so that clinically meaningful differences are not missed.

For example, if comparing two treatments (X and Y) in a pragmatic approach, the researcher will want to know by what margin does one treatment regime surpass the other. This pragmatic approach is concerned with reducing the probability of preferring the inferior treatment (an error of the third kind), whereas, in an explanatory approach, it is important to avoid concluding that treatments X and Y differ when they are the same (an error of the first kind), or that treatments X and Y are equal when they are not (an error of the second kind).

Choice of data

Perhaps the greatest challenge is to sift out what data to collect. There is a temptation to collect masses and masses of data in some mistaken belief that more data is somehow representative of the whole person. It is important to collect multiple data sets which are indicators of therapeutic influence, but these have to be analysed at the end of the trial. The challenge then is to define how the criteria which are used for evaluation are related to the treatment intervention, and one with another. The variables measured by the experiment in this way are the *dependent* variables.

The panel which assesses your applications will want to know why you have chosen particular measures or indices.

In assessing the effects of a treatment regimen we may use several diverse criteria: regression of a tumour, decrease in pain, return to work or mean survival time compared with a given prognosis. Return to work may be an important variable as identified by the patient, but it offers no biological information. Regression of tumour size may be biologically important but this may have no effect upon survival.

It is therefore important to develop an instrument for measuring clinical change appropriate to the study. Explanatory studies will seek to find separate criteria. A pragmatic approach will look for a single index which can be used to indicate therapeutic efficacy.

It may be that the aim of the research design itself will concentrate on developing an index. This may be in the form of a questionnaire, or a battery of measures. In constructing such an increment you will be able to use your own expert knowledge, the clinical experience of colleagues, the clinical literature you have reviewed and the experience of patients. It is essential to bear in mind how patient status will change in relationship to the therapeutic application, and that your instrument measures all clinically important treatment effects. (If you take this route beware! Questionnaire design and validation is a project within itself.)

What most of us seek is some sort of gold-standard measure which is both reliable and valid. Reliable in this sense refers to the consistency of a research instrument when applied to a stable population. Valid refers to whether those measures are genuine, i.e. do they measure what you say they are measuring? In addition the measure must be responsive enough to measure a small, but real, difference when one is present.

There are three main types of index which can be developed:

1 The *discriminative* index which helps to distinguish between individuals or groups where no gold-standard exists.

2 The *predictive* index which is used to classify individuals into predefined categories. This is evident in screening measures which identify specific individuals who will have a target condition or outcome. We see this in prognostic indicators or predictors of mortality.

3 The *evaluative* index which is used to measure longitudinal change in an individual or group on the given criteria of interest. Such an index can utilize both quantitative and qualitative data and is often used to evaluate functional change.

My aim when advising clients is to find and use at least one index which is well validated in orthodox clinical practice. This helps build a bridge to other research traditions. There are also a number of well validated and reliable self-report questionnaires. These are very useful if you do not have the resources to interview the subjects of your research yourself.

Data collection

It is necessary to say when the measures will be implemented, who will implement them, and design a form for data collection. In planning the collection of data, allow time for questionnaires to be filled in. If postal questionnaires are used, make an allowance for the follow-up of unreturned questionnaires, and be prepared to visit if necessary.

Ideally, if data is collected by more than one person then one person must be placed in a position to collate that data. Research is an obsessive activity. Data collection is tedious. Missing data is a calamity.

With the advent of modern computing methods it is easy to store and manipulate data. Putting data into a database or spreadsheet is relatively straightforward; getting it out again in a meaningful way is not. The statistical decisions which you made earlier, and your understanding of the relationships between sets of data, will be invaluable at this stage. If data is to be stored on a computer remember that someone has to enter that data and it will be necessary to say who will handle the data, and when they will enter the data. Entering large sets of data at the end of a project leads to error. Data sheets can be lost. Human errors from fatigue are common. It may be possible to consider direct entry of data to a computer with some form of data-checking routine built in.

It is important to describe how any specialist laboratory tests will be carried out, the nature of those tests and who will carry them out. Specialist testing is expensive and another potential source of error, so it is important to be clear about how valid or necessary such measures are. Some specialist tests can be therapeutic interventions in themselves and it is important to bear this in mind when designing the study and perhaps consider them as control variables. (A control variable is a potential independent variable which is held constant.)

Treatment variables

Treatment variables are the *independent* variables. They refer to the techniques of the programme of treatment you will use as a clinician. This will probably be the easiest part for you to organize. It is important that you say clearly what you will do, when you will do it and why you are doing it. For complementary practitioners working together it is vital that they achieve some standardization of practice while remaining true to their therapeutic discipline, thereby maintaining their own therapeutic integrity and validity. If your therapeutic discipline contains its own idiosyncratic terms it may be necessary to provide a glossary of terms within the application document.

When a control group is used then it is essential to define how, when and where they will be treated, even if they receive 'no treatment'.

If you are carrying out a clinical trial it will be necessary to incorporate some time when baseline data can be collected before treatment begins.

The time when treatment periods begin and end must be planned and recorded. Criteria must be made for when the trial period of treatment is to end, and when a 'follow-up' assessment is to be made.

It is also important to say what will happen to patients who are discovered to have new needs during the process of the study.

Administration of the study

Analysis of the results

If the data is stored on a computer, and the researchers understand their data, then a statistical package can be used to analyse that data. If statistical advice is sought at the beginning of the trial, and the trial designed according to certain principles, then the appropriate routines will be clear. With the implementation of statistical analysis packages on microcomputers, it is possible to view and analyse the data in a variety of ways. Such retrospective data analysis, sometimes called *post hoc hypothesizing*, is dangerous. While it may suggest new hypotheses and correlations between data, those relationships may be completely spurious. Analyses of data are only spurs to critical thinking; they cannot replace it.

When considering using a statistical package it may be necessary to enlist the help of a statistician to interpret the results. Many packages also have a graphics capability which will enable the data to be displayed in forms which are easier to understand than tables of figures.

Timetable of the study

In the process of making the previous decision you will have some idea of how long the study will take. The most common mistake that novice researchers make is to underestimate the amount of time necessary to complete a study. I shall assume that you have contacted the practitioners and referrers to be involved and gained their cooperation.

First, you will need to assess how long it will take to recruit the requisite number of patients. If you are recruiting patients with special characteristics through a seemingly cooperative referrer, check the time it will take to recruit a starting sample, assess them, and gain their consent. This information will also influence how many patients can be treated in a given period of time. If you are collecting data as well as treating patients, then the time you allow for your usual treatment session may be extended.

Second, plot the time it will take for all the subjects of the research to be treated and make a definite date for the trial to end. Ensure that any specialist testing will have been carried out by that date and the results received. Allow for any missing questionnaire data to be followed up.

Third, allow time to analyse the results. Initially data is 'raw' data. It can do nothing by itself; you as researcher must process it. Unlike patients, data is not self-actualizing.

For example, a client group of *Heilpraktiker* in Germany, while willing to collect data over a period of 18 months, were astounded by the suggestion that the analysis of the data and the writing up of the report would take at least another six months (in my opinion a conservative estimate). Originally they heard this suggestion as six weeks, and thought this also was too long.

Fourth, consider that the results must be thought about and then written up in some form for publication or as a presentation to your target audience. Because we are practitioners does not always mean that we are writers. If you are writing a joint report then allow time for arguing. A useful tip is to present your work at regular intervals to colleagues, and to the collaborators in your study at the end of the trial. This thinking for a presentation can help your writing, particularly if you record the presentation on audiotape.

Finally, if you are writing and working with colleagues, make sure that you have made a decision about who is to be senior author, or at least to have final say on the finished report, and who is to be accredited in the list of authors.

Ethical considerations

If your professional group has a code of ethical considerations for research then it will be necessary to consider them. Mention such a code of practice in your research application. If you are working with an institution then there will be an ethical committee which will need to see your research submission.

Your sponsors will want to satisfy themselves that you have obtained approval for your intended research from an ethical committee. While your sponsors may be flexible in their approach, local ethical committees may not be quite as well educated. The onus is on the clinician/researcher to consult with them and explain what he or she intends to do.

As soon as data is collected, and particularly if it is stored on a computer, then that data must be protected and made confidential. Similarly, if the research is to be written as a report, which potentially can be published, then arrangements must be made to maintain confidentiality and this must be stated in the application.

The consent of patients and cooperating practitioners must also be obtained. Be clear how you are to obtain this consent, and what information you will give to the patient in the trial. The rights of the patient to refuse to participate in, or withdraw from, the trial must be observed.

It is essential that any possible risks to the patient are made clear and harmful consequences removed. If an unorthodox practice is to be used then be prepared for what seem to be obstructive and awkward questions. As practitioners we take for granted what we do. Our normal decisions and practices can sometimes be misunderstood or misinterpreted.

For example, a news programme which juxtaposes concern about the spread of AIDS and highlights the use of needles by addicts, coupled with the debate about complementary medical practice, notably acupuncture, can indirectly raise issues about risks to the patient from the use of needles. If you are about to embark on an acupuncture trial, and are attempting to recruit patients from referrers who are only marginally convinced about cooperating, then such news can have negative consequences.

Any statements about insurance for professional indemnity and the limit of that indemnity can be included here.

Costing of the project

As mentioned earlier, research is greedy for resources and particularly for money. In a research submission you will need to justify your needs and also satisfy your potential sponsors that the request is valid. Ask for enough. Do not underestimate your requirement.

The principal considerations are:

Staffing costs

(a) The salary of the investigator(s), and the hidden pension and N.I. costs over a given period of time. Allow for annual increments.

(b) Secretarial costs.

(c) Specialist consultancy services for data handling, statistical advice and analysis and research supervision.

(d) Specialist consultancy services for patient assessment.

Treatment costs
Any tests will need to be costed, particularly when carried out by an external agency, and the cost of treatments or medicines will need to be considered.

Handling charges
Most sponsors will support an institution rather than an individual. Such institutions will often charge a handling cost as a percentage of the funds received.

Administrative costs
There will be accommodation charges, telephone bills, stationery needs, printing requirements, postage and overheads.

Travel costs
Visits to expert informants, visits to follow-up patients.

Hardware costs
Any specialist equipment which must be rented or bought.

Computing costs
It may be necessary to purchase software for computing or to have that software adapted or written for your trial. If you have access to a computer centre, then that centre may charge for such support.

Library services

Searching for references in the literature, collecting literature and photocopying literature is costly. Sometimes it is necessary to break these costs down into yearly requirements.

Personnel

For the main personnel working on the project it is important to include curricula vitae, and their appropriate clinical and academic qualifications. Some sponsors require you to nominate a key person to oversee the work. If you are using an external supervisor then his or her qualifications will need to be included.

Research experience can be included in this section. Hopefully, lack of experience should not preclude the clinician from a research grant,

External thinking	*Application*
Have a good idea Decide to research Find time and negotiate possible changes	AIMS OF THE STUDY
Try out ideas on friends and colleagues	state hypotheses
Identify target audience	
Identify sponsors	
Gain statistical and methodological advice	consider PILOT STUDY
Search, collate and read literature Write literature review	BACKGROUND TO THE STUDY
What type of study? How will subjects be chosen? What sample size?	STUDY DESIGN
Identify dependent variables How will data be collected?	
Identify treatment variables	
Gain statistical and methodological advice Statistical routines and methods	ANALYSIS OF RESULTS
	ADMINISTRATION OF THE STUDY
Consult colleagues	Timetable of research
Contact ethical committee(s)	Ethical considerations
Contact specialist agencies	Cost project
	Personnel
	Curriculum vitae

Fig. 29.1 A guide to preparing a research application.

providing the sponsor is satisfied that there is adequate research supervision. Otherwise it would be impossible to gain research experience. With the dwindling resources available for research through academic institutions, we are in danger of seriously damaging our research tradition in Britain. However, by taking research out of the academic environment we have a chance to promote research training for clinicians within the context of their own practice. This approach is not bound by traditional thinking and should enliven our scientific medical culture.

Submitting the research

Send the completed design with a covering letter. It may be that you can submit your design for a preliminary review before a formal submission to a full committee. Be prepared to revise and negotiate a little. Most big committees meet only once or twice a year so it is important to find the final date for submission.

Conclusion

If you can incorporate all these considerations then the research itself should be easy. Applying for funds is the worst part. It takes a lot of work and organization with no guarantee of results.

Remember that research takes time; personal time, reading time, thinking time, and time away from your routine practice. It is prudent to negotiate such changes with your friends, colleagues and family.

Be clear about the intended audience for your research.

Research is expensive. It may be worthwhile investing in preliminary research planning which would include a brief review of the literature and statistical or methodological advice.

30 Conclusion: are you ready to begin?

David Aldridge

We have read in the preceding chapters that there are many ways to do research. Underlying any research lies the activity of careful data collection, linked with an underlying hypothesis, stimulated by a good idea which has inspired the researcher. Complementary medicine will be subject to clinical trials. The methods used for those trials can be selected from a range of possibilities, although it will be hard to escape from the demand for controlled studies. It is hoped that the novice researcher will have gleaned some information about where they can begin in their own search in clinical practice.

Even with the best intentions and precise planning, clinical trials can go astray. We recently carried out a trial using music therapy as a treatment for twelve developmentally handicapped children. To overcome ethical objections, all children received music therapy. Children were randomized to either treatment, or a waiting group. The allocation to a waiting group would have been normal practice as all twelve could not be accommodated in our clinical capacity. The paediatrician involved was blind to the treatment allocation of the children when the tests were applied. However, several problems arose. First, it was difficult to find twelve similarly developmentally handicapped children. Second, the randomization randomized the lowest pre-test scorers to one group and the higher scorers to another. Third, at the first test the mothers of the non-treatment group invariably found a way to ask the assessor, who was blind to the treatment allocation, when their child would have music therapy. Fourth, three children could not complete the trial for various reasons, which was natural as the research was carried out over a nine-month period.

In addition, during the course of the therapy one child was found by the music therapists and the kindergarten staff not to be mentally handicapped as described by his medical notes, but suffering from a profound hearing handicap. Thus, he was excluded from the trial as he had to come to terms with his artificial hearing aids. While emphasizing the benefit of music therapy as a diagnostic tool, it was yet another difficulty for the successful running of a trial. One autistic child seemingly failed to develop according to the well-validated child development rating scale which we were using, yet her musical abilities flourished, as did the satisfaction of her parents. Rigorous data collection helped us to salvage important elements of the work. The important point is that no plan survives the test of reality.

We have read earlier that social science research methods also have much to offer, particularly as they encourage the researcher to stand back and look at the content of what they are researching within the context in which those ideas occur. However, there are pitfalls to social science methods. It is all too easy, and I write here as a social scientist, to end up writing only about methods,[1,2] or about the context of health care delivery,[3] or about the meaning structures of practitioners[4] without really getting to grips with clinical practice at all. The health beliefs of our patients, I suggest, are a more urgent priority than those of the practitioners.

The new researching paradigms, while raising the awareness of potential researchers and challenging us as practising researchers, have inflated the currency of debate while adding little to the stock of practice. It is possible to meet would-be researchers who know the paradigm parameters and their limitations from the literature, yet have never done any research. If we want to learn to swim, we must at some time enter the water and try it. Reading about swimming, and thinking deeply about swimming on dry land, attending conferences where well-known swimmers of past and present make an appearance even, is of little value once you are in the water. The experience itself teaches. If you have an experienced swimmer in the water with you then they can help. So it is with research; there is no substitute for doing it, and having experienced help to call on is imperative.

Similarly, new paradigm research encourages participation. Yet what appears to emerge from this participation is that the academic partner is the one who writes up the research (often in a highly elaborated technical language), who gets the academic qualification and title and whose name appears on the paper, no matter how egalitarian his or her intent. Furthermore, the content of the work, which looks at the practitioners and how they come to agree on treatment policies, or how their political consciousness may change, has only a tenuous link with the patient. That a negotiated language between practitioners based on research into multidisciplinary practice has a benefit for patients seems reasonable, but demonstrating this in research is difficult. In short, social science can end up looking more at itself and the researchers than at the patients.

What social science survey methods may bring is an understanding of the health economics underlying the delivery of complementary health care. Regardless of the therapeutic mode in use, a systematic assessment of complementary health care as delivered to a given community, or systematically delivered to matched populations, would provide a strong argument for the acceptance of alternative forms of health care delivery. With the potentially overwhelming health care demands of the elderly in the next century we need now to investigate forms of health care which are less expensive and have the potential for prevention.

I suggest, then, that for the future we need:

1 Longitudinal studies of health care practice (including cost-benefit analysis) using matched controls. For those who argue against the ethics of control groups, the matched group allows for the treatment application to be delayed or staggered. In those situations where we really do not know whether our initiatives work or not, the matched control allows a particular clinic to work in its own particular way, but then compares that clinic with another working with a different outlook.

2 Coordinated single case designs combined with developing the existing statistical analyses of time series data. When we can provide a statistic of significance related to the physiology of the patient demonstrating a change correlated with an intervention then we will have a methodology suitable for clinical practice in general.

3 To extend our currently scanty knowledge about the link between health-seeking and health-making behaviour in patients and their families. Furthermore, we know little about how patients relate the knowledge of their own bodies to the forms of medicine which they seek, and the implications this has for their therapy. Similarly, we know little about what people are willing to spend in terms of their health care.

4 The urgent collaboration of workers throughout Europe to build potential data sets, to share methods and coordinate our knowledge. The art therapies in Europe have initiated a world communication system which allows them to share bibliographical data and professional information. We can quickly find other interested clinics for research, potential placements for our students and read research reports not yet published. In addition, it is possible to compare curricula between training institutions and prepare for the open market in Europe. This should also be possible for complementary medicine. In Germany, there is a government-funded centre for the centralization of information concerning complementary medicine. A part of the work of that centre is to examine research submissions regarding the application of unconventional approaches to cancer treatment. This centre guides the applicant in the writing of proposals, offers appropriate methodologies, and suggests sources of grant funding if money is not available from government sources. Several centres so linked throughout Europe would provide a beneficial resource for the practitioner wishing to engage in research either as an individual, or wishing to join a group. (It is also essential that such centres actually give out money for research, with an intellectually generous attitude, and not sit on the money waiting for an orthodox safe design as occurs with some research councils. If research is to be pioneered it requires pioneer funders.)

As a final personal note I would want to warn the would-be researcher of the perils involved in research. Sometimes it feels that I am writing in exile from a foreign land. That is no reflection upon my German colleagues who have been both generous and tolerant. Yet, the experience of challenging the establishment in England was a painful one, no matter how supportive my immediate colleagues may have seemed. Peter Reason's important article[5] about power and conflict in multidisciplinary collaboration at a health centre missed out the power and conflicts issues involved in what research approaches to take, how that research planning was dependent upon the allocation of grant funding to the whole project, and the paradigm split between the research steering committee, the senior practitioner and the senior research fellow at the time. Even researchers who emphasize looking at all levels can have blind spots. Research in complementary medicine can damage your health. It is vital for any researcher to ensure that not only the financial support for research is available, but also that the social and emotional support is there. While I am sceptical about the feasibility, although not the ideas, of the new paradigm research proposed by Peter Reason,[6] I would recommend the course he runs which challenges the would-be researcher to understand why he or she wants to research, or the current researcher about the personal emotional, biographical and spiritual content of that work.

Finally, while we research, write and publish for complementary medical journals, it is a major challenge for us that we write in a language that is understood by other professionals. Medical journals and periodicals are willing to listen to criticism and new ideas. I do not subscribe to the idea that we can only change from within. That is the way in which orthodoxy subverts its dissidents. But to change or influence from without, we have to communicate in a language that can be understood. When we wish to work together for the benefit of the communities in which we work, then 'within' and 'without', in the context of suffering and distress, are concepts which we can abandon.

References

1   Aldridge, D. Aesthetics and the individual in the practice of medical research: a discussion paper. *J Roy Soc Med* 1991; **84**: 147–50.

2   Aldridge, D. Single case designs for the clinician. *J Roy Soc Med* 1991; **84**: 249–52.

3   Aldridge, D. The delivery of health care alternatives. *J Roy Soc Med* 1990; **83**: 179–82.

4   Aldridge, D. Making and taking health care decisions. *J Roy Soc Med* 1990; **83**: 720–3.

5   Reason, P. Power and conflict in multidisciplinary collaboration. *Comp Med Res* 1991; **5**(3): 144–50.

6   Reason, P., Rowan, J. *Human Inquiry*. Chichester: Wiley, 1981.